PhotoTherapy Techniques

PhotoTherapy

Exploring the Secrets of

JOSSEY-BASS PUBLISHERS
San Francisco

Techniques

Personal Snapshots and Family Albums

Judy Weiser

For sales outside the United States, contact Maxwell Macmillan International Publishing Group, 866 Third Avenue, New York, New York 10022.

Manufactured in the United States of America

The paper used in this book is acid-free and meets the guidelines for permanence and durability of the Committee on Production Guidelines for Book Longevity of the Council on Library Resources.

Library of Congress Cataloging-in-Publication Data

Weiser, Judy, date.
PhotoTherapy techniques : exploring the secrets of personal snapshots and family albums / Judy Weiser. — 1st ed.
p. cm. — (The Jossey-Bass social and behavioral science series)
Includes bibliographical references and index.
ISBN 1-55542-552-6
1. Photography in psychotherapy. 2. Psychotherapy—Audio-visual aids. 3. Photographs—Psychological aspects. I. Title. II. Series.
RC489.P56W45 1993
616.89′16—dc20 93-3622
CIP

FIRST EDITION
HB Printing 10 9 8 7 6 5 4 3 2 1 *Code 9355*

THE JOSSEY-BASS SOCIAL AND BEHAVIORAL SCIENCE SERIES

This book is dedicated to my husband, Bob,
and to those special others in my life
whose photos I hold closest to my heart...
stilled moments of time, cherished forever.

Contents

Preface

"If you still have my photograph, then I'm still safe in your heart."

She knew exactly what she wanted: "Over there, beside the tree, with the ocean in the background." She looked at the scene to arrange it in her mind (and camera viewfinder), and then traced an *x* in the dirt with her foot to mark the exact place for the friend holding her camera to stand. "Wait until I'm ready and I pose with my arm around the tree. When I smile, take the picture, but don't let any other people get in," she directed. And her friend tried his very best to record what she asked. Watching all this from the hotel balcony, I was struck again, as I had been many times before, by the preciseness of people's expectations regarding photographic records of their special moments. I was also rather concerned for the woman's friend, who was expected to produce the perfect image that would later be used as proof of that much-enjoyed vacation.

I wondered what would become of this single snapshot: Would it have a treasured place in her home as a memory of holiday time spent with a friend or be instantly rejected because it didn't turn out "right" (as she had visualized it)? Would she like how she appeared in the final print or perhaps find that it instead reminded her of her mother (ugh!)? Would this picture perhaps bring to mind associated memories of other places, people, and times in her life, connecting related experiences, or would it serve only as an icon of one isolated happy time amidst later disillusionment? Was she at all conscious of such potential significance of her chosen moment of time-stopping? Did she understand that the reality in the finished print had its importance more in her heart than in the emulsion-covered paper? Did she stop to recognize that her interpretation of it was only one of many possible versions? Was she aware that she was being watched, and would this awareness have made any difference in that scenario?

It is just such hidden components in the lives of ordinary snapshots that add to the meanings within their borders, yet it is these "secret" aspects that most often remain out of conscious awareness of the photo's maker or later viewer. Many years ago I began to notice how people's conversations about their own personal photo collections would produce factual and emotional information that I had not been able to find out by asking them direct questions. I also discovered that the same thing happened when people viewed my photographs hanging on gallery walls. I would sometimes even hear people arguing about the meaning of the photograph in front of them, having made opposite assumptions about why the photographer originally took the photo or included it in the show.

It was often possible to engage them in casual conversation about the photo, and as an artist, I was fascinated to hear what they were seeing and feeling in response to an image that I myself knew very well, but which they obviously were perceiving very differently (especially if they didn't realize I had created it). I began to realize that there would never be a way to clearly predict what people might "get" from one of my photos or what emotions might be evoked in them as they interacted with it. The part of me that is a therapist was intrigued by all this silent communication "accidentally" embedded along with the visual details of the photo.

My initial conception of photographs as art objects had led me to these experiences where the pictures were serving instead as nonverbal communicators, regardless of any potential artistic merit they might also contain—and this book now presents the consequences of this transition as it attempts to give readers "a better picture" of ways that different kinds of ordinary photographs can be used as powerful tools in the hands of those providing therapy or counseling. The artistic components of people's snapshots quickly become irrelevant as the therapist begins to probe the inner meaning that each photographic catalyst holds for the person perceiving, taking, posing for, keeping, or even only remembering it.

A BRIEF HISTORY

When I then decided to start using clients' ordinary personal snapshots and family album photos as stimuli, I discovered that their responses to my questions about their pictures permitted connection with unconscious and deeply-buried memories, thoughts, and feelings that my verbal inquiry on its own had been unable to reach. Using the symbolic communication that is naturally embedded in the photographs my clients responded to, created, posed for, or collected, I noticed that they began to contact feelings and information in ways they were simultaneously unaware of and yet totally familiar with: talking about the ordinary informal snapshots and album pictures that were already part of their daily lives. Because of these realizations, I began to develop a more formalized interrelated framework of techniques based on this spontaneous informal process of "photo explorations" that often happens while people casually discuss their personal photos (especially those they appear in).

I first tried these techniques when counseling several hearing-impaired First Nations children (*First Nations* is the term used for Native Americans in Canada), and the results were very exciting. When asked to write an article about the work (Weiser, 1975), I was asked to come up with a title for this process. I chose the name "PhotoTherapy," trying to emphasize an equal balance of its two parts by using two capital letters. I thought that as a result of this publication, I would soon be famous; I thought I had invented a new field all by myself.

About six months later, I received an invitation to the first International PhotoTherapy Symposium in Illinois. Ideas of fame quickly disappeared, but I explained my work at that first conference and met dozens of other therapists who presented their own similar versions of these photo-counseling combinations; it was obviously an idea whose time had come. A quarterly journal began publication, an international association formed, and a 1983 publication of a book called *PhotoTherapy in Mental Health,* edited by Krauss and Fryrear, provided many of us with the opportunity to write about what we had been doing.

A decade later, professional activity, media attention, academic publications, and collegial networking have all increased. A few of us began offering training to other therapists who wanted to learn more about using photo-based therapy techniques, and in 1982, the PhotoTherapy Centre in Vancouver, Canada, opened as a resource, training, and networking base for the field. The Centre includes an open library that contains several hundred articles, books, and numerous videotape recordings of "live" case sessions that are maintained for use by students and practitioners.

AUDIENCE

A wide cross-section of people have attended public or professional presentations on PhotoTherapy as relevant for therapeutic practice or for more general applications. These audiences have included not only the expected mental health professionals whose work involves conducting therapy or related counseling activities (psychologists, marriage and family therapists, psychiatrists, art therapists, social workers, and so forth), but also those from secondarily-related backgrounds, such as special education teachers, English as a second language instructors, summer camp personnel, clergy, and so forth. There has also been a lot of interest expressed by theorists who apply concepts of visual literacy, cross-cultural studies, and nonverbal communication to social learning or classroom situations, as well as anthropologists and sociologists interested in the way visual information is coded, represented, and placed in context, as well as many people involved in the photographic arts or those involved in their teaching or critical theory. And finally, there has been a lot of curiosity expressed by the general public, people who may not necessarily be having psychological problems themselves, but nevertheless want to explore more about their own lives as reflected back to them by their photos as a way of enhancing their self-knowledge and personal growth.

This book, though written primarily for the first group above, will still certainly be of interest to all the others listed. It may prove especially useful to art and expressive therapists, whose theoretical foundations are based on the concept that symbolic art expression gives form to feelings that otherwise might resist translation into conscious or verbal investigation. This is a book for demonstrating serious therapeutic process, which is an activity best done by those properly trained to do so. Yet I am certain that anyone else interested in visual communication or self-exploration and the ways personal photographs can be asked to share their embedded secrets will also find it interesting and personally useful, even if only for themselves rather than for professional work applications.

PhotoTherapy as presented in this book is a set of techniques for already-competent therapists to add to their professional repertoire of counseling skills when involved in the work of helping others. This book is not written to teach therapy per se, but rather to teach already-trained professionals how and why to make use of these additional tools to permit them to do their helping work a bit better. It is up to readers to adapt PhotoTherapy to the types of therapeutic model and client difficulties, populations, or settings they prefer to work with. For readers not already trained in therapeutic skills, these pages can still be very useful, but you are cautioned that you must also have professional training in therapy itself if you wish to try using them with anyone other than yourself.

A question that often arises in regard to PhotoTherapy is whether you have to be a skilled photographer to do really good PhotoTherapy work. The answer is no. Professional training in the art of photography has often turned out to be more of a handicap than an advantage because esthetic concerns about image composition, tonal qualities, zone system, formulas for deconstruction, and so forth, get in the way of spontaneous therapeutically focused responses to photographs as communications and emotional stimuli.

In my clinical therapy practice I treat photography as a verb as well as a noun, as an active agent of change as well as an object to reflect on, as very direct emotional communication as well as art; therefore ordinary personal snapshots that are blurry, wrinkled, "poorly" composed, and so forth, are just as useful as those made for artistic reasons. Thus, therapists who are amateur hobbyists, or even those who have never taken photos, would likely be just as good at incorporating PhotoTherapy into their repertoire of counseling skills as those trained in the photographic arts.

In addition to being a therapist, I happen to also be an artist, a "full-fledged" photographic artist whose work is shown and sold in galleries, and so I have frequently reflected upon my photographic work as being able to provide me with much insight into my own inner processes. However, I want to very clearly state that I consider my most primary "art" (that is, the main outlet driving my creative passions and giving form to my inner feelings) to be rooted more in the creating and doing of successful therapy. Doing therapy, and doing it well, *is* my art. My specialization is helping people, and photography is one of my main languages for communication with the subconscious when words alone are not enough. This itself is an art, and readers don't have to be official "artists" in any other discipline to do well with PhotoTherapy techniques.

RATIONALE

Over the past decade, many mental health professionals sought further training in using PhotoTherapy techniques, but as interest grew, it became evident that one person alone (or even in combination with other colleagues) could not possibly personally train every individual interested, especially as so much of learning how to apply PhotoTherapy techniques in your professional practice must be accomplished by first experiencing them personally in order to comprehend their potency.

Although the 1983 book about PhotoTherapy contained an excellent conceptual introduction, it only detailed what various therapists had individually done using PhotoTherapy techniques in their particular practice or setting and thus really provided no practical advice for readers to learn how to actually get started doing PhotoTherapy themselves. *This is the reason for this book:* to make available a practical guide giving readers fresh ideas (with reasons to support them) and activities to try out for yourselves as well as with your clients, because I believe the best learning is internalized from personal experience. It provides a structured framework combining theoretical foundations, richly illustrated technique explanations, plus a significant amount of practical suggestions and "how to get started right now" exercises to try for yourself first, and then later to use with your clients.

A brief note should be added here about what this book is *not.* Some theorist-authors (notably, Akeret, 1973, and Lesy, 1976, 1980) base their entire practice on the assumption that they already know what people's photographs are about, and that they can instruct readers to decipher a photograph much like a book. Similarly, many postmodernist art theorists and critics suggest that it is possible to decode and mentally take apart the visual "texts" of photographs according to preestablished rules for interpretation (for example, Burgin, 1982; Roskill, 1989; and Roskill and Carrier, 1983).

I do understand that it may be possible to at least partially explore some embedded meanings in this manner, but only if you have advance guidelines (including a specific awareness of the privileges of power, culture, gender, race, and so forth) that will enable you to understand and translate according to those given rules. Nevertheless, in such cases, your "truth" will still be only relative to the reality of the person who authored those guidelines—and thus may be totally irrelevant to someone else whose value system is altogether different. So this book will not give readers lessons on how to go read the meanings of someone else's photographs *for* them; rather it will show how a collaborative therapist-client approach to the journey into the image can permit people to bring to light their own previously unconscious associations and feelings about the picture.

By the time you have finished the book, you will have learned the "why," "what," and "how" of PhotoTherapy techniques, and hopefully also made some enlightening personal discoveries along the way. If you are a therapist wanting to then begin working with these techniques, I would hope that you will have also learned that perhaps, instead of "walking in your clients' shoes for a day" to better understand their lives, you might metaphorically step behind the lens of their cameras in order to see what (and how) they see; to pose for them according to their directions of how a person "should" look for a portrait; to reflect with them on the meanings, feelings, memories, and thoughts stimulated by a photographic image; to explore their albums or photo-taking projects with them as they explain why they took certain photos in particular ways (and what, if anything, was missing that should have been in those pictures). You may also serendipitously encounter valuable insights into their families and their values by looking with them at their family albums and exploring with them the subtle nuances of their nonverbal behaviors as you see how they were captured unknowingly or in posing. Finally, if you ask them for their reactions to photographs you yourself have taken, you may discover anew how uniquely different and special each human mind truly is.

In this book, I have used a framework for presenting the techniques that corresponds to each position a person might take with regard to a camera: for example, as the subject, having a picture taken of yourself by someone else (who arranged or chose the moment to capture); as the photographer, doing the picture-taking (of others, scenery, objects, or whatever else catches your eye); as the photographic director, posing for a photo of yourself, but making all the choices involved (including control over the moment the shutter is pushed); as the "curator" of the photos in your own personal collection that have special meaning for you, such as those found in albums, on desktops, or on the walls of your home; and finally, as the reflective viewer looking at photos of your own, shown to you by others, or "found" in magazines, gallery exhibits, in greeting cards, and the like.

OVERVIEW OF THE CONTENTS

The major chapters in the book present the different PhotoTherapy techniques from much the same perspective: what happens when you view any photo (*photo-projective techniques*), your interactions with photos of yourself when you had all the control over the image's creation (*self-portraits*), photos taken of you by other people, whether posed or spontaneous, but where those others made all the decisions about timing, content, and so forth (*photos of the client by others*), photos taken by you, including those "taken" by gathering photos or photo-reproductions that other people may have created but which hold special meaning for you (*photos taken or collected by the client*), and finally those photos put together for the purpose of documenting the personal narrative of your life and the various family and other contexts from which you have developed (*album and photo-biographical snapshots*). Each technique chapter includes numerous anecdotes that illustrate various clients' experiences with it, and each is followed by a sampling of recommended "starter" exercises or activities.

Before these more detailed technique chapters, Chapter One gives some theoretical background and context for the rationale of the techniques, and then Chapter Two provides an overview that not only gives a brief introduction to each, but explains how they really are more an interrelated and interdependent system than discretely separate, individual steps of some particular fixed linear progression. I have not attempted in this book to provide the full developmental history of PhotoTherapy, nor any comprehensive literature review, though I do mention particularly relevant sources occasionally when I believe them important. A philosophical tome of many pages documenting others' findings is not my aim. It is one thing to read a book about therapy and something altogether different to actually start trying techniques out with a live client, and this book is definitely oriented toward the second option!

Similarly, although I emphasized earlier the additional value of this book for art therapists, there is not room in this book about PhotoTherapy for much in-depth discussion of the purely art therapy elements of exercises or examples given in this book. There are already numerous texts available about art therapy itself, some of which are listed in the Recommended Readings, should readers wish to learn more about these components of the client's expressions.

After the general introductions of the first two chapters, the remainder of the book contains primarily practical information, illustrations, and suggestions about each technique involved.

The *photo-projective techniques* in Chapter Three make use of the spontaneous associative process of connecting visual stimulus with conscious and unconscious meaning, quickly affirming that there is more than meets the eye when a person views any ordinary snapshot. At its most elemental level, seeing is believing. Both metaphorically and literally, we see what we believe and we believe what we see—the two are basically inseparable. *Seeing* is a word frequently used synonymously with *understanding*. This chapter establishes the foundation for all remaining PhotoTherapy activities, in that projective interactions with photos take place within all the others as well.

Readers are shown various ways to engage clients with photographic imagery and ways to structure therapy based on the questions posed during that process. Several examples are provided of people's responses and how these are integrated into the overall therapeutic progress. The chapter ends with a lengthy transcription of one person's encounter with one image over several sessions conducted over many months. This illustration is the longest anecdote in the book and is accompanied by commentary that explains my reasons for asking those particular questions.

Chapter Four, about *self-portrait techniques,* is the second major technique chapter because of the therapeutic primacy of self-oriented issues (such as self-esteem, self-confidence, self-acceptance, and other self-perceptive reflections). "Self-portrait" PhotoTherapy techniques focus on the client perceived as a distinct individual identity as removed from surrounding familial or societal contexts. Here the self is addressed as perceived directly by itself, hopefully to obtain a better sense of objective self-awareness, and the two chapters following this one then deal with the self as a separate individual as perceived by others and as perceiving others.

This self-portrait chapter details the various kinds of self-portraits clients can make spontaneously or in response to the therapist's assignments. Suggestions are given for both the process of creating self-portraits and for what can be done with them in active discussion after they have been created (and, if desired, elaborated on with various art materials, words, collaging, or three-dimensional work).

One key section demonstrates the kinds of questions that can be asked about any format of self-portrait, and I have selected for detailed presentation one of my favorite exercises whose questioning format demonstrates how I would orient questions to the client now holding one of these photographic assignment results. The transcripts used in this chapter's final examples in fact follow exactly this same questioning format model, so that readers can observe how the "live" processing of self-portraits can proceed in real experience as well as how differently one exercise can be interpreted and activated, depending upon the client's needs and the therapist's goals.

Chapter Five is about *photos of the client taken by others.* Some colleagues include photos others have taken of clients as part of the general category of self-portrait work and photos relating directly to self-image and self-perception. However, I prefer to teach "photos of the client taken by others" separately and distinctly from "self-portraits" due to the differential power issues around a photograph being made of a person in situations where the process was not fully under his or her own, independent control. (I also make a similar kind of differentiation about the technique discussed next, *photos taken by the client.*)

This chapter does *not* teach readers to examine photos of clients and then make pronouncements from an external viewpoint about the meaning of their faces, postures, bodies, or other accompanying photographic details. Instead readers are shown how to use photos of clients as starting points to find out more about their life and their feelings, along with discovering more about how they perceive themselves and their nonverbal communications to others. The chapter attends to the visual contents of photos clients appear in, as well as all the extra information that happens to appear in the photograph along with the person's image. There is also discussion about the relevance of the photographer, the person responsible for that photo's existence, whether he or she asked the client to pose or instead spontaneously captured the client on film.

Because this chapter and the following one are closely related to photographic self-statements, I have not included more lengthy transcripts or case studies in them. Rather, this chapter uses several briefer anecdotes to illustrate a variety of ways that photographs of the client taken by other people can provide PhotoTherapeutic benefit.

Chapter Six is about *photos taken or collected by the client.* As noted above, I also treat this technique separately because, although all photos are in some ways metaphoric self-portraits in their personal selectivity of focus and attention, clients are rarely conscious of this; thus their photographic selections indicate what kinds of images they have felt worth noticing and keeping. And sometimes it is the events surrounding the moment of picture taking that give the image its strongest emotional meaning, rather than the actual visual contents inside the frame. This also applies to photographic images taken by other people that my clients have collected, often simply because they liked them. These kinds of photos were "taken" by selective accumulation rather than pushing a shutter, so clients may not perceive these as being self-reflective visual statements until later encounters with them.

This chapter discusses uses of photos clients have taken or collected, both those brought into therapy already existing, as well as those created in response to assignments given by the therapist. It also suggests ways these visual artifacts can be used later for exercises concentrating on partializing or prioritizing goals, values clarification, and other multi-photo activities. It concludes not with a client illustration, but rather with a personal reflection by someone who directly experienced one such in-depth exercise working with his own photos (plus one invisible one), and who shares how it felt to journey through its many steps.

Album and photo-biographical snapshots are covered in Chapter Seven. The concept of "self" was worked with as an isolate in the previous three chapters. This chapter completes the PhotoTherapy picture by considering the "self" of the family—the family unit as a self, a distinct identity apart from just the sum of those individuals who form it by virtue of birth, affiliation, choice, or whichever type of "family" is being identified with—as well as what this means in terms of one of its members being my client. Either way, self as isolate or self in context, an externalized and objectified self-identity is really its own myth and its own construction. Readers can learn the advantages of using both in family work when comparing the family story created by the album's keeper with versions of the same photos as defined by the people appearing in them (or left out!). I also note the isomorphic parallels in considering any album as itself being a systemic level of photographic organization.

This chapter blends a framework drawn from family systems theory with a discussion of how to apply its concepts to both reviewing existing family photos (or missing ones) with clients, as well as activities that can be done to reformat these according to specific assignments. The role of the album keeper (the family story's narrator) is also explored and documented in several anecdotes as being illustrative of several systems-based positionings. There is also discussion of how these can be used in situations requiring discovery of personal support networks, for life review summaries with those facing end-of-life issues, with abuse survivors, and other special applications.

As this chapter discusses the value of clients reviewing their own family photos for both secrets and discoveries of systemic undercurrents, I thought it might be beneficial to use for the anecdotal illustrations of this chapter a thorough album review done by a person who also happens to be trained in systems theory—in this case, myself! Thus readers will find the major illustrative example for this chapter to be a retrospective reflection of my own family's album as divided into sections organized according to systems theory concepts, such as pattern repetitions, intergenerational and triangulation dynamics, gender role expectations, differentiation/fusion, and other key structural elements.

Chapter Eight ends the book with a brief discussion of other related aspects of PhotoTherapy that are important to all readers, therapists or not, and ties the book together in a comprehensive interweaving of applications useful for all.

Following the final chapter, readers will find both a Reference List and a Recommended Readings section that together provide a comprehensive listing of additional literature readers can access directly or contact me for locating. Both demonstrate the wide scope and variety of these techniques as documented in actual application.

My goal is that this book be a practical and functional distillation of information about PhotoTherapy that will guide readers in beginning to use these techniques as soon as they have finished reading it and experienced the recommended "starter" exercises firsthand.

For further information about references listed, networking contacts, author addresses, or for any other information or feedback, including informing me about your own findings or ideas, readers are welcome to write me at the PhotoTherapy Centre, 1107 Homer St., Suite #304, Vancouver, B.C., Canada, V6B 2Y1.

ACKNOWLEDGMENTS

Many thanks are due to those whose help made this book possible: to all those students who asked why and how and thus precipitated my decision to write the book; to my good friend, Terry Goodwin, for patience and endurance through hours upon tedious hours of proofreading and videotape transcriptions as well as many comments of helpful criticism; to Laura Morrison for also transcribing videotapes; to both David Krauss and Joel Walker, my PhotoTherapy colleagues and dear friends, whose thoughts on the subject parallel mine so closely that we often seem to "breathe the same air" when teaching or writing; to Susan Robinson (known in my earlier writings as "Debbie F."), who was the patient recipient of some of my earliest attempts to actualize these ideas; to all those who have trustingly released their personal photo-anecdotal stories for use in these pages; to my parents (who still love me despite my revealing many personal details about my childhood life and snapshots—most of which they have demanded I tell readers "aren't really true"!); to my editors Rebecca McGovern and Xenia Lisanevich, to the Canada Council, and to two other financial contributors who wish to remain anonymous, for their belief in (and financial support of) my efforts to pioneer this field and who thus have literally bought me the time and confidence to complete this book.

I want to express my deepest appreciation of the very special friendship offered me by Billy Rodda, whose inner strength, loving support, and complete trust have permitted us to journey through some of the most validating (and amazing) PhotoTherapy experiences of my life. And finally, I want to acknowledge the special importance of my husband Robert Ostiguy, whose infinite patience, continually forgiving temperament, and totally unconditional love throughout the writing of this manuscript (as well as throughout my life in general) are appreciated far more than mere words (or even photographs) could ever fully tell.

The Author

Judy Weiser is director and training coordinator of the PhotoTherapy Centre in Vancouver, Canada. She received her B.A. degree (1967) in psychology and anthropology from Rice University and her M.S. degree (1970) in education (specializing in counseling) from the State University of New York at Plattsburgh. She is a licensed psychologist and registered art therapist who focuses her clinical and consulting practice on the nonverbal, and particularly visual, aspects of communication and behavior, including cultural and gender differences relevant to therapeutic, intercultural, educational, and rehabilitation situations.

A consultant and therapist in private practice, she specializes in teaching mental health professionals how "ordinary" snapshots and family albums can be used as effective therapeutic tools. In addition to giving numerous lectures, workshops, courses, and skills-training intensives across North America, Europe, and Great Britain, she teaches for the Graduate Program of the British Columbia School of Art Therapy in Victoria as well as the Creative Therapy Program of the College of the North Netherlands in Leeuwarden. She is listed in the Canadian Register of Health Service Providers in Psychology. She is an occasional consultant for Kodak and is the Canadian Liaison to the Board of the International Arts-Medicine Association. Recently she was appointed to the Editorial Board of the *Journal of Medical Humanities.*

In 1982, her PhotoTherapy training program was awarded distinction as one of the top twenty programs in the world by the International Visual Literacy Association (of which she is a past board member). She has been featured in a variety of publications and media interviews, including *Life* magazine, *Maclean's, New York Times, National Globe and Mail, USA Today, B.C. Photographer, Child,* American Airlines's *In Flight,* Kodak's *Montage, Canadian Living,* and *PhotoLife.* A past Canada Council Explorations grant recipient, she has appeared numerous times in local and national print, radio, and television productions, describing and demonstrating the uses of PhotoTherapy. In 1989 she was featured in a two-part special program about photography for the Canadian Broadcast Corporation's television program "The Journal." Past editor of the journal *Phototherapy,* she has authored numerous articles and several book chapters on the uses of photography as nonverbal communication in cross-cultural as well as general psychotherapeutic settings, and with particular populations such as women, adolescents, or people with communication impairments.

A therapist and trainer for over twenty years, she originally concentrated on work with culturally different, disadvantaged, disabled, or marginalized populations, particularly hearing-impaired First Nations people, as well as on systemic approaches with families experiencing physical, sexual, emotional, or substance-related abuse issues.

For the past decade she has specialized in helping people with AIDS-related emotional problems (including HIV-positive persons, long-term survivors, and their families, lovers, and friends), along with grief counseling and work with various AIDS Memorial Quilt projects in Canada, the United States, and Great Britain. She is on the advisory board of the NAMES Project–Canada as well as coordinator of the Vancouver affiliate of that group. She is the ongoing chairperson of the HIV/AIDS Study Group of the American Art Therapy Association and is on the board of the Deaf Outreach Project for AIDS Vancouver. Her publications on AIDS-related topics have appeared in the *Art Therapy Journal, Vancouver Sun,* and *Gallerie Magazine.* At the request of the U.S. NAMES Project in 1990, she wrote their national emotional support worker training handout, which is also used in several other countries.

Fluent in a variety of Deaf Sign and nonverbal symbol languages, she is also a professional photographer. Her works have been presented in many gallery exhibits and in numerous photographic publications.

PhotoTherapy Techniques

1 Photographs as Therapeutic Tools

Photographs are footprints of our minds, mirrors of our lives, reflections from our hearts, frozen memories we can hold in silent stillness in our hands—forever, if we wish. They document not only where we may have been but also point the way to where we might perhaps be going, whether we know it yet or not. We should converse with them often and listen well to the secrets their lives can tell.

The mind can only absorb information through the organs of sight, hearing, smell, taste, and touch. Since about 80 percent of sensory stimuli enter through our eyes (Hall, 1973), sight-based information is crucial to our understanding of what we encounter. Thus there is a strong visual component to our experiences, and to our memories of them. Moreover, meaning doesn't really exist "out there" apart from us, but rather in the relationship between the stimulus object and the perceiver. It isn't just beauty that is "in the eye of the beholder"; our idea of reality itself is based on our perceptions. If we notice something, it is because it has some kind of meaning for us. If we don't notice it, it hasn't stood out as distinct; in some ways it doesn't exist for us at all. When we first perceive an object, it is already etched with our personal meaning. That meaning is impossible to remove; it is permanently fixed in our memory.

Different people will interpret the same sensory stimulus in different ways, based on who they are and the background factors that influence what they do or do not notice. The basic units of visual and other data will be more or less the same for everyone; for example, each person looking at a photograph might see a woman dressed in a red shirt and jeans, with curly dark hair, and so on. What these facts mean, however, depends primarily on what each perceiver brings to the photograph.

Things or people we don't notice are likely those that are not significant to us; differences that make some difference in our minds will likely be those we pay attention to. (Was there a photo on a previous page? What color is the cover of this book? Is there background noise as you read this question?) In the act of perceiving, we partially bring into being that which we later accept as "reality." The meaning we think we are getting from a visual stimulus (seeing a person, seeing a photograph) is primarily *created* by us during our process of perceiving it. Important components in how we create that reality are our personal sets of perceptual filters, personal symbologies, and unique "inner maps" or frameworks for logical thinking. These factors shape the practice of photography on many levels, from influencing which pictures we take to affecting which ones we like or remember years later.

The postmodernist art movement is based on the concept that there is no one universal reality that can be objectively observed by all spectators. Rather, postmodernism posits reality as totally relative and conditional upon human perception of it. People's experiences of reality actually construct its meaning for them, and their eventual definition of it will be based on their deconstruction of that meaning.

Constructivism holds that there is no neutral knowledge; all perceptions are given value and context by the perceiver. Knowledge does not relate to facts but to assumptions about life; all we can know about an object's reality is its surface appearance, as we selectively perceive it. Therefore its meaning is personally, socially, and culturally constructed during the process of making sense of it to ourselves, including later verbal explanations or artistic representations about it. Similarly, photographs can then also be considered constructions of reality rather than objective recordings of it, owing in part to the choice of a moment to depict and the subsequent imposition of a frame around the fragment we select from the "whole picture" available to the eye.

Deconstruction deals with how objects are interpreted by viewers. Just as constructivism suggests that there can be no single fixed reality, deconstruction denies that objective meaning can be decoded from a given image or object. Ideally, when we examine art or life from either of these perspectives, we become more aware of how our own unconscious has contributed to meaning formation and how language—both verbal and nonverbal—mediates significations.

In therapy, as people attempt to unravel layers of meaning beneath even familiar persons' ordinary behaviors or conversations, they can begin to recognize how feelings unconsciously connect to thoughts or words, and how some people can manipulate others' emotional responses by using "loaded" images or words to construct visual or verbal messages. In this sense, postmodernism can be seen to have evolved from existential and phenomenological theory, all three of which provide a theoretical framework for understanding how people get meaning from photographs.

The postmodernist view that meaning is selected through the filters of the individual and that a different meaning can be taken from an image by every person who perceives it holds true in all human interactions with external reality. These ideas have great import for therapy, which deals with people's understandings about their lives and identities.

Most of us think, feel, and recall memories not in words directly, but rather in iconic imagery: inner, silent thought-pictures (sometimes accompanied by kinesthetic or other cues), and visual codes and concepts. All of these make up the mental maps that we use when later trying to cognitively communicate about things, whether using words or artistic symbolic representations of them.

A snapshot seems to me a simultaneous representation of the thinking and feeling parts of people, and thus, it is very difficult to distill a simple objective observation or direct correlation of meaning from its initially spontaneous origins. Feelings are transient unless a camera catches their behavioral or affective manifestations; it is only their visual traces that appear on film. Trying to "read" a photograph like a book results in problems similar to those of wave-particle theory in quantum physics, where the act of observation automatically alters what is examined, changing it from its natural, unobserved state. A camera does not just record; it also mediates. Cultural, ethnic, sociological, gender, and other types of filters cannot be removed from the person doing the observing or interpreting, and so the meaning extracted from any photograph is personal and idiosyncratic, and often not the communication intended by the original photographer. As each viewer's response is based on unique individual perceptions, the meaning of the photograph therefore exists as an unobservable, though not necessarily random, combination of possibilities that occurs only in the interface *between* that person and the image itself.

HOW PEOPLE RESPOND TO PHOTOGRAPHS

If you stop to think about it, a photograph is a rather curious thing. It's a piece of very thin paper that we perceive three-dimensionally, as if alive, and as if existing right now. The moment we look at, inside its borders, is "now"; we are *there,* within the space and time of that image, as if really physically there ourselves. Our mind does not separate viewing the visual contents of a photograph from viewing those visual facts themselves; it is a transitional object that bridges without our even realizing this is happening. Looking at a photo of our relatives of a hundred years ago, we conceptually process the image as if we are seeing them alive in front of us at that moment, and we are right there, across from them, looking on. Our mind achieves a cognitive leap that equates looking at the photo with being in the actual scene. Thus we feel certain that the camera did not, and could not, lie, because it obviously took a picture of what was really happening right there, right then, right in front of it. Except, the camera didn't take the picture; a person did.

Someone once told me a photo was paper with "emotion" all over it; of course he meant emulsion, but the malapropism stayed with me. Photographs are indeed emotionally charged, as if electromagnetically etched, and we can never view our personal photos dispassionately. In fact, these small pieces of paper are empowered far beyond their apparent value; their significance resonates to and from people, over the past and into the future. Emotions connected to the subject matter become transferred to the photographic representation of that subject as a type of stand-in for the real person, place, or thing. It is natural that people respond to these visual artifacts as if they were full of life.

A photograph, then, has the special quality of being simultaneously a realistic illusion and an illusory reality, a moment captured—yet never fully captured. We use film to stop time, which cannot be stopped. These aspects are crucial for an understanding of why (and how) PhotoTherapy works: it permits the complex examination of a slice of time frozen on film as a "fact," and it also allows an endless variety of "realities" to be revealed as each viewer responds to it differently. Every snapshot has stories to tell, secrets to share, and memories to bring forth.

The person who takes a picture is trying to make a permanent record of a special moment (it is special because the perceiver sees it as such; perhaps no one else would). If the picture turns out "right" it is because it satisfies the photographer's expectations; if it doesn't, he or she will likely have some idea about what was missing or "wrong." The photos people take (or collect as postcards, posters, magazine or calendar pictures, and so forth) can tell something about them. These photos were taken or gathered because they mattered. As a collection, they constitute almost a mirror-reflection of their owner, in that we usually won't keep photos around that we don't like or that don't matter. The ones that are most special to us express many things about us and our life that we might explain. We only need to be asked good exploratory questions.

When people pose for photos, even those they take of themselves, they usually have certain ideas about how they should look in the final picture, and these reflect their expectations about how they should be perceived by other people in real life. Asking them questions about photos of themselves can be a good way to find out how they evaluate themselves.

The visual contents of the photographic image itself are important, but the meaning of these contents to each person encountering them is also significant. A photo will "mean" differently to the person who took it, to each person in it (whether posed or captured unaware), any person later viewing it (regardless of their familiarity with the subjects of the photo or the photographer), and certainly any person who keeps it as part of a permanent collection or, perhaps more important, a family album. (Family albums have their own private lives and reasons for existence.)

Frequently, in PhotoTherapy processes, clients' explanations of the meaning of a snapshot turn out to be far less significant than their explanations of why what they know is true and how they know that it is true. A lot can be revealed as a person delves into what a photo is about emotionally as well as what it shows visually. No matter how large the photograph, it is never more than a detail of an even larger picture of life in space and time. Its significance grows as we learn more about its context. Clients who are able to regard their photographs as starting points rather than end products, and who can use them to initiate questions and explore feelings, can learn a great deal about themselves in the process.

THE POWER OF PHOTOTHERAPY

Throughout our lives, we store information for later recall without any words coming into use. We may use words later to try to translate back to others the thoughts and feelings that we understand "wordlessly" from inside ourselves, but the words we use are only an attempted representation of that inner meaning, not the meaning itself. Each of us uses an inner language to categorize reality and code our experience of it so that it is accessible inside us, but raw experience isn't necessarily translatable into words for full description. Photographs, however, have the power to capture and express feelings and ideas in visual-symbolic forms, some of which are intimately personal metaphors.

The symbols and visual representations that appear in photographs are clearly a language, but one that an outsider may not understand without assistance from the person who produced them. Language constructs reality, yet language is not always solely verbal. Artistic representation is a language, and certainly it communicates as well as words about our thoughts, feelings, and relationships. When we become aware of our visual (nonverbal) literacy—and understand fully that it differs for each of us—we can begin to appreciate the extent to which decisions, expectations, feelings, thoughts, and memories are based on nonverbal stimuli and meaning-making and are thus directly connected with our sensory perceptions.

In summary, most of what we absorb in everyday interactions with life is not verbally coded when it goes into our brains and is not accessed that way when we want to refer back to it. Information only shifts into verbal language when we are trying to make something that is inside our mind comprehensible to the mind of someone else. Thus it should be no surprise that communicators—teachers, therapists, and others whose work focuses on inner meanings—need to make use of nonverbal means of expressing and sharing meaning, such as music, dance, the visual arts, and definitely photography. All the various arts therapies and expressive therapies are based on this concept. Before considering how PhotoTherapy both is and isn't art therapy, it will be useful to discuss how PhotoTherapy can fit into the spectrum of therapeutic models and techniques.

Within the therapeutic context, I believe it is impossible to think of a client's problem as being the effect of any single cause. A person experiencing a problem in a given situation is not only part of that situation but also partial creator of its definitions and potential; thus the person cannot be expected to view the problem from an objective "outsider" position, nor can the person's therapist be expected to fully understand it from an outside position, looking in. Also, while effects may accompany causes, they do not, in reverse, define them.

In my work with clients, I prefer to see cause and effect not as a linear sequential connection traveling in only one direction at a time, but rather as synchronistic or intuitive movements that are just as valid as cognitive or logical ones. Thus, to paraphrase Rhyne (1990), I have ceased to be single-minded and have become instead "pattern-minded"; I find that chaos or systems/cybernetic theories are much more useful models for understanding the complexities of people's problems than those based upon linear causality. This in turn has influenced all my other activities, from theoretical lecturing to conducting therapy to planning my weekend calendar; similarly I try to get my clients to understand that they live "more than one-octave lives" (personal letter from Shaun McNiff, February 9, 1990).

I'm a therapist who prefers to use all the tools I can discover for helping my clients: hypnosis *and* dream review *and* Gestalt "empty chair" or role-playing, *and,* of course, also art therapy and PhotoTherapy techniques—when any of these seem the most sensible and promising approaches. But I don't do the same thing with every client, nor do I force the same identical sequence or selection of PhotoTherapy techniques onto each one, as if following a prescription list. Instead, I fit the amount of PhotoTherapy involvement to each individual client's particular needs. If one technique doesn't turn out as effective as hoped, I try something else. I don't use all the techniques all the time, and the extent to which I join them with various art therapy or other applications will vary markedly, depending on each client's unique needs and goals. Because of this I also strongly resist using the term "PhotoTherap*ist*" because any good therapist isn't going to stick to one single approach or technique, any more than a photographer would always use only one lens or an artist just one color from the palette.

In working with people who are having emotional and communication problems, with others or inside themselves, I need to know about them as individuals, apart from family or work contexts, but I also need to gather information about the client's enmeshing and contexting relationships. PhotoTherapy is an unusually effective way to approach that information, with both self-related photos and family relationship ones playing important parts.

For me, PhotoTherapy involves at least two phases: what happens to clients during the active work component of the PhotoTherapy process, and also (possibly more to the therapeutic import of it all) what happens as they begin to later synthesize, understand, absorb, reflect upon, and emotionally process all the "fallout" from that doing of the work, the viewing of the results, and all that evolves from the entire process. Anyone who has ever chosen to go take photos or review the ones taken previously has likely encountered the natural process of self-exploration and personal development that the medium of photography can provide. This is photography *as* therapy, and many amateur photographers have experienced its benefits. All photography can be therapeutic, though the effects tend to be more concentrated when assistance is involved. With photography *in* therapy, the primary emphasis is on the therapy, wherein the therapist directs the client's involvement with photographs and photography as treatment progresses. This is all reminiscent of the argument about whether the focus for art therapists should be art-as-therapy or art-in-therapy; my response is always a confounding but simple "yes, it's clearly both."

Some of my colleagues in psychotherapy find it sufficient for their clients to experience, remember, emote, viscerally understand, or re-create. In my experience, clients seem to benefit greatly by progressing to self-witnessing and reflective validation. This also helps them bring their experience into a cognitive, and usually verbal, framework, which they can then use to further integrate and build upon what they have experienced emotionally.

I believe that for people to benefit from therapy, they need to experience both a cognitive awareness and an emotional experiencing of the role of past events, memories, thoughts, and feelings to fully grasp the effect of the past on the present. Both the mind and the heart, both insight and cognitive framing are necessary. One or the other alone is necessary but not sufficient for success. Memory is part of the body as well as the mind, and thus in reconnecting people with their feelings or doing something to help them change, we cannot work solely with the brain. Nonverbal and sensory-based techniques seem the best choices for working with those parts of ourselves that are essentially unconscious and that use a primarily symbolic nonverbal language of representation and communication. For these reasons, therapists who want to help people with deep-rooted problems need to use tools that can reach those nonverbal, and primarily visual, components of our unconscious domains, such as art therapy and PhotoTherapy.

PHOTOTHERAPY AND ART THERAPY: SIMILARITIES AND DIFFERENCES

Some theorists have debated as to whether photography is indeed art. Some view photographs as only the products of mechanical documentation, involving no creative personal input from the artist. They say that photographs may well be communications, but that they are not "pure" art. Having to decide whether photographs are art *or* communication can only serve to delay their use as both. This dichotomizing issue is not relevant for therapeutic purposes, where both easily coexist simultaneously. It seems a bit silly to argue whether photography is art *or* communication, when art *is* itself communication, and all communication *is* a form of art expression itself! I certainly agree with a systems/cybernetics approach to art therapy practices (Landgarten, 1981, 1987; Lusebrink, 1989; Nucho, 1988; Rhyne, 1984; Riley, 1985, 1988, 1990; Sobol, 1982, 1985).

In that PhotoTherapy has become a popular topic for study, among art therapists in particular, I think it is important to discuss the implications of art therapy theory and practice for the understanding and application of PhotoTherapy techniques. I do not see the two as being mutually exclusive, nor do I find any argument between them.

There is a long-standing debate as to whether art therapy is a set of techniques that all therapists (psychologists, family counselors, psychiatrists, and so on) can learn to use, or whether it is a separate model, with a distinct underlying conceptual basis. Good arguments can be made on both sides, but it is not my purpose or intention to attempt to resolve them here. My own position is that PhotoTherapy is not a separate model, but rather a set of interactive techniques useful for all therapists regardless of their preferred theoretical modalities. To me they are integrally interrelated, reciprocal subsets of each other, even though sometimes very different in product or process owing to their being very different media. They both work on the basis of giving visual form to feelings and making the invisible more visible, a type of "unconsciousness raising" (Martin and Spence, 1988). Krauss (1979, 1983) provides a detailed comparison and contrast of the two, and a summary of some of his points appears within the following discussion of the similarities and differences I have experienced.

Symbolic representation is the only language we will ever have for expressing and communicating thoughts, feelings, memories, and other inner experiences, even though it necessarily mediates and filters those experiences in the process of describing them. All art therapy is based on the idea that visual-symbolic representation is far less interruptive and distortive than verbal translations of sensory-based experiences, and that we not only often project unconscious meaning through such metaphoric communications from deep inside but also tap into those areas while simply reacting or responding to symbolic imagery produced by others. Krauss stresses that nonverbal personal symbols are immensely powerful because they arise from the unconscious to indicate their own existence; he refers to them as the actual source of our consciousness. When we look at photos or artworks we have produced, or review our responses to seeing them, and when we explore the themes and patterns that emerge when we do so, we are able to learn about our own unconscious by bypassing the verbal translations that also provide good hiding places for rationalizations, defenses, excuses, and other protections.

In art therapy, clients usually produce images spontaneously; these symbolic communications arise directly from the unconscious. Sometimes the many levels of metaphoric signification in these images are readily comprehended, but usually they serve only as a starting place. Although the "art" of art therapy may not be "real" art, it is personally coded expression in nonverbal form; similarly, photographs are in some ways private communications to and from the self, regardless of any serendipitous artistic merit.

Krauss (1983) makes this observation:

> Although both art therapy and phototherapy utilize the methodology of pictorial projection, it would seem initially that they do so in very different ways. Art therapy relies on a client's internal concerns to emerge from the unconscious through the process of a drawing, spontaneously produced by the client, and external stimuli, light, or content, need not be available at the time the client draws a picture for an image to appear in the drawing. . . . Photographs, on the other hand, will be taken at the place where the physical content actually exists [or its symbolized form appears or is arranged to appear]. A photograph of a house will use as content some physical representation of a house. Since art therapy is dependent on externalized internal subjects, and photo-

> therapy is dependent on internalized external subjects, it appears as though they deal with different aspects of personal symbolism [p. 53].

Many art therapists stress the importance of the client actually making the symbolic images as being often more valuable than the other components. This illustrates one central difference between the two approaches: making images is only one facet of PhotoTherapy, and not necessarily a central one. Another difference is the familiarity and comfort level that most people have with the medium of photography. There is an element of ordinariness to taking and discussing snapshots that is usually not evident in making or commenting on artistic creations.

Similarly, attribution of a work of art is usually part of its meaning. Rarely do we view a piece of art without realizing that it expresses the personal viewpoint of its maker, yet somehow we see a snapshot as a factual image that anyone going by with a camera could have recorded. In PhotoTherapy, therefore, speculation about the goals, needs, or desires of the originator can be built into the investigative process with snapshots in ways unavailable with other art media creations. Indeed, because the creator of a photograph can be so readily detached from the image, PhotoTherapy can easily be done using photos not originating with the client, which is not common in Art Therapy practice (with the exception of collage work).

Art therapy usually seems to focus on the finished product, paying less attention to the concept or development of the image. In PhotoTherapy, the process is more balanced; the photographic print is often the least important element, while the criteria used for selecting the plan, deciding what to do in creating the photograph (where, when, who, why, who for), and so forth, are important and merit exploration. Therapeutically "working" the finished print is an important component, but just as often it is used to precipitate questions that carry discussion away from the photograph.

Krauss points out the additional value of factual documentation provided by so many personal snapshots: "The availability for utilization of personal and family photographs . . . provide[s] a rich source of projective and physical data that could not be obtained any other way. They provide background information about a client's relationship to the world outside of therapy [including their family members and how they relate with one another as captured by a camera rather than words]" (1983, p. 53).

Using photographs, we can see a fairly close proximation of the same way we present ourselves to others, rather than the reversed image we see in the mirror. We can also see ourselves in profile or from the back, and also as part of larger groups of family or friends. In art therapy, portraits of ourselves are strictly personal subjective representations; PhotoTherapy provides considerably less subjective images created by a mechanical device.

Finally, I find no parallel in PhotoTherapy for the developmental stages of art making that some art therapists believe to be crucial for measuring progress, improvement, or arrested stages. Photo-snapping skills don't really change much with age, other than perhaps that we learn to stand more still or to consciously compose more sophisticated contents (if that is our goal). I have seen some serious metaphorical photographic communications from eight-year-olds and autistic teenagers and some technically poor or confusing ones from adult professionals. So developmental stages of art-making abilities are not strongly relevant in PhotoTherapy work.

2 *The Five Techniques of PhotoTherapy*

The basic techniques of PhotoTherapy are directly related to the possible relationships between person and camera or person and photo. These are (1) photos taken of the client, (2) photos taken by the client, (3) photos of the client by the client (self-portraits), and (4) biographical snapshots, often of groups of friends or family, in which the client may or may not be included (parties, weddings, family gatherings, and so forth). Each of these four is represented by a major technique of PhotoTherapy, but there is a fifth one that is more a part of the others than it is separate unto itself. This final technique is what I have called the "projective" technique, in that it deals with the ways and reasons that a person gets any meaning from any photograph in the first place.

The projective component of understanding photographic meaning underlies all interactions between people and snapshots. Projecting meaning onto photographs (and anything else our senses encounter) is integral with our looking at them. Photos simplify by partializing life and help slow time into units of meaning that people can study. In describing and reacting to photos, people are frequently able to reach pockets of strong feelings that are usually covered by cognitive barriers such as denials and rationalizations.

PhotoTherapy techniques permit clients to bypass conscious verbal controls and monitors, as well as allow their unconscious metaphoric and symbolic (nonverbal) languages to emerge. Using the camera works particularly well for people who find other visual arts too demanding or too risky to try.

More details about specific applications can be found at the end of this book in both the References and Recommended Readings. Some citations reference the attempts of various colleagues to map the PhotoTherapy territory conceptually in order to structure a framework of reference for research or teaching (for example, Cooper, 1984; Fryrear, 1980; Gooblar, 1989; Krauss, 1979; Loellbach, 1978; Nath, 1981; Smith, 1989). A review of these will reveal how difficult it is to try to separate into discrete and clearly boundaried subsets techniques that are really intrinsically interrelated. Additionally, several therapists have conducted multistage comprehensive programs that regularly and successfully involved using more than a single technique at a time or from session to session (see Brenneman, 1990; Hogan, 1981; Krauss, 1979; Mann, 1983; Marino and Lambert, 1990; Reid, 1985; Smith, 1989, 1990; Weiser, 1975, 1984c, 1985, 1989; Zabar, 1987).

Krauss (1979) recommends a four-component framework for private practitioners in which clients are asked to bring in a current photo of themselves, a photo of their current family, a childhood photo, and also one that represents them symbolically. Stewart (1978) has produced a multitechnique workbook for his clients that includes relating realistic and fantasy images of self and family. Other therapist-authors documented the use of different techniques with one client in longitudinal applications lasting several years, where one facet has given way to another as the client need mandated (for example, Weiser, 1983a, 1983b).

Numerous articles and graduate theses discuss working with all the many techniques inclusively (some of the best of which are Amerikaner, Schauble, and Ziller, 1980; Burckhardt, 1990; Carpenter, 1986; Coblenz, 1964; Cooper, 1984; Cosden and Reynolds, 1982; Craig, 1991; Evans, 1989; Gallagher, 1981; Glass, 1991; Gosciewski, 1975; Graham, 1967; Krauss, 1979; Lambert, 1988; Levinson, 1979; Muhl, 1927; Nath, 1981; Peck, 1990; Reid, 1985; Smith, 1989, 1990; Stewart, 1979a, 1979b; Trusso, 1979; Turner-Hogan, 1980; Tyding, 1973; Wallace, 1979; Weiser, 1983a, 1983b, 1984a, 1984b, 1988a, 1988b; Williams, 1987; Zakem, 1977a, 1983, 1984). Finally, radio, television, and print media reportage may be useful for readers who want to examine PhotoTherapy's history or accomplishments as translated for the general public's understanding (such as: Brody, 1984; Cohen, 1983; Elias, 1982; Fenjues, 1981; Hagarty, 1985; Hathaway, 1984; Lipovenko, 1984; Medina, 1981; Morgan, 1974; Morganstern, 1980; Nierman, 1989; Palmer, 1990; Poli, 1979; Proudfoot, 1984; Robotham, 1982; Sevitt, 1983; Sheehan, 1988; Sherkin, 1989; Tomaszewski, 1981; Weal, 1979; Wilcox, 1990; Zakem, 1977b).

In addition to the major PhotoTherapy techniques useful for most psychotherapy situations, there are numerous related applications, among them video and active darkroom techniques, that can aid the therapy process. Readers will find several citations on video therapy listed in the Recommended Readings and may contact the author for additional references. Blended combinations of photographic and other artistic media can be useful to those trained in art therapy, and these may be tailored to specific uses in related fields, such as cross-cultural counseling, proxemics studies, special education, and so forth. There are also numerous possible applications for different age populations, diagnostic groups (schizophrenics, adolescent offenders, abuse victims, bereavement groups), and settings (agencies, group homes, hospitals, day-treatment programs). The literature also addresses the timing of different PhotoTherapy applications during the therapy process; for example, during intake, diagnosis/assessment, in-session treatment, out-of-session periods, termination, post-treatment follow-up, and so forth.

The scope of this book precludes further discussion of most of these applications of PhotoTherapy techniques, but there are numerous listings in the book's Reference and Recommended Readings sections specifically attending to each of these. Readers are strongly urged to use these sections as resources for information about the wide range of additional PhotoTherapy applications.

1. THE PROJECTIVE PROCESS

Much of what we think we see is instead actually coming from us. This, in a word, is the projective process that happens in response to photographs, things, or people—known and familiar to us or never seen before. The projective technique uses photographic images to elicit emotional responses, whether or not accompanied by verbal description. Any type of photo can be used, including the client's personal snapshots or someone else's, or pictures found on magazine pages, postcards, calendars, album covers, greeting cards, or even photocopies of these images. We look at a photograph and what we see is someone's representation of something important to them. But we will always take our own meaning from it, which may or may not be what the photographer intended. As we try to figure out the photograph, we mentally scan it, instinctively deconstructing it to get it to make sense. In constructing our meaning of it, our inner representations of that photo, our personal constructs, will be the only reality that we will ever be able to know of it.

It may remind us of something or someone else; it may bring up associated feelings; it may start us thinking. We use it not as a finished product but as a beginning, a stimulus or catalyst for our projections of meaning. We project ourselves and our uniquely personal interpretations onto it. In this sense, the projective PhotoTherapy process is similar to numerous other traditional projective instruments used in psychotherapy and art therapy, such as the familiar Rorschach inkblot test, the Thematic Aperception Test, or various draw-a-person or house-tree-person projective drawing assessments. However, there is no interpretation manual provided for evaluating projective responses to photo stimuli; they are accepted for their content rather than their correctness. This aspect of the process means that therapists need to be sure that answers always come from the client, who is only being guided by the therapist's questions. It is also important to keep in mind that a response doesn't automatically mean something significant in diagnostic terms; there must be repetitions or patterns in clients' responses before any significance can be supposed.

Thus when looking at snapshots taken by or of clients, at their albums, or at photos by others that they have found to be personally meaningful, therapists should be interested more in the "why" and "how" of these pictures than the "what." Because there can be no wrong way to interpret a photo and every answer is right for the person stating it, the projective process is a tool for developing self-awareness and self-empowerment. Projective PhotoTherapy techniques can be an especially good starting place for work with clients who have been long used to having their responses devalued or doubted, as well as for people who want to gain a better understanding of the unconscious processes that direct their lives.

What a person notices will always mirror the inner map that she or he is unconsciously using to organize and understand what the senses are perceiving. This continual process of attention and clarification, if reflected upon self-consciously, can also help reveal the value system and belief structure underlying clients' cognitive constructs. Therefore one of my main goals of therapy is to try my best to discover the criteria clients are using to distinguish relevant differences so I can better comprehend the uniquely personal maps or frameworks with which they make unconscious decisions.

I want to become more aware of the personal codes they use to signify and store meaning for later recall, as well as to learn more about what exactly connects their conscious thoughts to the associated spontaneous reemergence of previously unrecognized or unremembered feelings and memories. Such an awareness can provide a framework whereby clients can learn more about these parts of themselves that ordinarily are not observed and thus not consciously examinable. If they can become conscious of them, then the feelings connected with these stimuli can become better integrated and acknowledged (and if desired, changed).

There is an additional benefit from having people focus on their reactions to photos, and this relates more to interpersonal than intrapersonal process. The earlier comments about there being no single right or wrong way to perceive or react to a photo can easily be rephrased to refer to how people react when encountering each other in person. One person encounters another; expectations and personal perceptual filters of both persons collide and try to mutually adjust. If there is to be communication between two people, then there must be shared meaning to base it on. If one party to a dialogue is not what the other is used to encountering or is expecting to meet, their reactions to each other may reflect projections about each other that have no basis in fact, but rather arise solely in response to the threat of difference itself. This can make it hard to communicate about something they supposedly hold in common.

If people can become more aware that difference does not automatically signal "better" or "worse," the common defensive attitude that "if I'm right then you must be wrong because there's no other option" can cease to have valid meaning. And if differences between people cease to be threatening and become instead a basis for appreciating the range of possibilities available in the world (or within a family), then being different can be seen as enriching rather than problematical.

Consider the situation of many people viewing the same photograph of a person very different from all of them. Each will be likely to perceive the photo's subject a bit differently, depending on their own smaller differences from each other. Each person's perceptions about that photo's subject is indeed true and correct for that particular perceiver, even though possibly radically different from those of its other perceivers. If they can consciously recognize that all of them hold different truths about the photograph that are equally valid, they may begin to see that they need not feel threatened the next time they encounter a real-life person whose opinion or appearance is very different from theirs.

In my work with clients from traditionally marginalized, politically disenfranchised populations, I have found projective PhotoTherapy techniques to be particularly helpful in exploring those usually invisible differences that matter crucially to some people, but that others may not even notice. Projective PhotoTherapy techniques can also be an important tool in helping clients evolve into their own unique identities while maintaining their places and contexts in their families and with others, who may be threatened by those emerging differences.

Clients' problems are often based on their actual experiences clashing with their inner expectations of themselves and others; how things *are* seems to conflict with how they think things *should* be. Expectations are the standard against which our perceptions are measured. Our disappointments are usually direct reflections of expectations that are governed by strict rules as to how life or other people ought to be. When clients are able to "own" the parts of their problems that derive from their expectations, they can often relax the rules they live by. Projective PhotoTherapy techniques can be helpful in this process, as they can help people recognize the sources of their assumptions and expectations.

Internal images, idealized and protected from the tests of real-life experience, are difficult to challenge or change without the client's desiring that change. Cognitive dissonance theory (Festinger, 1957) suggests approaching desired change by getting clients to a point where they can see that change might actually be beneficial, useful, and desirable. Projective PhotoTherapy techniques are useful in probing people's unconscious value systems, which dictate their expectations for themselves and others. In making these concepts conscious, we influence whether change can be initiated from within.

People don't change just because somebody else tells them they must, unless they either want to, or at least accept the reasons that they must by acknowledging that they see the world differently than others see it. Using projective PhotoTherapy techniques, you can demonstrate that several people can look at a photograph and get radically different meanings, messages, and feelings from it. This is a comparatively painless way to begin to consciously acknowledge that there can also be more than one correct way to encounter a person or experience. There are reasons for people's differences in perception, and dialogue based on projective perceptions can help clients recognize them.

PhotoTherapy is an especially apt tool for helping clients understand that what others see in them may be different from what they feel they are inside themselves, and that they project to others whatever they believe themselves to be. Projective techniques combined with self-portrait PhotoTherapy can help clients to reflect about their processes of perceiving and to separate definition-by-others from self-definition.

In general terms projective PhotoTherapy techniques can greatly assist people to focus on previously unconscious parts of themselves, learn to analyze how and why they are getting certain meanings from perceptual stimuli or others' verbal messages, and become more sensitive to nonverbal and emotional cues. When clients learn to notice and clarify deviations between the signification intended by the sender and the message perceived by the receiver, communication is improved and disagreements better resolved.

2. WORKING WITH SELF-PORTRAITS

The term *self-portrait* loosely encompasses any photographic presentation dealing with the perception of oneself by oneself, whether actual or metaphoric. Self-portraits differ from other pictures of us in that the creation of a true self-portrait is not affected by anyone else. They are pictures of us—of our bodies or of something that we feel stands for us. We have control of all aspects of image-making, from beginning idea to finished image. Because they are pictures of the self, made by the self, they have the potential to be powerfully self-confrontational and undeniable.

It is rare that we take the time to really look at the way we present ourselves to others and see the ways we visually communicate the physical, mental, and emotional aspects of our being. Photos we make of ourselves, without any outside interference, allow us to explore who we are when we know no one is watching (or will later be judging). This connects with self-empowerment and freedom to create ourselves, without limitations or expectations inflicted by others, and to find out what we really seem to be like.

We can only be aware of ourselves to the extent that we can self-reflect; our existence at any moment is a summary of selective memory and, within the distortive nature of that process, also a partial fiction created only by what we can know of ourselves and have introjected from others. Self-portrait PhotoTherapy techniques can give us a look at the self as an external entity, as a separate person. When this happens, it is instinctive to compare the external self with one's internal image, which is often idealized. Discrepancies between the two frequently generate inner tension, and usually an internal unconscious process arises to resolve the inner dissonance. The concepts of objective self-awareness theory (Duval and Wicklund, 1972) emphasize the therapeutic value of seeing oneself as if from another person's viewpoint. With the use of self-portrait photography, this becomes quite literally possible. Such theories are beyond the scope of this chapter to review in any depth, but they point out how central the concept of self and the ability to self-reflect are to the whole practice of psychotherapy.

Photos of ourselves can be a safe way to self-confront, meet denial head-on, probe limitations, and reach beyond them in self-directed, manageable steps. Self-portraits provide a way to separate from what we may not like about ourselves and find room to strengthen our self-images apart from perceived limitations. This is often further aided by combining relevant projective techniques with self-portrait work, because even when clients are examining their own images in a snapshot, they are nevertheless still projecting and selectively filtering what they see.

Sometimes self-portraits represent only one component of the self. Using PhotoTherapy techniques, people can identify and express parts of themselves. These can then dialogue among themselves or confront the person they are parts of—all nonverbally, if verbally is yet too theatening. Much of self-portrait therapy's benefits derive from the fact that it permits quite direct emotional confrontation. Visual information about the self often doesn't encounter the same barriers, defenses, rationalizations, and repressions as verbal information does.

Self-portraits permit clients to explore the various possibilities of their identities, particularly through self-portrait assignments designed by the therapist. I have often suggested to clients that they take a picture of themselves looking as they think they'll look when their problems have ended. Within this assignment there is a message: there is an end; you can achieve change; seeing that image helps make the possibility real. Other assignments include making a self-portrait of "the you your parents will never be able to appreciate," "the parts of you you like the best (or least)," "how you would look if people did find you attractive," "the you your mother always wanted," and so forth. Each assignment has a therapeutic purpose; each photographic response answers nonverbally many things that words could never encompass on their own. In clients' discussions of the images afterward, explanations of a photo's content, process, message, and meaning provide contextual details that were often previously unconscious and inaccessible to conscious contemplation. Since issues of self-esteem, self-awareness, and self-confidence are so critically central to most therapy, self-portrait PhotoTherapy techniques cannot help but be important tools for seeing oneself more clearly.

As with all client-initiated photographs used in any of the PhotoTherapy techniques, self-portraits can involve just the "live" photographic moment (spontaneous decision aided by the immediacy of a Polaroid camera) or they may be made away from my office as a self-initiated assignment to be completed and created according to the client's own plan. As is true with all PhotoTherapy techniques, these photo-responses can also be combined with other expressive media (art materials, mask work, photocopied reworkings, collage, sculpting or movement, and so forth) for additional unconscious symbolic enhancement, as later examples will illustrate.

There has been a large surge of interest over the past decade in examining gender-based issues (and sociopolitical consequences thereof) as well as differential photographic representation of gender. This has been accompanied by a burst of photographic activity in both self-portrait and family-album work, particularly, though not exclusively, by women, many of whom have carried their discoveries into the therapist's office for exploration. Clients have found it very useful to compare their own images of themselves with those made by others, particularly by photographers of the opposite sex (especially if these are also family members), in order to explore gender-based dynamics that have unconsciously guided, influenced, and also possibly restricted, their lives. Even if clients find there is nothing about themselves they wish to change, it is still important for them to recognize that their identities have been constructed to participate in the sex-roles they have assumed.

Self-portrait work has proved to be particularly useful in helping women strengthen, or begin to emerge into, their own identities. Also, some important therapy using self-portrait interventions has been done with people from various disenfranchised or marginalized groups, who must frequently deal with consequences of having their lives defined or manipulated by others. Certainly this is relevant to individual and family definitions of sex roles and expectations that affect clients who are trying to gain possession of their own inner images.

Many photographers, such as Levey (1987, 1988, 1989, 1991), Martin (1987, 1990, 1991), Newberry (1990), Spence (1978, 1980, 1983, 1986, 1989, 1991), and Martin and Spence together (1985, 1986, 1987), have concentrated on photographic self-discovery techniques aimed at encouraging their subjects to collaborate in exploring gender-based issues, family expectations, and feminist-based personal growth development. Their subjects have been encouraged to use their self-portrait photography, family albums, and visual reconstructions as reflective-therapeutic processes. More important for readers of this book, they have also worked jointly with the subjects' therapists to help their mutual clients reflectively explore images of self discovered in self-portrait and family reconstruction.

3. WORKING WITH PHOTOS OF CLIENTS TAKEN BY OTHER PEOPLE

Photos taken of us by other people give us a chance to see the many ways that others may perceive us. They allow us to examine what it is about us that matters to others in our life and compare this with what we think is, or should be, most important about us to them. If we have posed for the photo, it shows our posing behavior (to the person gazing at us through the lens). If it is spontaneous—a candid shot—then often a different self is captured.

Photos are a good means for exploring the power dynamics in our relationships with the people who have photographed us. As each photographer "takes" another person's picture, the terms *subject* and *object* acquire additional meanings in terms of subjectification and objectification. It is interesting to consider which person's picture signals the most truth to us about ourselves and to explore what that may signal about whose reality is the most accepted as being true (and who can therefore be trusted with the photographic equivalent of one's self. Sometimes photos of a client can be effectively compared and contrasted with self-portraits made to show their "true" selves when unobserved or not being constructed by someone else's gaze through the camera's lens.

4. WORKING WITH PHOTOS TAKEN OR COLLECTED BY CLIENTS

Photos that people take, including those that have been assigned, are a form of self-expression. What is important to a person is reflected in the pictures they have found personally meaningful and thus kept or collected. A client once told me she felt "the picture taking her," rather than her taking the picture, in that many times she has looked at photos she had spontaneously snapped and found much more depth than she had realized at the moment of pressing the shutter.

Many things can influence a person's decision to snap a picture: their goals, hopes, desired outcomes, and how these are connected into visual language for meeting these uniquely personal criteria. If the snapshot didn't work out as they expected, then it can be equally useful to explore what went wrong and what this means, along with what they think might have made it turn out successfully.

A careful probing of moments people select to record can bring forth factual and emotional information, consistent themes and interests, personal metaphors and symbols, including those not fully present in their awareness at the time of shutter-snapping or photo selecting. Photos clients take or collect become metaphors of themselves or intimations of perceptions not yet in their conscious awareness. It is frequently illuminating for people to simply compare the subjects of pictures they took in past years with what is catching their eye currently, and to probe both sets of images to discover what they say about thoughts and feelings. This means of nonverbal retrospection permits the self to inform itself directly.

Taking photos spontaneously can be quite enjoyable and a source of creative communication. Having clients bring in a large collection of photos they have taken or gathered and then asking them to tell me about these images, has proven to be an excellent nonthreatening way to get to know them. Everything they tell me has potential significance, and thus I am honestly interested in hearing anything they might wish to tell me about the contents of the photos, the circumstances of their being taken, the reasons for their being kept, and so forth.

In a more directive vein, assigning clients to take photos or collect them can lead to answers to emotionally laden questions. Such assignments do not have to be tightly focused; fishing with a wide net often brings in a better "catch." Photographing what affects you can give you a bit more control over its unknown or unexpected aspects; getting it outside yourself can give you a better vantage point for exploring it safely. Photographing permits you to compare the expected and the actual, and to discover that in some situations there are choices available if you are willing to risk the consequences of initiating them.

Assignments I have given include asking people to take pictures of things they wish they could change in the world or themselves, of the person they are who no one really knows (the secret self), of people close to them, of family, of strangers, of barriers, of plans or hopes or dreams, or perhaps metaphoric equivalents that would describe them without their bodies appearing in the photo. I sometimes have had success asking clients to photograph what they were not permitted to tell others, secrets they don't want to share, or things they hope I don't ask them about; clients are often willing to provide such information visually.

Taking pictures is never a totally innocent act. People can be objectified, subjectified, colonized, or collaborated with in photographs, but they can never just be "taken" without an element of themselves and the photographer being changed as a result of the encounter. Most people who take photographs as a hobby are rarely aware of all the multiple layers to the simple act of snapping someone's picture, but the layers are always there for later deconstructive probing.

5. WORKING WITH FAMILY ALBUM AND OTHER AUTOBIOGRAPHICAL PHOTOS

Photographs in family albums and other types of photo-biographical snapshots require a separate category of PhotoTherapy techniques, even when the photos are of or by the client and even when they are self-portraits. Indeed, a person's collection of album snapshots is a form of self-portraiture. The selection of images, their organization, presentation, and particularly their personal meaning for the client can contribute many additional layers of significance and information to the client's personal explorations.

Techniques involving family photos deal with the self of the client as constructed by the person's particular family, roots, background, surroundings, and interconnected systems, relationship patterns, and the messages and expectations communicated across generations. As such, techniques involving autobiographical pictures and entire albums can be useful for examining the self from a perspective not offered by techniques mentioned previously (which deal mainly with who the client is when no one else is "in the picture"). With this technique, we can learn more about their role in the complex system that has surrounded them since birth. Albums build a pattern over many years that can be examined as a nonverbal expression of the family's interrelationship dynamics and power alignments.

Family albums are usually made for record-keeping, as talismans against the vagaries of time's passage, and as proof that people's existence and relationships with others have mattered and made some difference in the world. Among the pictures kept in albums there may be a few posed portraits from ceremonial events, but more often they are filled with snapshots that reflect quickly chosen moments of real life as it was passing by. Such pictures lend themselves to studies of what daily life was like in the years represented by the album.

Because these are photographs, rather than paintings, the viewer unconsciously grants them a quality of "factuality" that does not accompany painted portraits. We see photos from the past as true depictions of how life really was at that time. We forget that they present a version of family identity, especially of its female members, which may not reflect ordinary daily life. A family's photographic history documents what has meant a lot to that family; photos that didn't make any difference to the album keeper simply weren't included.

Photos kept in permanent form as an album can be differentiated from those discussed previously by the significance of the arranged groupings and even by the aspect of permanency. The common image of an album is a leather-covered book of pages holding photos that tell the story of someone's life, but family history photos may also be kept on refrigerator doors, in wallets, on office desktops, and so forth.

Album collections usually consist of photos of people and pets (and sometimes places) that matter enough to be kept forever. Inclusion in such permanent collections is not for the stranger or disliked person; rarely will the keeper of an album keep a photo in it of someone he or she hates. We hold onto those artifacts with the most intense personal meaning connected to them: images of places, people, or times that have strong feelings embedded in them. These are the pictures that would leave a hole in our heart if they got lost. Indeed, photo albums and family photos are often mentioned along with family bibles as being the items most missed by people who lose their homes to fire.

Having such a collection also incidentally provides proof that there are other people to whom we matter, too; people who are our natural support group and who love us even when they may not be liking us very much at that moment. Or, at least, the album has been constructed to present that image for public consumption. Sometimes the true family relationships are not those portrayed in the idealized pages of an album. Much depends on who is in charge of selecting photos for the family album and whether your own personal collection would be significantly different.

There is nothing quite like asking a client, "In this album you've brought to me today, which photos aren't true? Which are lies? Which show the family as it really is, when not posed to look good? What photos are you hoping I don't ask you about? Which photos would you remove or change radically if you could rephotograph them *your* way, according to your past memories of family life? You've told me about who all these people are, but now could you tell me about the relationships I see expressed *between* them?" Therapists trained in family systems theory find a wealth of information in family albums to stimulate questions about alignments, triangulation, double binds, issues of differentiation or fusion, and so forth. Therapists who are not approaching therapy from a systems model can just as easily look at the visual contents of photos and ask questions about physical proximity, facial affect, body language, regular inclusion or exclusion of people, as well as the visual data presented (or selectively left out) about the person's life and relationships.

And finally, simply probing the concept of "family" through viewing the places of honor in a client's album can produce information and emotion regarding the client's sense of place and feelings about belonging, as well as who the family would consist of if composed by choice rather than blood linkings. "Family of affiliation," "family of association," and "family of choice" are all terms of significance to therapists who wish to understand a client's contexts beyond family of origin.

If clients don't have real albums, they can easily be instructed to create stand-in versions through found imagery and elaboration of existing images. Rephotographed images, photocopied reworkings, collage, and equivalents can all be used to form a photo-biographical collection.

COMBINED APPLICATIONS

Like any truly interconnected system, the techniques of PhotoTherapy interrelate more than they stand apart. Many therapists have combined the ideas behind certain techniques with very creative specific assignments; for example, having people construct their own version of their life story *their* way and build an altogether new "old family album"; photocopying self-portraits and then collaging them into scenes in other photos; requiring a family to take a roll of photographs together, deciding by consensus what to include, when to press the shutter, and so forth; using photos as masks to speak through (or for). At all times, *both* the image (along with the circumstances surrounding its making) *and* the process of discussing it connect to the therapeutic goals and have joint therapeutic import; both the visual contents and what they mean emotionally need to be collaboratively explored by client and therapist.

The negative space within the photo can also be explored, and any image can be turned 90 degrees and 180 degrees to see it anew from differing positions (which helps view the overall forms and spaces more than the details). All such manipulations can be done with both singular snapshots and collections of many together; this is particularly useful to those Jungian, Gestalt, or systems-oriented therapists trained to notice form, pattern, figure-ground dynamics, and so forth.

Sometimes what is missing from a snapshot is more important than what is there. Sometimes what clients don't tell is more significant than what they do, and sometimes seeing, which is itself a selectively filtered process, is also a way of *not* seeing. What is missing from images sometimes defines a powerful reality. PhotoTherapeutically oriented questions need to be framed so that possibilities are opened for the viewer to see what is absent (or not noticed at first) as well as what is present in the picture.

An example of such existence-by-absence was demonstrated to me by a client who said she suddenly became aware of the total absence of any photographic recordings of her family's series of African-American housekeepers throughout all the years of her childhood. Her family kept albums that recorded important events in its own life, but though these women were in her home all her waking hours as a child, she couldn't find any evidence of their existence in family photos. It wasn't that these women were away when the pictures were taken. They simply weren't perceived as being equally real people who formed any significant part of the family's identity.

The various media involved in visual arts can be combined with PhotoTherapy to great advantage. Clients might express themselves onto snapshots directly by using grease pencils or other noninvasive art-expressive applications. They might attach the photograph to cardboard, paper, or to other tangible images such as magazine pages, mirrors, even themselves, and then further "decorate" these receptive surfaces by drawing, painting, making composite collages, or attaching other materials—ribbons, glitter, lace, buttons, organic materials such as flowers, leaves, hair, and so forth, or even words and other images cut from magazine pages.

Figures or faces in photos, or cutouts of the figures made into paper dolls, can be attached to objects, stuffed animals, background scenes as if on stage, or applied to objects in sandtray work, integrated with clay or plasticine constructions, stuck onto fingers as finger puppets or onto puppets themselves, or in forming storybooks or illustrating poems. Faces can be asked to speak; speech balloons can be drawn above their heads and filled with words, as in comic books, or they can "speak" additional snapshots or material snipped from magazines. These projects can be done singly or put together to form narratives or even frames for videos or movies.

If a photograph is too special to use in such manipulation, photocopies of it can easily be made. The client can then make new images by cutting and pasting, enlarging or reducing, and by using the contents to construct a new picture. In this way clients can reconstruct presentations of previously undocumented memories or make their own version of their family album, personal narrative, or life story.

Such combinations of PhotoTherapy with art therapy or other expressive media techniques are productive when these involve clients' images of themselves, and are also successful when using metaphoric symbols of the self, such as clothing, representational objects such as the person's bicycle, favorite cup, bed, books, eyeglasses, and the like, or photos from family albums or other photo-biographical collections.

Photographs made with instant cameras have additional potential, in that the image on the top surface (the one usually seen) can be worked with as one visual reality, and its backing layer can be carefully peeled and removed to achieve a "shadow" image. Also, an image can be cut out to produce positive and negative (solid black) images. This can be particularly useful, for example, in Jungian therapy when therapists want to contrast the ego component of the self (that which can be known and is "in the light") with the "shadow" component (that which is invisible, unknowable, and usually thought of as more a part of the collective, rather than individual, unconscious).

Collage, in the art therapy or PhotoTherapy sense, is the use of numerous images attached all together on one background so that together, they form a whole image that is itself a picture or message in addition to the visual contents of its individual component parts. A collage can include photos, photo-reproductions (magazine pages, photocopies, and the like), as well as additional enhancements such as writing or drawing onto the created image itself. Collages can be free-form creations having no restrictions or can be accommodated to specific goals. For example, a collage on large sheets of newsprint might be made to represent a certain theme or component of the self. Attached to a long sheet of shelf paper, it could be unrolled as a scroll to illustrate a time-oriented narrative.

Clients can lie down on large pieces of paper, and have someone outline their bodies, then fill in the outlines using art media or photographic images. They can hold up the collaged form next to the real person and take an instant photo, which can be used in work with issues relevant to body image, self-representation, subjective and objective impressions of self, and so forth. These techniques can be useful with a variety of clients' problems, including eating disorders, self-validation, and objective self-awareness.

Expectations and the selectivity of memory can be addressed by having clients take photos and then, while waiting for the prints to be developed, sketch from memory, with pencils or crayons, the images they have just photographed. When the prints are ready, they can be compared with the images the clients drew. Rarely will the drawings include absolutely everything that appears in the photographs.

Clients can simplify complex images (metaphorically, issues) by using a large sheet of white paper in which a small rectangular hole is cut. Moving this overlay around on top of the image permits encountering it part by part so that the client interacts with manageable segments. This kind of partializing can provide a way of excluding unnecessary "background" and not only highlight salient components but also, in some cases, discover which ones they are. This technique teaches clients by analogy how to gain some control when life problems seem overwhelmingly complex.

If you want to really focus in on where the essence of any photograph is for you, try the following procedure. Partialize the image by covering different large and small areas of it with your hand or a piece of paper, asking yourself "If I cover this part of the image, does this photo still have the same overall feeling or message for me?" If you move around the whole image, covering both tiny details and large sections, at a certain point you will inadvertently cover up something that changes your "gut-level" feeling for that image. That covered-up "something" has demonstrated itself to you as a key emotional focal point of that image for you, and its symbolic conciseness speaks clearly about its own powerful condensation and distillation of significance. Without it, the particular emotional meaning of the photo is gone (it has changed or disappeared). When you uncover it again, the feeling or meaning will once again be there. This is one easy way to help clients identify the areas of an image that are the most critical, and probably most emotionally laden; the process works equally well for us therapists, who may find ourselves strongly drawn to snapshots for reasons which we may not understand, as is demonstrated in the example below:

Something about a photo of myself and my husband (see photo 2.1), taken when we were just beginning to date each other and still very tentative about our relationship's commitment, kept pulling strongly at my attention. Somehow it seemed to signify that a more permanent relationship was being established between us than I was certain that I wanted.

Trying to figure it out, I used the cover-up/partializing technique presented above to find the elements in the snapshot that were broadcasting this to me. It turned out that the key was in the way I was holding his one finger with my whole fist, as a small trusting child might do. That was the key image, but there was still something nagging at my mind that seemed to say there was more to that finger signal. A year later, when we'd definitely advanced to the "couple" stage and been married, we visited my parents. My mother pulled out the family albums to show him my childhood in pictures, and there on one of the pages was a snapshot of my two parents, just returned from a fishing trip, photographed in a playful, spontaneous mood (see photo 2.2). In that image I discovered my mother holding my father's hand in the identical gesture.

That image announced itself into my consciousness with the "aha!" of sudden meaning: of course he and I would live happily ever after; the gesture had already told me so unconsciously. Obviously, I had seen the earlier image many times before, and so it therefore had long been part of my unconscious storehouse of images connected to happiness, security,

Photo 2.1

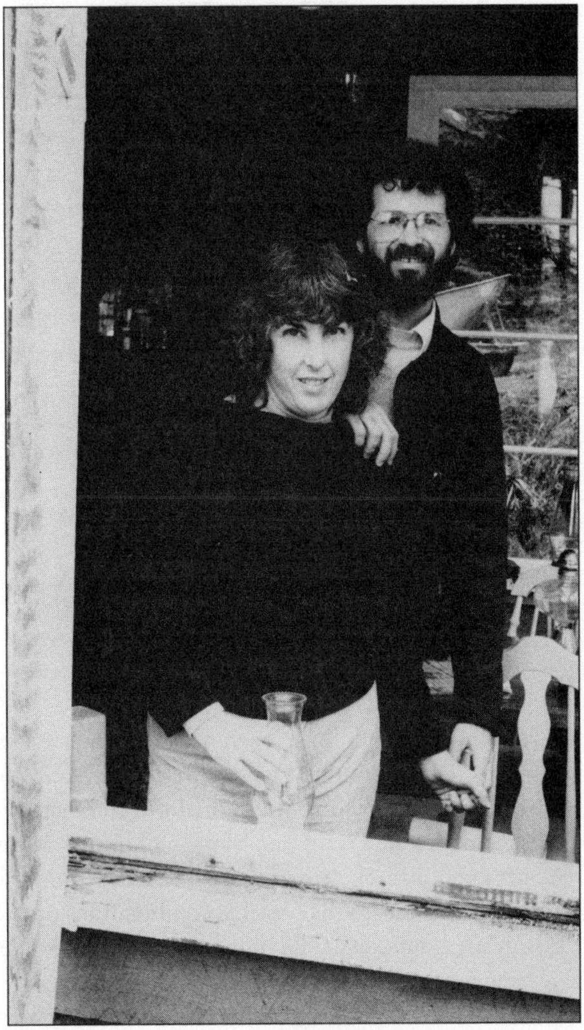

and my willingness to trust being spontaneously happy with someone. But I certainly was not consciously aware of its particular existence, and had someone referred to the photo of me with my husband-to-be and asked me if I'd ever seen that pose before in photos of other people, I am sure

Note: This and all other photos in this book, unless otherwise specifically credited under a particular photograph, have been taken by the author and are copyrighted by her. No reproductions of any photographs in this book are permitted under any circumstances.

Photo 2.2

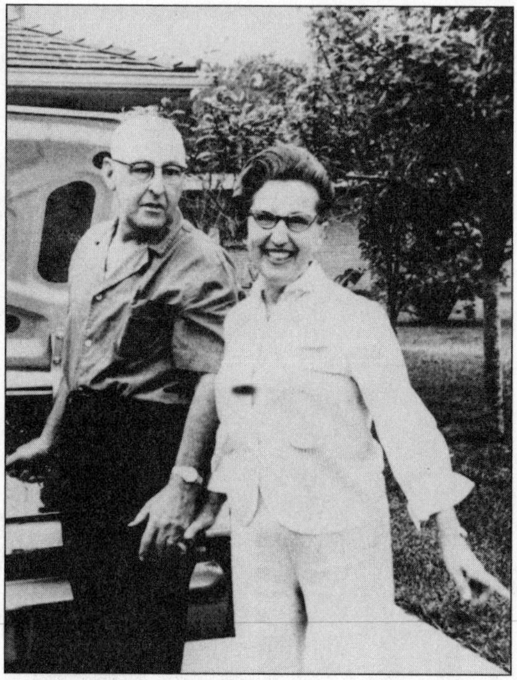

my answer would have been no. Had I not rediscovered that decades-old snapshot on the album page, I would have only known that he "felt" right, and that that feeling was somehow connected to the finger holding. A therapist would have had to probe far back in areas deep below my own personal awareness to try to find that connection.

The limits to the possible combinations of PhotoTherapy and art therapy are boundless. The only restrictions lie in the therapist's imagination, preparatory training, and similar self-limiting constraints. Certainly therapists who would ask clients to use art materials to elaborate upon snapshot stimuli should first accomplish training in those art therapy processes they are likely to precipitate. Not to do so would be to cheat your client of additional levels of possible communication they might be expressing without realizing it, because if this expression is unconscious to them, and if the therapist also doesn't notice it, then for practical purposes, it simply isn't there. Photos 2.3 to 2.6 provide some examples of snapshot-based art-elaborated expressions that my clients or workshop participants have produced, often adding written contexts as well.

Photo 2.3

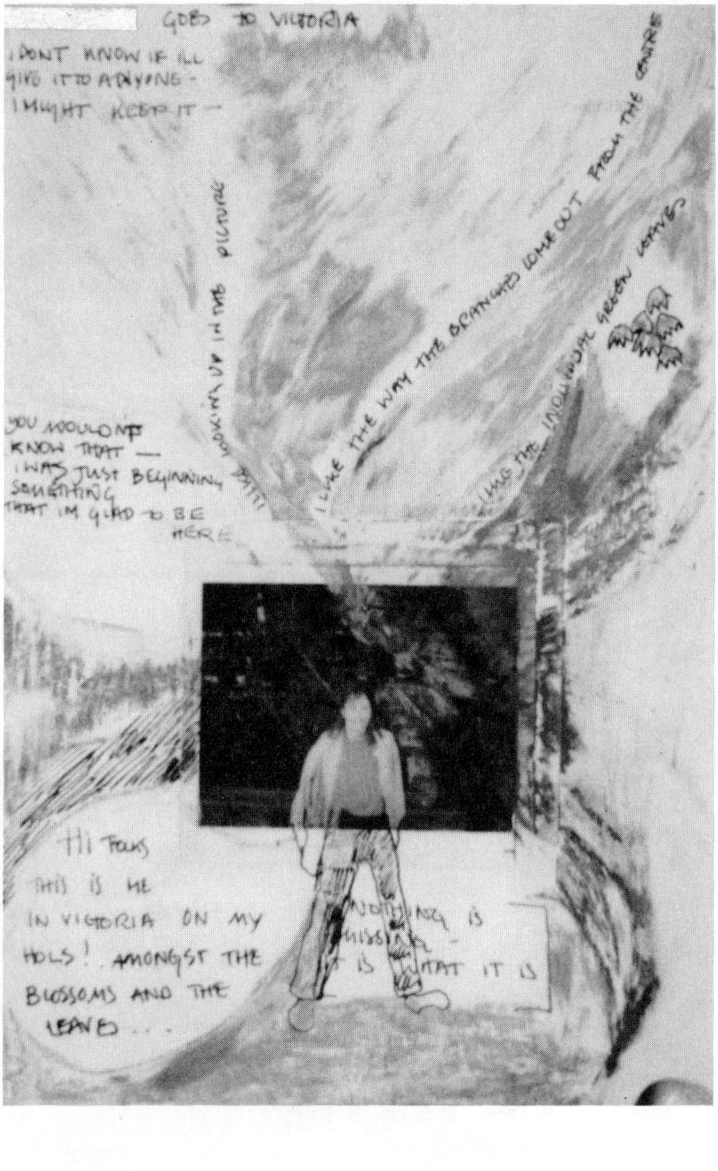
GOES TO VICTORIA
I DONT KNOW IF ILL GIVE IT TO ANYONE - I MIGHT KEEP IT -
I LIKE THE WAY THE BRANCHES COME OUT FROM THE CENTRE
LIKE THE INDIVIDUAL GREEN LEAVES
YOU WOULDNT KNOW THAT — I WAS JUST BEGINNING SOMETHING THAT IM GLAD TO BE HERE
HI FOLKS THIS IS ME IN VICTORIA ON MY HOLS! AMONGST THE BLOSSOMS AND THE LEAVES . . .
NOTHING IS MISSING - IT IS WHAT IT IS

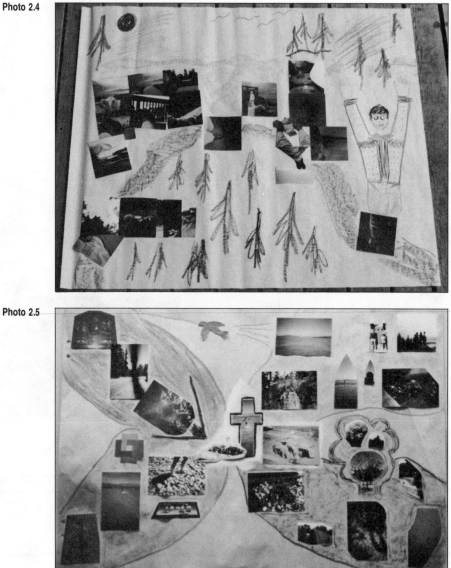

Photo 2.4

Photo 2.5

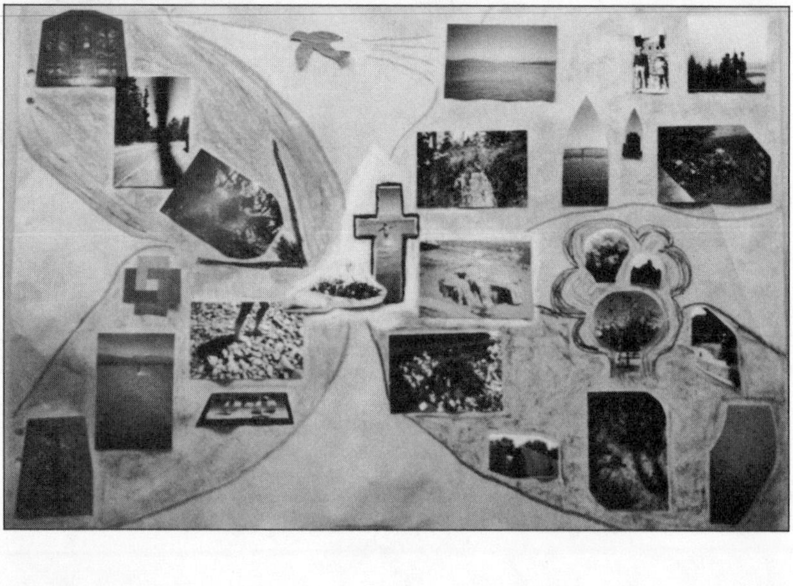

I think it would be very difficult to have to decide whether expressions and representations like those shown here are PhotoTherapy *or* art therapy, or to have to choose one or the other type of technique to help a client. Far preferable is knowing enough about both kinds of techniques

Photo 2.6

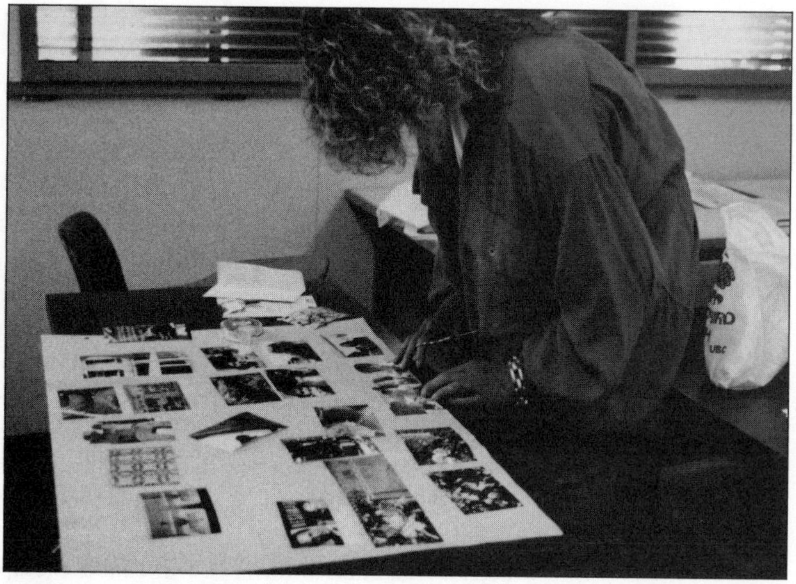

to make use of them when they are relevant, as they are all parts of the larger therapy picture.

CAUTIONS AND GUIDELINES

At its most basic level, PhotoTherapy is what happens when people and snapshots get together to communicate back and forth in a therapeutic setting so that the information and insights that are brought to light can be noted, fit into the helping framework, and be consciously and cognitively reflected upon. Obviously, a very similar interaction process happens quite spontaneously whenever people and snapshots get together, regardless of whether a therapist is there or not. The difference is that while those kinds of "accidental" photo explorations can, and often do, take place without any guide, therapeutic facilitation can help people reach into areas not commonly encountered in daily conversation about personal snapshots. PhotoTherapy without the therapy is just photography, no more and no less. For effective PhotoTherapy to take place, a competent professional therapist must be present who has the knowledge to use the techniques adequately and ethically and the experience to understand how to make use of what to others may sound like ordinary random comments about photos.

The "what" of PhotoTherapy seems rather elegantly simple: clients and therapists focus their attention on photos taken of clients or by them, their self-portraits and family snapshots, and use these artifacts, along with the projective and interactive processes involved in examining and interacting with them, as starting points for therapeutic dialogue and client introspection. However, the "how" of PhotoTherapy—how you do it—is significantly more complex, as PhotoTherapy techniques are intended for open-ended interactive applications, yet they remain situationally idiosyncratic in terms of individual clients' unique needs.

The "why" of PhotoTherapy—why it works so well—is a less obvious, but nevertheless extremely essential, component in the use of these techniques. It is important that before beginning to use these techniques as therapy-assisting tools, readers understand the various cognitive and emotional processes that they facilitate, and why they can succeed at such deep levels. Such knowledge will enable therapists to decide what to use for the best "fit" with clients' unique situations and particular difficulties.

PhotoTherapy is not as simple as saying "use album reconstruction to help reempower abuse victims," or "use self-portrait work with such clients to help them reframe their self-description as 'abuse survivors' and thus have therapeutic change as an accompanying consequence," or "use projectives to reenter those preverbal years where early trauma is blocked from memory," and so forth, as if each is independent of the others. It is not that these ideas won't work; they do, and quite well. It is just that things aren't so linearly simple that a single technique can be matched with a single diagnostic category or problem in a one-to-one correlation. In fact, most interconnect in both theory and practical application.

While this entire book discusses what PhotoTherapy is, I also want to state clearly what PhotoTherapy is *not* (or should not be). It is not a closed methodology of steps and procedures that must be followed in a particular way, or matched with certain situations according to certain rules. It is not a structured, finished package that must be used only as I explain it, nor done only exactly as I have done it. Rather, PhotoTherapy is most successful when practitioners recognize the flexibility and selective applicability that the techniques offer and use them as an open-ended interrelated system of adjunctive tools applicable in numerous situations. In teaching therapist trainees and workshop participants, I explain how to ask good PhotoTherapy questions; I do not tell students which ones to ask when, according to some fixed list.

In applying PhotoTherapeutic techniques, photographs should be externally or objectively analyzed very sparingly, and defined (in absolutes) not at all. PhotoTherapy isn't about interpreting other people's photos for them. Therapists need to resist the temptation to overgeneralize or overinterpret from just one or a few photographs. The idea is to keep the focus off the client and on the photo, as clients will far more easily tell you about the picture than themselves. Your role is to ask questions; the client is the person who is to make the discoveries and find the personal truths (though we therapists can share our opinions if we clearly "own" them).

In using PhotoTherapy techniques, the process of interacting with the snapshots becomes at least as important as the image's content itself (and usually more so). Nonjudgmentally listening to, observing, and probing client responses to photographic stimuli is the primary therapeutic role. The therapist must refrain from making assumptions about a person after viewing only a few of their snapshots, but initial questions can be asked and responses noted and held in reserve until more observations are collected. Themes or patterns of visual images will begin to appear so repeatedly that they will seem to be demanding to be noticed, and recurring symbols will emerge often enough that therapists may start to formulate connections and want to base further questions on such observations.

I should clarify here that not all of the anecdotal case examples in the following chapters are taken from my psychotherapy practice alone. Some are from therapeutic processes that took place in the intense experiential portions of various lengthy training sessions I have given in which other therapists were the participants. At the "meta" level of personal-experiential training of therapists in using these techniques, the work is identical to clients' experiences in the process itself, as therapist-trainees will use their photos to search inward and explore feelings much the same way as their clients will.

In such training situations, I often demonstrate a technique by role-playing, having myself act as the therapist and one of the participants serve as my client. More often, I have them pair off with each other for long (and private) practice sessions approximating the length of their usual counseling appointments. In these mock counseling hours, they take turns serving as the therapist and the client so that the technique can be actually used in simulation of real-life process. That is, participants work with their own photographs as if they were clients discovering firsthand what this process can uncover; then later we review and discuss what happened.

Frequently one or more of these experiential dyads is videotaped (at participants' request) for later review, as it is difficult to be involved in interaction and at the same time observe one's own behavior. Many of these tapes are available for viewing in their entirety at the PhotoTherapy Centre, should readers wish to examine more than the short excerpts used in this book. Also, as only a few examples of client-produced photographic artifacts (such as art-enhanced self-portraits, collages of reworked family albums, full layouts of photo-narrative metaphoric constructions, and so forth) can appear in this book as illustrations, readers who wish to examine others of the several hundred of these kept on file at the PhotoTherapy Centre are encouraged to contact me for viewing arrangements.

As the kind of "live" work mentioned above is therapeutic whether the participant is a client or in a workshop setting, I have not noted any differentiation between these types of sessions in this book. However, I do wish to make it clear that all persons whose specific situations are discussed in this book have approved the material depicting their experiences, and in all cases except those where people have specifically requested I use their real name, I have disguised identities to protect against their recognition.

The ethical issues surrounding PhotoTherapy are much more complex than those for regular psychotherapy or art therapy, and the ethical and legal ramifications—such as photographic versus therapeutic issues of confidentiality, proper release forms and reassurance guarantees, ownership of clients' photographic materials, and so forth—should be of serious concern to readers planning to incorporate PhotoTherapy techniques into their psychotherapy practice. For more information about ethical and legal considerations, see Weiser, 1985, 1986a, and 1986b. For ramifications of these in terms of conducting PhotoTherapy research, readers may contact me directly.

As I mentioned before, PhotoTherapy is an idea that occurred to many therapists simultaneously. Although I personally created most of the exercises given in each chapter, a few others have been adapted from other colleagues' original versions. For example, my "Space Station" exercise (accompanying Chapter Six) has been adapted and revised from an earlier exercise ("The Mars Trip") first shown to me by Stewart (1980), which itself had at least partial origins even earlier in the work of Harbut (1975) as well as Anderson and Malloy (1976). My adaptation of this exercise is presented in this book as a clinical tool; however, a related version has also been used by Zakem (1990) in an attempt to form an objective research-assessment tool, and various revisions of the therapeutic version have frequently been used by both Krauss and myself since the early 1980s as clinical training tools.

Thus it can be seen how many therapists have pioneered this field, and several of us have used the benefits of our experiences to train others, personally adapting (and in most cases decidedly tailoring) the exercises originating with others to meet our particular teaching needs—and I expect that our students will go on to retool them further. Most of us have freely shared our ideas about what best facilitates a particular kind of conceptual learning, and we have learned much from being each other's students. I have tried throughout this book to give proper credit to colleagues for ideas or activities not originally my own, but sometimes it's difficult to track an exercise back through its various forms to its originator.

The exercises described in each chapter are matched to the primary technique involved, but as they really are an interrelated system of applications, all also usually involve some of the other chapters' techniques. *Therefore I strongly recommend that readers finish the entire book before pausing to try out exercises from any particular chapter.* And although I have no objection to readers copying an exercise that is particularly useful for work with your clients (as long as any copies credit this author as their source), the contents of this book are copyrighted, and reproduction in any comprehensive or bulk form is not permitted. If readers are in doubt or want to seek wider permissions, please contact me.

One part of my operating assumptions about psychotherapy is that one should never put a client through process that one has not first experienced for oneself. Before starting to use PhotoTherapy techniques with clients, I believe therapists must first personally experience the surprisingly powerful feelings that these activities can elicit. This caution of "doing unto yourself" before beginning to "do unto your clients" is a very serious one, and I am certain that once you start trying them out you will soon see for yourself what I mean. Readers are cautioned to treat these experiential exercises carefully and make certain that enough time is scheduled to complete them fully. They frequently reveal just the surface of a very deep pool of unconscious or buried memories and feelings, which, once uncovered, tend to push the rest of the way up. The exercises that end each chapter should not be treated lightly; that these techniques work so intensely and powerfully is part of the reason for their success.

Readers not already trained as therapists should be cautioned that, although I have written for ease of comprehension, these directives and suggested implementations can precipitate intense emotions and powerful cathartic release. The various techniques and recommended experiences should not be attempted lightly, but should be taken seriously as tools for use by someone who has enough training to be able to competently handle any emotional process they start. Of course I cannot restrict what readers do (nor would I presume to have this much power), but carefully experienced, these exercises can lead to strong insights and emotional communications from oneself; I just hope readers not professionally trained in therapy will not be using this book to open something in other people that cannot be voluntarily closed again.

Therefore, I strongly urge all readers, regardless of professional training, to first try each of these exercises out on themselves several times before ever beginning to use them with clients. You might want to pair off with a professional colleague and take turns as therapist and client in role-play. If a partner isn't available, perhaps read the steps into a tape recorder and listen to them at your own pace, advancing to the next question only when you are ready for it. Facilitating your own insights is not always as easy as it sounds.

The exercises are not intended to be substitutes for actual therapy, and must not be employed as such. At the same time, readers must be aware that emotional issues and unexpected feelings are often stirred up as a result of trying them. If readers anticipate that any major difficulties might arise while involved with these exercises, I strongly suggest that you not attempt them, as I cannot be responsible for any consequences that might result.

HOW TO BEGIN

I have set up the office where I practice to nonverbally signal that photography is part of my life. Although I work alone, rather than in an agency, clinic, hospital, or other setting, and usually only with individuals, couples, or families, rather than groups or inpatients, some of my tactics may serve as suggestions for adapting any therapeutic setting to encourage PhotoTherapy activities. I have personal photos of special people all around me, above and on my desk, and a few framed special pictures on the small tables near clients' seating areas, which I hope signals a relaxed homelike environment where clients may feel comfortable.

Additionally, two walls of the waiting area are covered (above chair level) in approximately eighty 8-by-10-inch unframed photographs mounted on cardboard and hung with their edges touching. These are snapshots that I have taken as creative artwork rather than personal life-markers or with therapeutic goals. These are primarily black-and-white because that is the medium I prefer; color ones would have done just as well for this purpose. These "wall decorations" are of people, places, children, objects, and abstract forms, and they are not organized in any formal sense at all. This area is the first part of my office that clients encounter, and it is rare that they do not comment on these photos. It is therefore very natural to suggest that they look at these for a few minutes while I return a phone call, gather my notes, or make some other excuse, giving them some time alone with the images before we officially begin talking.

I always tell new clients that I would like PhotoTherapy to be part of my work with them, if they agree to this, and giving them a chance to casually scan the photos for five minutes or so is a good informal, non-threatening introduction to the idea. Then I show them how this can itself be a starter by means of projective work by asking general questions like "So, what do you think of all these?" or "Anything up there particularly catch your eye?" Accepting any answer as a conversation starter, I explain that I regularly use photos as part of my tools for helping people, that sometimes I ask people to bring in their family albums or favorite snapshots to give me a better idea of the faces that go with the names I am hearing or to flesh out details of their past that they may be telling me about, and that this photo work can sometimes include their taking a few snapshots, making informal self-portraits with my office Polaroid camera, and other activities.

I give them a summary that presents PhotoTherapy in very personal and familiar terms, saying something such as, "You can learn a bit about me from looking at the pictures I've taken, and I can learn some about you from yours. We can talk about them and think we're talking about the photographs, when it's really us we are discussing. I cannot ever tell you what your pictures mean any more than you can tell me about my own on the wall. Until I ask you to tell me about yours I only have my own opinion, which may interest you, but certainly doesn't prove anything. I can tell you how I see your pictures, what they suggest to me or my feelings in response to viewing them, and offer that to you, but there is no way that I can assume you would or should have the same perception or intention regarding that image. We can look at your snapshots and family albums and imagine what each image's truth might be, but we can never know for sure, because the importance of who is in it, or the meaning of each scene depends on who is in it, taking it, or looking at it later. Your own snapshots may be yours, but I can guarantee you that they definitely have new stories to tell you." I stress that it is entirely up to them whether we use PhotoTherapy techniques and that they are completely free to refuse to do any or all of these and instead just work with words alone. I suggest that they consider trying the activities for the first little while on the condition that I will drop the idea if it makes them the least bit uncomfortable.

I discuss thoroughly with them—and also give them a signed statement explaining—that all photos taken of them or by them during therapy are theirs to keep and do with whatever they please, although I may from time to time request that they permit photos (or copies of them) to stay in my office until we are finished "working" with them or promise to bring them back should we need them again if they have taken them home. We negotiate about their comfort level with all these possibilities, and I usually begin showing them how PhotoTherapy can work by demonstrating projective techniques.

I might make a choice of a photo on the wall that seems "safe" to me to begin with, or I may ask questions to prompt them to pick one. "Is there anyone up there you'd like to meet?" "Which of those places would you rather be instead of here today?" "Is there one photo up there that you might wish to take home with you if you could?" "Is there any up there that reminds you of someone you know?" And so forth. After talking a while, I stop them to demonstrate just how easily we have started to converse when the topic was not about them directly. Then I usually pause to share with them the sorts of information I think I may have learned about them just from the few sentences they've said thus far. I point out that I know my perceptions are not always correct and ask them to let me know about any errors I make. In correcting my mistakes, they tell me even more about themselves.

This approach models questioning techniques used in real therapy, and gives clients an introduction to the power of PhotoTherapy techniques without their having to risk being personally vulnerable. The techniques are not kept hidden from the clients. Rather, I explain directly, just as I have here, what they might expect in therapy itself. I frequently offer to let them ask me questions about my photos, so that we can explore some of my reasons for making them or choosing them to hang in the office. These behaviors mirror ordinary patterns of social conversation, and by reversing the roles clients can see how natural it is for people to share their inner selves by talking about things they have created or collected. This also signals my attitude about power balancing in therapy: I let the client have as much respect and security while in my "power" as I can possibly provide them while still getting my work done (which from time to time may nevertheless involve challenging them or pushing their emotions a bit).

I then usually explain that they have just experienced the way I use ordinary photographs for starting therapeutic conversations, and that although I may later choose to initiate a different technique, such as self-portraits or album reviews, or ask them to bring in a selection of pictures torn out of magazines, that the questioning style itself will remain essentially the same. When we officially contract at the next session I include PhotoTherapy as one of the terms they have the option of agreeing to or not. This gives them a week to think about it, and me a week to ponder where we might begin.

Asking Questions

In actually beginning to work with a client, there are some general recommendations I believe important for readers to keep in mind. These suggestions have more to do with how you might ask clients questions than with what you ask them about. Many times when people are asked direct questions, they are unable to reply with prompt succinct answers: they may know something but not be certain enough to risk a firm answer, they may know the answer but have inner fears about the consequences of telling, or they may know but be unable to tell in words alone.

In questioning people, we are to some degree prying. Prying information out of people, even if we are certain it might help them, can result in their feeling rushed, threatened, or even violated. Our manner and the wording of our questions are crucial to the client's comfort level and willingness to open up. It helps if clients understand that we know that some details may be difficult to bring forth or painful to look at. It is reassuring to clients to be reminded that they are in charge of what gets said, and that the photograph can be a stopping-off place, a bridge between the inner and the spoken, or something that can sometimes speak for them, if they will guide it.

When I work with PhotoTherapy techniques, I may ask clients to speak about a photograph, try to remember one and describe it, talk to it, or even construct a dialogue back and forth with it being an equal in the conversation. I may have them ask it questions or imagine that it is asking them some. I may ask them to place it in front of their own face to speak to them, or across their face like a mask and have it speak for them. I may have them hold two images, one in each hand, and have those two photographs speak with each other or to the person holding both. I have made use of these sorts of procedures, similar to Gestalt "empty chair" techniques, not only with photographs having people as their focus, but also those having other subject matter. (I have observed ponds talking to ducks, lamps talking to street corners, chairs talking to windows, and so forth.)

I might ask clients a question based on a photographic stimulus, and have them answer by finding another photo to serve as a visual, and thus metaphorical, reply. If clients tell me they don't know the answer to one of my questions, I ask them to pretend for a moment that they do know that answer, or I ask if they did happen to know it, what do they think it might be? Once freed from total responsibility for the answer, they can usually bring forth a spontaneous reply that will be therapeutically useful.

I ask clients questions to get information that can help me help them. I may want to know something and have to get to it indirectly, by moving slowly, step by step, listening, and noting significant comments. Regardless of the subject of the photo at hand, I ask what thoughts and feelings and memories are stirred while the client ponders the image. I ask about what it seems to mean and what seem to be the most significant or obvious elements in it, which sometimes turn out to be components of the image that I would never have noticed.

I ask clients to hold the edges of the border and imagine stretching them wider and higher, "looking" for what else was in the reality from which this snapshot was taken. Sometimes I even suggest they "step over" into the image itself and "walk around" in there while telling me what they are seeing and feeling. I might ask them to imagine the rest of the 360 degree physical or social environment that existed at the moment the shutter was tripped, or to imagine being the photographer and turning around to see what else or who else is behind the photographer.

I use time much the same way as space, suggesting that clients imagine what may have happened right before or right after the moment of photo taking (or weeks or years before or after). For example: How might that scene be different now than when the photo was taken? Where might the people in the picture have gone after it was taken? What were they doing before it? Do you think they wanted their photo taken in that way, or would they perhaps have preferred something different? And so forth. I might ask a client to imagine dialogues between the subject and the photographer at the time the photo was made and now. I ask about how the client thinks the people or objects in the photograph might be feeling, what they might be remembering, thinking about, or wanting to say.

I might ask clients to imagine taking or finding other photos to make this one part of a longer series. I might ask them to recommend a title for it, decide whether they themselves might have chosen to take this picture (and if so, why), or to consider who they might wish to give the photo to as a gift (and what that would signify nonverbally). They might be asked to consider making an enlargement of just one portion of the scene, and choose which part would be the most important for doing this.

But throughout all of this kind of question-asking, my focus is not only on the clients' answers but also on absolutely everything else that is going on and being communicated nonverbally—posture, speed of response, muscle tension, facial expression and color, pauses, silences, and so forth. My goals in this are to compile the patterns by which clients uniquely communicate the unspoken and to notice what issues or discussions trigger what sorts of emotional communication nonverbally. These clues will help me to recognize their later signals as they communicate emotionally what is happening inside themselves.

I might interrupt a dialogue by suggesting the person stop, as if a "pause" button had been pushed on our live process, and pose right then for a quick snapshot to better explain what he or she means. This could involve actually taking an instant-print snapshot, or just showing something to the "camera" in my mind. I might assign them to go out and take photos on a topic that I believe they need to explore further without the usual protective layer that verbal inquiry can provide. I might ask them to find images from the print media, such as magazine ads or story illustrations, that will help them show me what they are trying to convey. I might use videotape and photographs interactively, so that people can see themselves as others usually see them, watch the nonverbal parts of themselves while they are discussing a family album, or check discrepancies between body and speech when feelings are being explored during our conversation. The idea here is that if you see a photo made of yourself for yourself, it becomes very real and is difficult to argue with, rationalize away, or attempt to deny.

I try to avoid asking clients questions that they can answer with a simple yes or no. It seems much more effective for me to ask questions to which they must supply more extended answers. For example: Why do you think he said that? How did it happen that she stood there? or Could you please tell me a bit about this picture? I often use open-ended sentences for clients to complete, like filling in a blank. I may ask them to suggest questions we might want to ask the photograph. Even appearing to be confused myself and asking them to add clarification to "help" me can be very useful.

I try never to push my clients beyond the levels of meaning that are true for them at that particular moment. If I think there is something they might be missing, some underlying connection or possible symbolic content, I offer it as one possibility among many for them to consider as potential additional alternatives. They do not even have to respond to these. However, if it has made an unconscious connection for them, that thread will reemerge later. I might request that the client silently rearrange some of the family photos on a table to get a different "picture" of family relationships, or perhaps have the client pose for an instant-print self-portrait in a different posture than usual. Trying out such alternatives can result in new revelations suddenly clicking into place.

Taking Pictures

PhotoTherapy may involve taking pictures weeks in advance of a session as well as immediately and spontaneously in-session. The type of camera used will dictate whether pictures are ready immediately or whether the client must wait for prints to be developed. Both processes have advantages. Immediate feedback is good if the client's attention span is short or you want to catch some immediate action or emotion and feed it back at once to help the client cognitively integrate that behavior or affect. Immediate self-confrontation in instantly available images is good, but so is the supposedly more "objective" perspective gained by viewing images of the self later, from a more removed position. Waiting for instant prints to develop can begin to teach delayed gratification; however, for those who can or should learn more about waiting, a delay of a few days or hours instead of minutes can be useful.

I keep referring to a client or a "self" to do PhotoTherapy work with, but because I base a lot of my therapy work on systems theory, there is another level that readers who prefer that model might want to consider when evaluating PhotoTherapy applications. Since the family unit may itself be viewed as an interrelated, independent entity that is in many ways a discrete "self," it may be successfully approached PhotoTherapeutically using self-portrait techniques "one level up" hierarchically. For example, clients can be asked to provide a family self-portrait, photos taken by family consensus, or photos of the entire family that visually express the personality of the family as a single identity.

Staying Flexible

That there are so many demonstrations of success in the following chapters may make it appear that using these tools will always produce successful insight or catharsis. Please be aware that, as with any other psychotherapeutic techniques, PhotoTherapy cannot produce consistently wonderful results. If your approach doesn't seem to be working, you should try something else, and if words alone will produce the desired information, you don't have to "PhotoTherapize" the client just because you like the tools.

Sometimes the best thing we can do for our clients is nothing. Sometimes the best communication we can speak is silence, and the best thing to do PhotoTherapeutically is to just leave people alone with their snapshots, sitting alongside them as they look, but not intruding as their inner dialogue evolves. By this I do not mean leave them alone in another room and go off for a coffee-break! Rather, make your presence that of a "silent witness," allowing clients and their photographs to converse and exchange feelings; share in that experience without altering its nature too much. Too quick a therapist-initiated closure or reflective summary, and the work will not succeed as well. Too directive and clients never become aware of their own innate abilities to heal themselves or accept themselves unconditionally, which will leave them dependent on others, including therapists, far too long.

The power of these techniques to effect good results under even the most difficult circumstances was clearly demonstrated to me in a recent opportunity I had to discuss PhotoTherapy "live" on national radio. The interviewer, four thousand miles away, sat with a list of questions and (unknown to me) a snapshot of his daughter. We began discussing the field in theoretical terms; suddenly he asked me if I could show him how I worked by commenting on his photo. I thought this was an excellent challenge for testing my claims about being able to work with images I myself could not see (and had not ever seen), and agreed.

I began to question him about the snapshot and then asked him to engage directly with it, talking to it, speaking for it, and telling me his feelings about it. His voice altered significantly into a tone that indicated he was experiencing a light hypnotic trance. He spoke softly, intensely, and spontaneously, revealing a more vulnerable human side of him than he usually expressed in his professional interviewer role.

He told me later he was surprised that he would ever share the things he revealed with a stranger, much less the entire listening audience across Canada. He expressed much deeper meanings than he had expected, and he said that this had greatly pleased him. As a recording of this interview clearly demonstrates, PhotoTherapy works, even when done on live radio, with a photograph that cannot be seen by the therapist!

Each of the chapters that follow presents a specific technique as individuated from the others as I could make it. Most therapists (including myself) who are experienced in using these tools may find it rather restrictive to work with only one technique, and find that in the midst of one, something arises that precipitates using another along with it. Examples of these interweavings and combinations of techniques can be found throughout this book.

ADDITIONAL POINTERS

Some of the points made in previous pages about the nature of photographic communication directly influence the methodology of PhotoTherapy. For example, in recognizing that a photograph cannot have any objective meaning separable from that of its creator and/or later viewers, we can see that there is no single right way to "discover" its meaning. Therefore, a single photograph cannot be read or decoded like a book by anyone, not even a therapist; rather we must recognize that every participant in person-photo interaction has his or her own (correct-for-them) viewpoint. Just because something may appear evident to me, the therapist, it is not automatically therefore correct. Similarly, we cannot ever know for sure what a photo's contents really mean; we can only work with what they suggest, cause us to recall, and catalyze in our emotions. Together, the client and I mutually focus on a photographic image and try to become more aware of any visual symbols that seem evocative. We jointly explore it and interact with it; we "work" it—and all the while we may also be conversing at many levels simultaneously.

Because they are visual metaphors for an actual moment or for the experiencing of "raw" feelings, personal snapshots and albums can assist us in remembering, confronting, imagining, and exploring complex parts of ourselves and our lives. What we perceive is filtered by how we felt or what we thought at the time we noticed it, and these factors will affect whether something was photographed or noticed at all. Therefore, it is not surprising to find that this can also work in the opposite direction, as a means of assisting people to reconnect with thoughts and feelings of the past as if they were being presently experienced. People can interact with snapshots by stepping into the frame's reality as if it were the present and take note of what feelings or thoughts spontaneously emerge.

When emotions are contacted through nonverbal means, they are often encountered suddenly or unexpectedly and therefore are frequently perceived as being much more "raw" than when they were originally experienced. Then they were filtered through a cognitive process or framework mapped by verbal constructs that helped the client prepare for their possible emergence. We may be consciously aware of the existence of feelings of grief, anger, or fear to the point of acknowledging that they are stored inside us, but it is altogether different to reexperience them. To be willing to go through such processes requires relinquishing conscious controls. This is not something most clients are initially willing to do, and thus they must be helped to recognize the need for letting go in the safety of the therapy session. Using photographs as a bridge to focus such emoting can help clients retain a small bit of extra power to support them through the process, allowing them to deal with intense emotions at arm's length.

While the client and I talk, supposedly about this photograph in front of us, I try to absorb all the other signals going on and try to encourage the client to do the same in self-reflection, both during the process and in "debriefing" afterwards. It helps to videotape sessions so that we can review the process; this allows for better tracking of all the many moments that may be lost to later recall. Videotaping is rarely available in most traditional psychotherapy settings, however. While we converse, although my clients think we are only talking, I am also trying to simultaneously take mental note of their many nonverbal body signals, such as posture, facial tension and color, hand configurations, gestures, restless movements, and any other physiological cues that people use to signal emotional states.

I try to notice which topics seem to produce strong emotional reactions and then try to return to these later in an attempt to reach some inner resolution, understanding, or catharsis by reworking the visual codes to restimulate the crucial moments of that process (or by connecting them laterally with other similar clues from related image material). Once clients engage with the image(s) in front of them, there is a transition into a state of attention between them and the image that is a light autohypnotic trance state in which I and the rest of the room become essentially nonexistent. Their conscious mind is occupied with trying to keep track of the conversation, while the rest of them is being stimulated nonverbally, participating in something much deeper, as additional emotionally related details are continually evoked.

This hypnotic state is most obvious to me when my client actually, and sometimes almost literally, enters into the image as if its contents were real and alive, right there, and they are talking with the people pictured or mentally moving about the scene as if everything inside its borders existed right now in three dimensions surrounding them. This "suspension of disbelief" can happen while using any of the various PhotoTherapy techniques, but it is particularly integral in activating the projective technique, which underlies all the others.

The arousing of intense emotions is very frequent in PhotoTherapy work, precisely because of this kind of disengagement of conscious controls over the deeper levels of memories and feelings. When clients actively and aggressively try to remember or recontact emotions through conscious attempts to directly probe, there remains some degree of power in the automatically protective censorship of the process itself. There needs to be an encouragement of what Wolf (1990) refers to as that state of ego regression that must be experienced in order to reach what can be called those more primitive places in our selves where our experiences were initially condensed into symbolic forms, particularly during our earliest preverbal years.

Long after their birth, children are dependent upon sensory-coded communications. This period of prelogical thinking, sometimes referred to as primary process, is mainly biologically mandated, and its consequence is that the experiences and reactions that form our early memories are not coded as words because that form of language is meaningless in those early years. Rather, they are directly absorbed sensorially, nonverbally, and unconsciously, and they remain stored in a portion of our minds that is difficult to access verbally in later therapy or other direct thought probings, primarily because word categories weren't used to store them there initially.

It is possible to state that until a person has a cognitive framework of language concepts with which to categorize her or his experiences of reality, that person could be said to actually possess no conscious mind at all, or at least no self-reflective consciousness, and thus live only in a reactive state. This point is very significant in helping clients who are urgently trying to reconnect with memories of trauma (such as abuse, fear, anger, phobias, and so forth) that took place at a very early age, but who find that they are simply unable to make contact with these things through verbal probing.

Therapists try to assist clients to bring to consciousness that which cannot be known to exist without it. To become better aware of those deeper levels, which may also reflect more universal collective archetypal imagery or emotion, clients must be able to unhook from conscious controls and defenses and move less directively. We really never do forget anything we have perceived, but some memories may be stored away out of our ability to find them through conscious means. In this way, memory is always selective.

Gestalt theorists explain "insight" as a discovery, through nonlinear thinking and noncausative reasoning, of unexpected underlying connections between things that were previously not considered influential to each other or not perceived as mattering. This seems to closely mirror the way art can directly communicate meaning and emotions to a viewer, especially through the means of isomorphic representation. It is no wonder that the word *insight* is now commonly used in psychotherapy to describe instantaneous moments of illuminating perception or sudden pattern recognition. This is why I like to trust apparent "accidents," "mistakes of perception," and other unexplainable connections that almost inevitably produce therapeutic revelations and catharsis if permitted to happen. Both Gestalt and systems theorists place a lot of trust in this kind of "aha" experience, which is also known as synchronicity. Trusting the possibility that uncertainty often later results in clarity mandates the simultaneous acceptance of both knowing and not knowing while listening to the "truth" the client is presenting. The more open to synchronistic and collective archetypal experiences therapists remain, the more conscious this deep potential can become for their clients.

For example, several times in my PhotoTherapy projective work I have encountered clients responding to abstract photographic images of mine, going through entire sessions discussing offshoots from their original reaction to an image. Never would I tell them that the entire time they were holding the image upside down from the way I had originally intended it to be viewed. My original intentions were irrelevant to the clients' perceptual reality at that time, and it was their versions of my photograph that first attracted them to it and began to stimulate internal material. It is even likely that, had they viewed my photo right side up, it may not have produced any inner connection for them at all.

Unconsciously embedded meanings and feelings are by definition unknowable at a conscious level. They are spontaneously encoded and unexpected in their reappearance. In fact, their reappearance is sometimes at the unconscious level; for example, if the emotions are reinformed at a nonverbal level, a person simply reacts without knowing why. This cannot be predicted, nor forced by therapeutic plan, but if both client and therapist remain open to these sorts of possibilities, they will inevitably happen because of the very nature of nonverbal symbolic communication and the powerful connection of memories with unconscious feelings. The best model for this kind of work seems to me to be one of supporting clients as they (re)discover information about their own lives, most of which they already knew but weren't yet consciously aware that they knew. This position of noninterpretation encourages the use of photographs for crystalizing "inner landscapes" (Doughty, 1988) and encouraging their emergence into a cogent reality for external examination.

Sometimes such resurrected memories are so traumatic that they cannot be dealt with consciously, and if they emerge too suddenly, they are often protectively reburied, leaving no conscious memory of their having temporarily surfaced. For example, during a projective exercise, one client found herself strongly drawn to an image of a small vulnerable-looking child sitting expectantly on an adult's chair (see photo 2.7). This was a snapshot I had taken of a neighbor's child. I thought it was cute, so I had included it in the collection of images on my office wall.

This woman had been telling me for weeks how uncomfortable she felt when being photographed, and that even when she wanted to have her picture taken for promotional business purposes, she inevitably stiffened and experienced vague feelings of fear or anxiety when confronted by a camera lens. Since she kept examining that child's photograph, I asked her to talk with it for a while. She kept expressing concern for the child's well-being and using reassuring, comforting words. As she seemed to believe the child was somehow endangered, I asked her to "move into" the image and become that child, though first checking to make sure she was actually willing to risk doing this. Hesitantly, she agreed, and then internally assumed that child's identity as she understood it. She also physically took on the child's posture, without being aware she'd done this. I let her sit in silence at first, so that she could feel the emotional space she was now in; then I asked her questions, as if she were now the child.

"How old are you?" I asked. "Two," she answered immediately. "What is happening right now?" I continued. "Someone is taking my picture," she replied, with a quavering tone in her voice. "Tell me more about that," I requested. "He's big and tall and has a camera pointed right at me, and, oh no, it's going to hurt, I think." Continuing this process of being the child, she revealed that "that man" who took her picture was to be feared and avoided. We explored more of that reality, and then I brought her back out into the present, making sure that she also consciously carried into the present her memory of the dialogue that had just taken place.

As coinvestigators, we tried to find out why the association had formed between the feeling and the photo-posing. I asked her to reconnect with the child's feelings for a moment, and then I inquired about whether she could remember any time in her own life when she had had those sorts of feelings. She suddenly remembered her mother having told her that in her early childhood she was so cute that she had been selected to pose for a calendar. The calendar pictures were of children making funny faces, each picture had a jokey caption that went with the face. But one day my

Photo 2.7

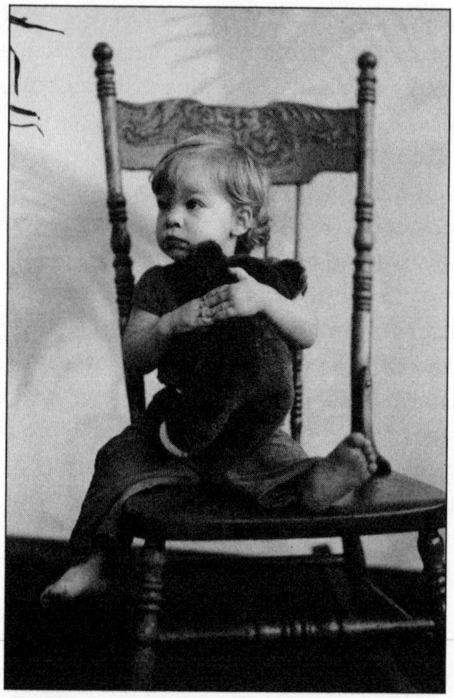

client's mother discovered that in order to produce these unusual faces, the photographers (all men) routinely physically and emotionally abused the children by doing things like sticking pins in them near their diapers or armpits, where the wounds wouldn't be noticeable, and teasing them by holding toys or candy just out of reach—so her "employment" was stopped.

Thus, in my client's earliest memory, long before she ever had words to communicate about such an experience, a strong negative emotion was bonded to the visual image of having a camera pointed at her. This memory was so strong as to still exist inside her thirty years later and so painful that it had not been permitted to become conscious. She herself was quite pleased to discover this information, long hidden inside herself, and expressed to me that she thought she would be able to be photographed now without any difficulty. As she had to move away soon, we had only one more meeting, so I could not verify if this actually became possible.

Interestingly, I spoke with her again two years later and reminded her of this incident, only to be told that she had no memory whatsoever of that previous "revelation" nor of our processing of the photograph of the child in the chair. She did mention that she still was not really comfortable being photographed, though she was much better than she had been a few years ago, but she was quite amazed to hear me recount what she had found out about herself in our discussion. It seemed that she had once again repressed conscious awareness of it altogether. To find out why she had done this would require more sessions, and as we could not arrange for them, this anecdote must remain unfinished. However, it demonstrates the power of the unconscious to protect us from material that might be too upsetting if it were to surface all at once, without any support for processing it into something less overpowering.

3 The Projective Process

Using Photographic Images to Explore Client Perceptions, Values, and Expectations

Any photograph presents selectively framed information. Each person encountering an image responds to both explicit and implicit messages, to the manifest and latent meaning, intention, and emotion embedded in its contents. As mentioned earlier, there are no simple clues for decoding snapshots' visual symbols. A person searching for the meaning of a given photograph will never be able to find the truth it holds for anyone else. In this supposed limitation lies the power of snapshots as therapeutic tools for accessing unconscious feelings, thoughts, memories, personal values, and deeply held beliefs.

Viewing any photograph begins an associative and emotional process in each viewer, and each viewer sees a unique reality inside the photograph's borders. Thus any single photograph can hold numerous meanings simultaneously. The borders of every snapshot form both a window into the image and also a window into the viewer's mind. The photograph's viewers create what they see by projection and imagination during the process of focused guided imagery, in this case a type in which both participant and guide can actually see and touch the externalized image of attention.

Personal experience is the best way to understand these concepts, so readers are invited to look over photos 3.1, 3.2, 3.3, and 3.4 now. Then explore your observations and reactions through the questions that follow. They are not unlike the questions that have worked well for me in therapeutic situations. Later in this chapter, you will find references to these photos in therapeutic discourse with clients. You will be able to compare

Photo 3.1

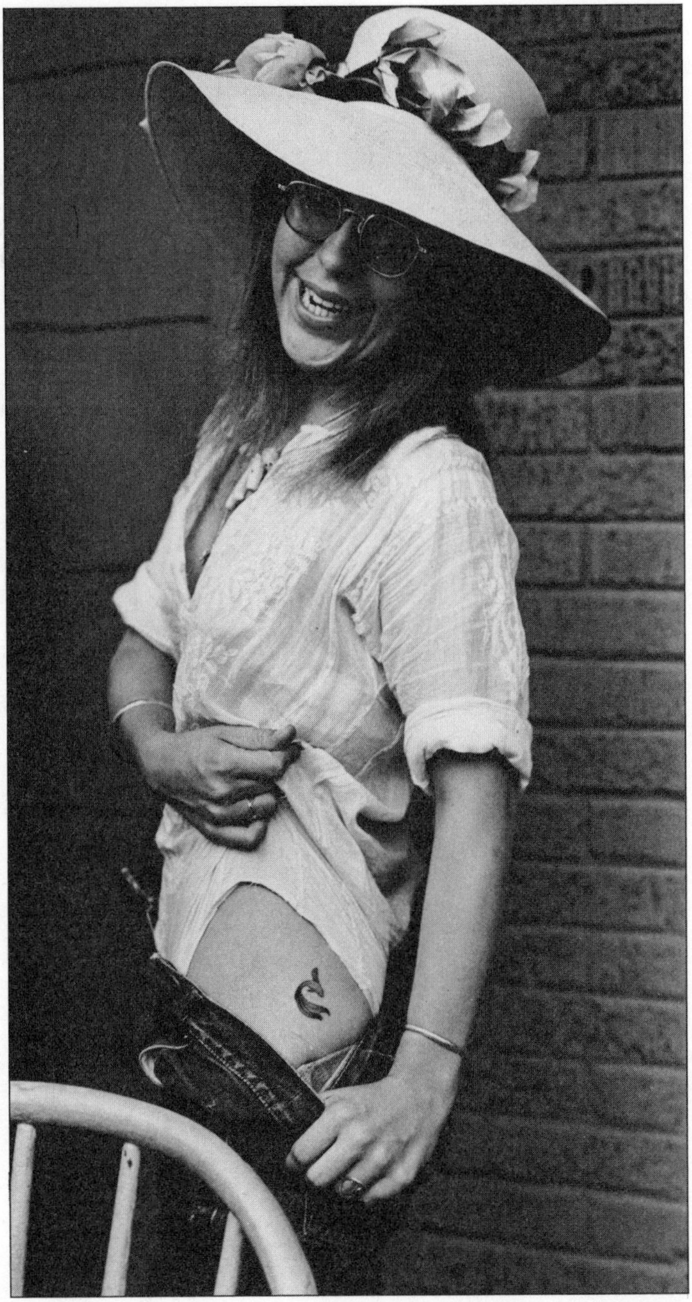

Photo 3.2

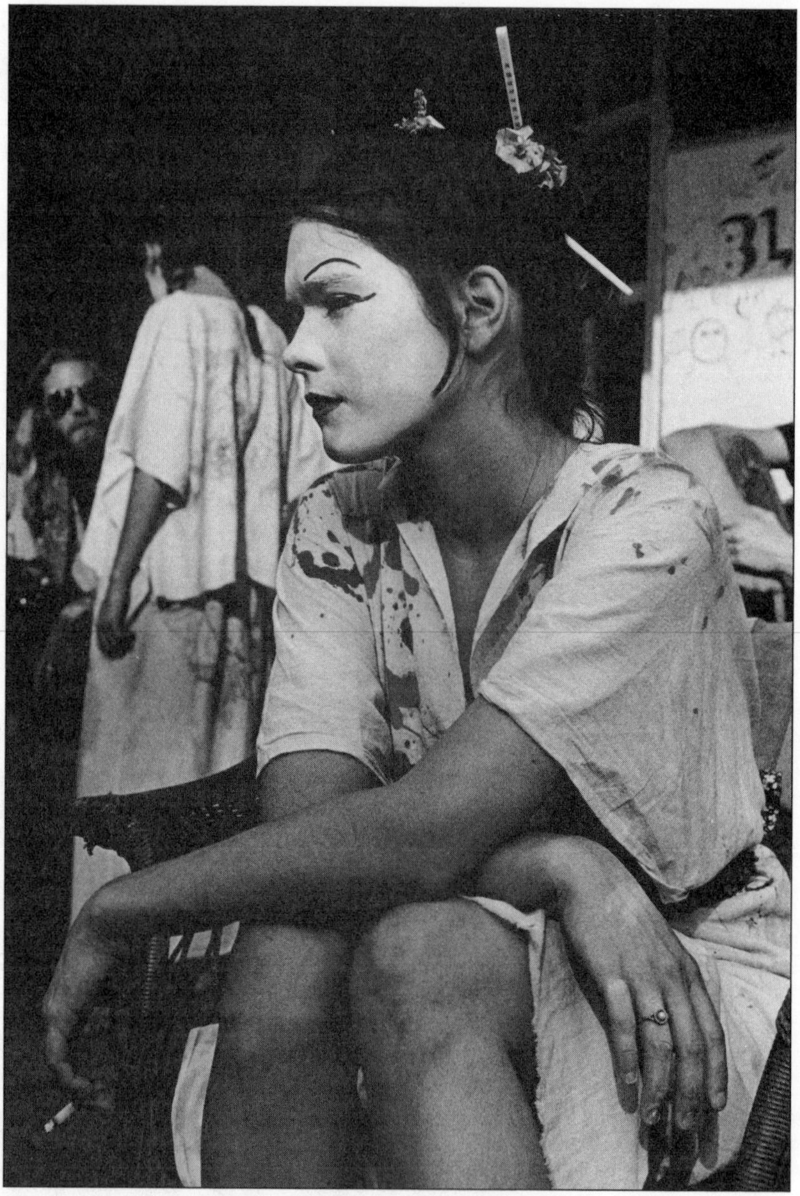

Photo 3.3

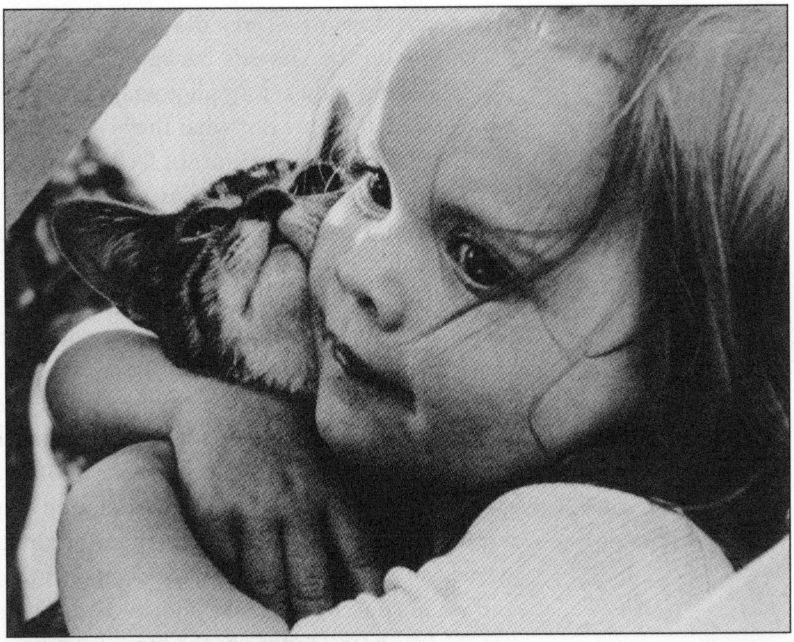

Photo 3.4

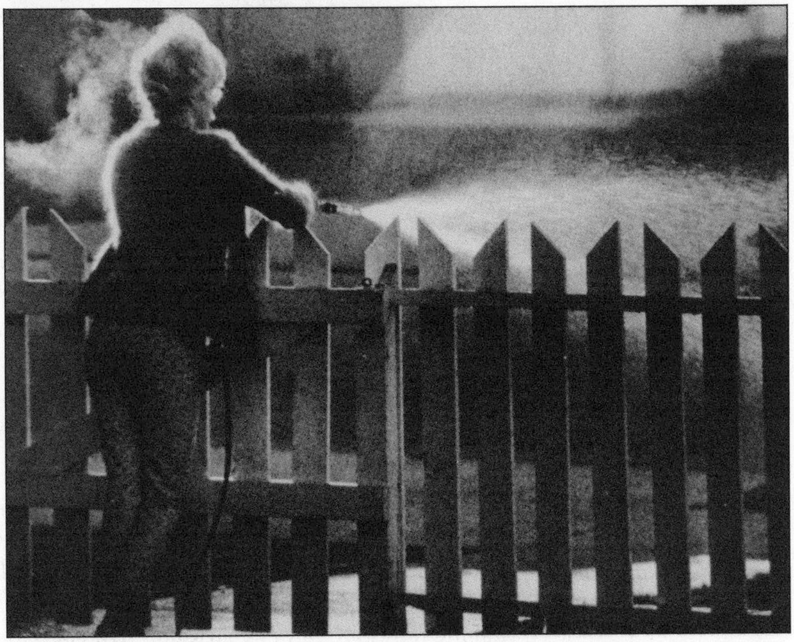

your perceptions with those of others and also see how meanings change, depending on the viewer's background and selective vision.

In looking at these four photographs, you probably tried to make sense out of them, to figure out what they were about or why I put them there, or perhaps you had some sort of feeling response to one or more of them as your mind instinctively free-associated. Try covering them up now and reconstructing each one from memory. Without looking at them again, think about what you might say or do to describe each image to somebody else. Then look again at the photos to match your memory with their true visual contents. What differences emerge between the details you remembered and the actual visual contents of each one?

The meanings you found and the feelings you responded with could only be your unique perceptions, and they may not be the ones I intended for viewers to have when I took these photographs (which you have no way of knowing). The meanings you found originated inside *you* as you responded to each image. In reacting to photographs—or to any part of everyday reality—we receive all the component information simultaneously, and we unconsciously make choices about what to attend to or remember. These choices represent the inner frameworks of values that map and prioritize what matters to us. These, in turn, affect the behaviors, expectations, rules for living, and other factors with which we measure and evaluate ourselves and others.

Is there one of those four pictures that you felt particularly drawn to when you first glanced at it? Is there one you perhaps would like to have on your wall at home? Does one remind you of your own favorite place or someone you know? Can you think of more details about each image that would give it more depth or context? Can you think of a story that would link all four together or imagine other images that could accompany these? (You will find that no words are needed for this kind of "visual essay.")

Did you happen to notice that all the people in the previous set of photos are Caucasian and female? If you are a Caucasian female, you probably didn't. However, if you belong to an ethnic or racial minority, you probably observed that people from non-Caucasian backgrounds were not there. Perhaps you noticed that there were no boys or men in the picture. A same kind of significance-by-absence has often happened as a result of the generalizations that a predominantly male-oriented society has traditionally imposed upon its girls and women. Until recent years have begun to reflect a change, females usually remained basically invisible as individual people. They were simply generically subsumed within the masculine pronoun and appeared in the public media when their use as manipulable objects was needed. Other minorities have also experienced similar exclusions to the margins of mainstream society (and thus of mainstream photography). Therapists must remain aware of such exclusions.

HOW THIS TECHNIQUE WORKS

Projective PhotoTherapy techniques involve both active and passive aspects of projecting, de-coding, de-constructing emotional content from stimulus images as the client is assisted in exploring their construction and association of meaning and feelings which they believe to be originally residing in the photographic artifact. This is true regardless of whether the viewer is looking at his or her own photos, album snapshots, self-portraits, photos belonging to the therapist, or pictures found in printed media.

Looking for the Realities in a Photo

It is certainly useful to attend to what clients present as being relevant or important about their lives, but I am equally interested in learning *why* they are telling me about or showing me these things. Why this, why there, and why now? Why are they making this connection? How or why do they go from one specific detail to that particular next one? When the probing has gone as deep as it can consciously, and when the client is at the point where they don't know how they know something but they are nevertheless certain that they know it to be true for them, this level of unshakeable certainty marks the core of their inner values which have been nonverbally absorbed as part of their very culture and family upbringing—producing the person they are. This inner and deeply unconscious value system is the basis of all their ordinary daily decisions, opinions, and judgments about themselves and others. These are the "shoulds" and "oughts" of their lives, and they filter their every interaction with the world outside their own minds.

As explained earlier, the idea of using photographs in my therapeutic practice evolved for me through finding that people continually responded differently to my own snapshots than I did (or expected them to). I began to recognize that having ordinary looking photographs around my office where people could see them might result in clients being able to share deeper parts of themselves and their emotions with me than I might have discovered through verbal inquiry alone. It seemed natural to collect a few dozen of my photos for my waiting room wall and use them actively as topics for client discussion and probing of thoughts or feelings they evoked.

For example, the father of a family I was treating for difficulties with their two teenage daughters viewed photo 3.1, of the girl showing off her tattoo. His reaction was, "Would you look at that!" "At what, dear?" the mother replied, and the dialogue continued:

"At that young lady pulling down her trousers in public like that. She ought to be ashamed."

"Good heavens, dear, she's just trying to show us her tattoo."

"Well it's indecent, that's what it is. I'd better not ever catch our daughters doing anything like that!"

"But, dear, she's showing less than if she had on her bathing suit. And besides, my bathing suit's not much less revealing, and neither is yours!"

"Well, yeah, but that's different!"

It quickly became obvious that we weren't talking about the girl in the picture but were instead touching on much deeper issues about young girls' vulnerability, parental expectations, and especially the father's attitudes about his daughters' sexual identities. To ask him what would have to change in that photo for the girl pictured in it to have been one of his own daughters, or to ask him what he thought that girl's parents should say to her about the photo, would be to enter into therapeutic process with him on levels that would involve the entire family's system of nonverbal communication of their values.

If the girl in the photo were actually one of his own daughters, we might role-play dialogue with her to explore, practice, and rehearse ways for him to get his message of caring across to that daughter, who was used to hearing his criticisms. If the father were to bring in snapshots from his own teenage years, these might help him remember how old-fashioned his own parents had seemed in regard to his teenage behaviors (and might also help him place the source of some of his own words). These are the sorts of therapeutic possibilities that often open up as a consequence of hearing someone "just chat" about a photo that happens to be hanging on my wall.

While I am very interested in helping clients deal with emotional difficulties in their lives, I am also interested in learning how the situation might change to have different consequences. Personal responses to such probes work almost entirely at nonverbal levels of knowing and changing, and photographic representations of potential realities can be very useful clarification tools. Conceptualizing what could change in a situation—to make it better, worse, less emotionally involving—helps clients realize metaphorically that alternatives are possible, and that their "truth" is relative to both its context and perceiver. It also helps clients to realize that they have some freedom to initiate changes and to safely explore possible consequences in their minds before initiating them in actuality.

Deep inside themselves, people often know what changes they need to make, but translating those ideas into words can be very difficult. Once the ideas become words, they can be consciously contemplated and manipulated, but then they have been removed from their direct raw power.

Once something is "out" in conscious view, it can no longer remain safely protected and defended (and thus avoided). It is much more difficult to continue stating that we are powerless to do anything about it. This is why so much of the most potentially powerful emotional material needing therapeutic focus usually remains so deeply protected inside the client's unconscious; it has so much power that sometimes they cannot deal with it without being quickly overwhelmed. Other times it stays down there because it is easier not to deal with it at all. In both cases, clients cling to the excuse that they are unable to change things.

If life is conflicted because of inner dissonance, things will "out" (emerge, reveal) themselves on their own, in contrast to when things "out" because people are consciously searching for them therapeutically. If something that has been repressed into the unconscious must out, it will repeatedly present itself, emotionally or nonverbally, until it is consciously acknowledged, much like the woman's buried memory of being abused by a photographer, described in Chapter Two. Emotional messages that emerge from deep inside can take symbolic form, as when you become aware of repeating patterns in your life or art, but only after their visual demands have made them obvious.

An example of this is demonstrated in the initially strong negative response a client had to the photo of the white-faced mime at the beginning of this chapter (photo 3.2). He had told me several weeks before of taking his son to the circus, but having to leave when the white-faced clowns came out. He had thought it was merely claustrophobia related to being in a crowd, but his son's disappointment had pained him, and we had tried to explore the incident. He mentioned that the "new" photo on my wall had the same effect on him: he felt panic and the need to flee. It took me a moment to realize it was a photograph he had commented on twice before as "sad" or "scary," but he no longer remembered having noticed it before, so he perceived it as being new.

He continued, "This photo really caught my eye. My first reaction was that I was back in Vietnam, and I was overcome with an emotional rush of sadness and decay. She is some kind of painted lady, a bar girl, torn and bloody, with the endless patience born of despair. No more tears left in her, so used up that no one would want her any more. The cigarette in her hand especially draws me. It's the currency of soldiers. It makes me want to cry." Once these thoughts were more conscious, he suddenly remembered two months previously when his children had been trying to choose Halloween costumes and he had "irrationally" forbidden them to put on face paint. Then he suddenly connected it all with the powdered lime dusted on children's bodies in a village he had helped eradicate. The meaning finally emerged fully, after repeated attempts to "out" itself. When the client was ready to consider them, those repeated efforts became clear parts of a pattern unnoticed until that day.

Sometimes, once an issue has become conscious, the client discovers that signals of the difficulty have long been evident in personal snapshots that have never been examined for the significance within them. I hear comments such as "I know there's something about those people that I should be hearing" or "There's something about that tree that's more than a tree for me, and I wonder why it pulls me so much." An excellent example of this is a client of mine, an amateur photographer who loved taking "people pictures," who discovered only months after deciding to file for divorce, that for the previous two years *none* of her photographs had included any couples whatsoever as subjects for her camera to capture. These sorts of discoveries all reflect the projective nature of people's interactions with the camera and its products.

A young couple's responses to the image of the child hugging a cat (photo 3.3) illustrates how a photograph helped two people become conscious of how their lives as children affected their marriage to the point of near-dissolution.

The newly married young couple came to me for counseling because "things just weren't going right." The wife was unhappy and disappointed, and although she was attempting to keep her sadness from her husband, it was affecting every interaction they had. He had just been promoted to a more stressful job and came home exhausted each night to her expectations and needs. He felt torn by all the demands on his time at work and at home, and as an only child in an undemonstrative family he had been unable to get to the root of his problems with his new wife, no matter how much time he spent worrying about this privately. When she had suggested talking it over with her mother, which was her natural instinct, his horrified response about sharing such private details with one's parents quickly squelched the idea, and she was left feeling even more isolated.

While sitting in my lobby making small talk before our first session, the wife found the child-hugging-cat picture to be particularly to her liking: "What a sweet, loving hug. It's all homey and warm and comfortable. They look so happy together, as if they are both purring." Her husband replied rather explosively, "My God, she's choking that poor animal! It can't even breathe. How can you call that love? It's pure suffocation! If she lets go, that cat will immediately dash away, and if she keeps grabbing at it like that every time it returns, it'll never get close. The only way it would stick around would be if she'd relax her grip and have the patience to wait until it approached her!"

She looked astonished at his reaction to the photo, and we quickly moved into using this event metaphorically to discuss some of their problem areas. It turned out that he had been coming home every night needing some time to be alone and make the transition from work to home. In contrast, she had been alone all day and eagerly awaited his return as the highlight of her day. From the moment he came through their front door, she "lovingly" attached herself to him, following him from room to room and never leaving him alone because she was so pleased to be with him. She admitted that she had been rather jealous of all the attention he gave to work. He, who had never lived with another person after leaving home ten years previously, was feeling suffocated, but not at all unloving. He explained that he just needed to have some regular time alone with himself. Although this was altogether foreign to her, she agreed to try for a week to leave him alone for half an hour after he arrived home ("loosening her grip" and giving him "breathing room"), even though this seemed to her to be very strange on the part of a wife. It worked very well, and they began to build on this experience to share different feelings in other problematical situations.

Thus using a photographic catalyst helps in ways that solely internal imagining or pondering cannot, in that it permits therapist and client to focus together on an image relatively external to the client's defense structure. As a result, somewhat intrusive questioning will be far more tolerable than if the client were to be directly questioned or challenged. However, if the couple and I had not happened upon the photograph of the child and the cat, I believe that issue would have continued to present itself in one manner or another (for example, in reviewing album photos or posing together for someone else's camera) until its emotional message was acknowledged and resolved.

Projective PhotoTherapy is a metaphoric process on many levels. Free association as a projective technique works because underlying connections are already there to be perceived, though not necessarily consciously. Earlier pages discussed how sometimes significance emerges through a previously unrecognized pattern. A careful journey through other people's snapshots can sometimes reveal a pattern as well, as the following example illustrates:

When a mother and her adult daughter viewed my photo of the woman leaning on a fence holding a watering hose (photo 3.4), they literally found themselves face to face with their differing perceptions of women's work, sex roles, and generational expectations. When discussing how the woman in the photo was probably feeling, the mother said, "She's so relaxed and peaceful—the kids are in school, her husband's at work, her chores are done, and she's finally got time to herself while she waits for them all to come home."

Her daughter replied, "What a terribly bored person she is! Look at her posture and her slouch. She's smoking and probably strung out on tranquilizers and living in a valium haze! An empty aimless existence, doing nothing and expecting nothing. Just the same routine day in and day out. No wonder she's so depressed!" This dialogue continued as they contemplated what that image meant inside their own value systems and expectations. This led to further discussion about the role of mothering, which was timely because the daughter, herself a mother of a child just starting kindergarten, had recently chosen to go back to work, much to her own mother's disapproval.

Photos as Representations of Ourselves to Ourselves

Whenever we interact with photographs—viewing them alone or talking about them with others, or even conversing with them—we find meaning being created in that very process itself. This is demonstrated by a woman's reaction to a photograph of a broken window in the wall of an old building (see photo 3.5).

She had picked this window as her self-portrait equivalent, saying, "It is definitely *me.* My outsides are tattered and my paint's peeling. Some of my windows are broken, so I'm not as protected from the wind and rain as I used to be. What you see when you look at me is my outsides, the boards and glass that are my shell. The windows that you're supposed to look into to see me better only end up as reflections of the person who's looking. The real me inside it all isn't visible until the glass is broken away, and even then it's in deep dark shadows. It's really painful to have that glass shatter, because it protected me for so long, but it's too much of a barrier now, and it kept people away. I want out now."

I made her a photocopy of that photo, and cut out the four window panes so that they actually became holes in the paper itself. The assignment I gave her then was to create self-portraits, to fill each opening, that would fit the image of the self she felt to be emerging. She used instant-print film to do one of the four right there in my office, went home to do the others because they required more planning, and ended up also using one photocopied from an old album snapshot.

She asked me to rephotograph the finished collage and she had that print enlarged to poster size. She hung it on her bedroom wall to be looked at each morning; it became her talisman for personal growth, and she felt no need to further explain it. However, after she told her husband her story, he wanted to take photos of her to "go along with" the collage, so that she could see her changing self from his viewpoint. She accepted his offer, and in their collaboration, they also entered into some deep and worthwhile dialogue about their relationship.

Many art therapists consider a drawing of a house to be symbolic of the family life of the person drawing it, particularly their emotional and physical childhood environment. I explored these possibilities in several verbal discussions with this client. Traditional archetypal imagery guided some of my queries on general levels and helped illuminate her personally defined perspective.

Projective techniques are at work when clients create self-portraits by

Photo 3.5

picking images, from a large collection of photographs or magazine pages, that seem to represent them, even if only in some symbolic sense. These do not need to be photos of people; in fact, clients often choose pictures of natural objects like trees, flowers, or animals, and even sometimes inanimate subjects like boats, hamburgers, or rocking chairs. A client's explanation of why a particular photo "seems to be about me" can yield

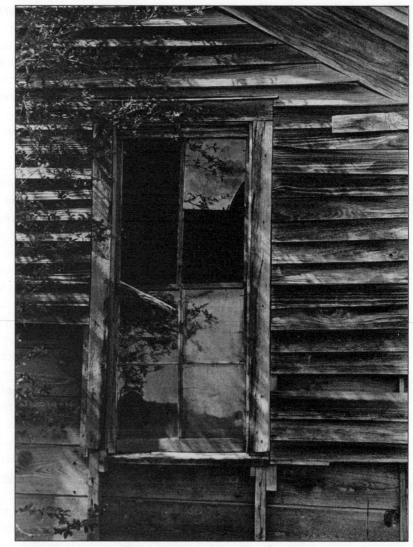

useful information about self-perceptions. To then, for example, combine this with having the client pose for a photograph along with that metaphoric self-portrait in a way that further illustrates their symbolic relationship could provide information which might not emerge from either one of these assignments done alone.

An example of this is illustrated by the response of a woman who selected photo 3.6 as a metaphoric self-portrait. Even though she had dozens of "people pictures" to choose from, along with numerous landscapes, still lifes, buildings, and abstracts, she held onto this one as she scanned all the others. Many art therapists consider tree imagery to symbolize the self or the client's personal emotional history. Most of my clients do not know this when they begin doing projective PhotoTherapy work, yet it is not uncommon for people to select trees as metaphorical self-portraits in both picture-taking and picture-selecting tasks. While this woman's choice of selection arose from her unconscious preferences, it clearly demonstrates how underlying archetypal imagery can emerge when the inner connection is appropriate.

She stated, "This is my symbolic self-portrait. I'm the tree holding my family together. My roots go deep and hold fast, and nothing can blow us over. I have a solid trunk and branches reaching out that can hold up just about everything. My children are those branches. No, rather, they sit on those branches and venture out like little birds to explore the world, but they always return home for support and nurturing. I take in energy from the soil and pass it up to them to use. I don't need to go anywhere. All I want is right here already."

Hearing all this, I had some concerns about her not mentioning her husband, with whom she had lived for fifteen years (happily, she had previously said). Since trees never move unless blown over, dug up, or cut down for timber, I was curious if she would want to stay rooted there forever, even when the birds no longer came back. In other words, who was she when she was not busy holding them all up? If she could be someone or somewhere else, would she find that option attractive or undesirable? Did she really like being "where she was at," being a tree? If she truly did, then of course that would be fine, but I felt it needed further exploring. So I began by having her place her own Polaroid self-portrait over the face of the person at the bottom of the tree trunk, and pictures of her children on what she saw as the tree's branches (I myself do not see any actual branches in that photo). I wanted to know how this felt. She said she enjoyed the experiment, but that something still seemed not quite right.

Photo 3.6

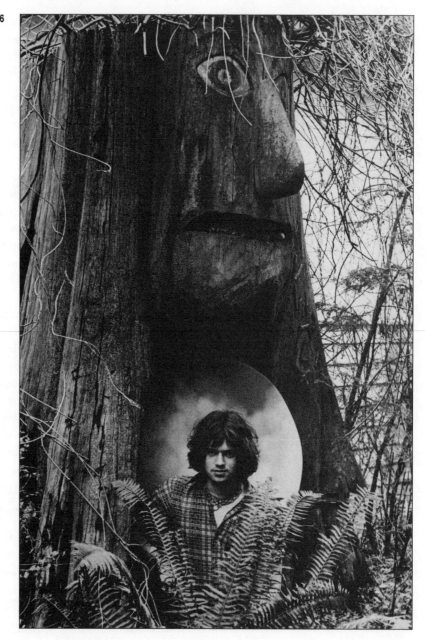

I suggested moving the photo of her own face off the person's face and onto the tree-trunk face, and she immediately agreed that this felt better and decided the 'self-portrait' was now complete. I rephotographed the collage and placed the new version on a large sheet of newsprint. I asked her to pretend that the big piece of paper contained the larger scene from which the photo had been selectively framed. I asked her to fill in this missing area (create it) however she wished, covering the entire sheet if that seemed appropriate. What emerged visually was more treetop, other trees (as if a forest scene), and other details. What interested me therapeutically was that the bottom was left blank. No roots were drawn in, and their absence seemed to signal that perhaps therapy ought to begin with issues such as fixity, commitment, desire to fully live the role she had idealized as wife and mother.

It was also intriguing to me that she continually "forgot" to include her husband in her photographic extrapolations or any conversations about the images. It was almost too tidy a story for me to believe when I found out that he rarely lived at home because he was a logger. Those are the moments when a therapist must refrain from making connections that seem too logically simple or deductively conclusive. However, the fact that he spent his life cutting down trees was an inescapable topic for careful probing in our discussion of their relationship. I was also surprised to find that in her childhood her family lived in a small town at the edge of a forest, and family outings into the woods were a frequently enjoyed activity.

Some therapists specialize in working with only those projective elements of photos that people have themselves taken, collected, or were assigned to take of themselves or the world around them. For example, Ziller and Lewis (1981) asked clients to take ten photos for each of four topics ("describe yourself, your family, your past, and your future"), or just to go use up a roll of film taking pictures of what interested them, to illustrate "who you think you are." Glass (1991), Krauss, Capizzi, Englehart, Gatti, and Reed (1983), and others have used a variety of photo-taking assignments to obtain clues about clients' inner value systems through noting how their choices of what to photograph suggest symbolic projections of the self. Fryrear (1982, 1983) does self-confrontation work by having clients, particularly adolescents, pose for self-portraits and then explore what has appeared on the film from an outside perspective.

Comfort (1985) was quite interested to find that when clients gathered pictures from printed media, any image they were visually and emotionally drawn to could be a significant projective focus for learning more about themselves. The stories people tell about their albums' contents are useful projectives in their construction of selective truth and some therapists, such as Entin (1979, 1980, 1981, 1983), use only the stories their clients tell in response to PhotoTherapy-based questions about album contents, and never use any other kinds of images.

Other Approaches to Visual Images

Although some of the previous anecdotes referred to photos clients encountered on my waiting room walls, I also have a second less formal source of images for projective work: a casual pile of my own hobby photographs is always at hand, ready for moving around on a large table in my office. There are about a hundred images of people, places, abstracts, buildings, nature, and anything else that happened to catch my photographic interest. This collection was originally prepared simply to help people feel comfortable manipulating photographs as touchable tools rather than treating them as art objects. They are somewhat tattered and stained from years of being handled, and I make a point of treating them informally. I usually toss the pile onto the table from a distance of several feet, so that the pictures spread out by themselves. This helps clients understand that the pictures are just paper objects that can be handled just as casually as note paper or playing cards.

I have no fixed rules for assigning clients' searches through them, nor for beginning questioning about these photos. Sometimes I ask clients to select a few key images along a theme I think will be useful. Other times we work with the entire spread-out collection, which can easily cover the eight-foot-square table. This is not a fixed collection; if a new photo seems useful, I add it, and if an image hasn't been worked with for a few years, I'm likely to pull it out. The only serious condition on my selections for this collection is ethical considerations regarding the subjects. I don't use pictures showing people's identity which would require special releases, and I don't include even "borderline" nonpublic images unless their subjects have given me their written permission. (Readers who want more information about legal releases and confidentiality requirements are invited to contact me.)

I may not ask clients to pick individual images, but rather to sort the collection into groups that seem to go together. This can serve projectively as nonverbal values-clarification work, especially when clients explain later what mental or emotional criteria they used to group and separate images.

Therapists who specialize solely in projective PhotoTherapy work may prefer to concentrate on only one style of questioning or one type of imagery. For example, Walker (1980, 1982, 1983, 1986) conducts effective image-based therapy using his own abstract, blurry color photographs. Others, including myself, prefer very specific contents. It is important to note that all kinds of photographs can work well as subjects for therapeutic inquiry; they don't need to be artistically "good" ones.

I often have clients try to find connections between their selected projective images and other photos from their albums, their self-portraits, or even memory or fantasy. We then work with these interactively by, for example, having a client look at a just-taken self-portrait and then find the photo from the "projective pile" that seems to fit with it, for comparative discussion. However, doing projective PhotoTherapy work involves more than looking at and talking about photos. The way images are interacted with can also be extremely significant.

How the Client Presents the Photos

When I ask clients to bring me some snapshots that show a certain topic that I want to examine, such as their home or their family, it is interesting to note how many or few pictures the client brings and how willingly this is done. The way people organize their presentation to me mirrors their inner mental pictures of those people or places. Even the inability to make choices can be meaningful in certain situations. I also take note of how quickly or inattentively clients show the pictures to me; whether I am given long intricate stories with each snapshot; clients' tone of voice, posture, or facial expressions when describing the photos; which images or people they consistently tell me a lot about or seem to want to skip; and other parts of the sharing process.

When showing their albums, clients frequently go quickly by photos of people they don't want to talk about or times in their lives that are painful for them to remember and discuss. I have done some rewarding PhotoTherapy work just by asking clients, before they even open their albums, "Are there any photos you removed from this album so that we don't have to talk about them?" or "Are there any photos you've brought today that you hope I *don't* ask you about?" After being reassured that they are free to not discuss those pictures, it's surprising how often clients will talk about those very images, simply because I gave them the choice of whether to do so or not.

Thoughts, memories, and feelings associated with viewing a snapshot usually arise unbidden, and yet they are frequently more therapeutically significant than the image examination itself. I watched a father and son look through a collection of my photographs, and though they didn't speak with each other a lot, I noticed an unspoken resonance in their movements. Gazing together at one of my peaceful landscape scenes, the father said, "Momma would have liked that one," and the son nodded in agreement, unable to speak easily because he suddenly had tears in his eyes. "Yeah," he whispered hoarsely, "I miss her when we see things like this." And they hugged tightly, both in tears.

All language is metaphoric, even visual-symbolic language. All metaphors are simultaneously multilevel and require thinking in a style that can encompass them. In addition, because metaphors (such as those in fables, myths, allegories, and photos) contain many levels of meaning, people can take from them the meaning they need, want, or are able to understand at any particular time. People seem to have a naturally protective process inside them wherein they take the meaning they need at a particular time (and need the meaning they are taking) and yet somehow naturally remain protected from getting in any deeper than they can understand or cope with.

The discovery of new levels constitutes learning, and we are nearly always more invested in a discovery if we make it for ourselves. Insights about our family histories are usually more powerful if we participate in their discovery. Insight can be thought of as seeing new meanings in old familiar stories—or photos; it is a way of reframing our beliefs, and this helps to precipitate change in us. We make new connections and associations, reconstruct a familiar story from a different viewpoint, or see it in the light of contrasting, but not necessarily contradictory, information.

WHAT TO DO

In their PhotoTherapeutic explorations of snapshots, clients begin to peel back the visual and emotional layers of meaning those images hold for them. All photographs contain personal/individual and collective/archetypal symbols simultaneously. In summary, therefore, projective PhotoTherapy techniques involve the use of a precise image or detail of an image to simultaneously understand a complex level of meaning by association, implication, and symbolic reference. All can be "worked" for more information.

Different Viewings at Different Times

It is important to keep in mind that a person's response to a given image will likely vary from encounter to encounter with it. We might view the same image quite differently, for example, before and after lunch, before and after learning something new about our past or hearing of someone's death, on a sunny day and on a rainy day; our responses to an image might be quite different, even though the snapshot itself won't have changed at all.

That such perceptions and reactions are so situationally dependent and temporally conditional is a positive component of PhotoTherapy projective techniques in that we can use this to help clients learn that their perceptions and reactions to life itself are influenced by what they bring to each moment. For these reasons, therapists need to be careful not to take too much significance from any one response to any single photograph, and to look for patterns of responses or sudden differences from the norm in assessing clients' comments.

I ask about the general contents to see which portions may have emerged as figure or ground for that client. What they haven't noticed, or have dismissed as negative "empty" space or background, is also of interest to me. I try to be aware of their natural instinct for "closure" (in Gestalt terms; that is, when they are making completions or interpreting conclusions that seem to me not so clearly resident in the image itself when I view it).

And when the client selects a particular component subject or feeling to focus on or discuss, I often ask for clarification to probe deeper and get additional information relevant to that person's life. Sometimes I sound positively ignorant in asking these kinds of amplifying questions; for example, "I'm not sure what you mean when you say it seems scary, so could you give me a few details to help me understand better?" or "You say that person's obviously upset, but I'm not sure I'd use quite that word, so would you tell me a bit more about what you think is happening in that photo, and more precisely what you mean by 'upset'?"

Sometimes I say something like, "Pretend I'm blind, and tell me what this is a picture of. What's in this image and what's the most important component," or "You're the one holding the image, not me. You can see it, but I can only see its white backing because you're sitting across from me. Please tell me what the picture is about, because I can't see the side you are looking at." A similar approach can be helpful as a general model throughout therapy: if clients ask me what I want to know, I usually reply by asking them what they think I want to know, and we start there, with them leading.

When I do eventually get to see the actual photo, I can note any differences in subject or emotional content between our two interpretations of the image, and we then discuss how our selective perceptions might represent differences between us. It can be empowering for clients to hold the meanings they perceive as true (for themselves), and at the same time see that there can always be more than one version of reality. This is a relatively nonthreatening approach to the idea that being "wrong" is relative, and that one can accept difference without demanding changes.

If I offer my perspective and clearly claim it as merely my own, it should not be threatening to the client's version. Then I can ask the client to help me understand why I am not getting it "correctly." When clients are in a position to help me, they have most of the power in our relationship. If, instead, they feel that I have privileged information or superior knowledge and am thus definitely right (which can only mean that their position is wrong), they may justifiably feel discounted, attacked, criticized, minimized, or judged. If that happens, they might retreat into not being willing to risk the vulnerability of sharing what they think or feel for fear of it being devalued or negated.

I often contribute neutral comments such as, "Wait a minute, I'm confused. You say that's a happy child, and to me she looks sad. Could we discuss this more? Where are you finding the clues in the picture that tell you that, because I'm obviously missing them. Why do you think it might be that you and I are seeing her so differently?" These sorts of questions help clients accept that although others may not always understand or agree with their perceptions, those differences don't necessarily convey a threat to their position. As they help me to see what they are seeing, I learn about the composition of their inner mental maps and how they frame their thinking. As they show me their own viewpoint, they begin to acknowledge it as their own, separate from mine and yet equally valid.

If we do not eventually find ourselves in perceptual agreement, then I am likely to say something like, "Well, you can see my position, and I can see yours. You are the client here, so let's work first from your perspective and then we can turn around and work from mine." That kind of role reversal gives clients some practice with the skills of leading a PhotoTherapy session, and those skills will likely be useful later as a means of improving their communication with others in their daily life whose positions may seem strange and in need of clarification.

Finding the Photo That Strikes a Chord

Most projective work begins with the client being asked to select one or a few images, from the larger collection, that will fit an assigned question; for example, which of my photos are their favorites, which one calls to them the most (which seems to "call their name"), which could be a metaphorical self-portrait of them (which seem most like them in tone or feeling), which of these photos would they have taken themselves if they could, which seems to most challenge them, which ones would they like to take home with them for a week, which ones express feelings that they have (or don't want to have), and so forth, including "negatively focused" questions, such as which photo do they like the least or feel least willing to talk about.

If our therapy work involves a lot of family issues, I might ask a client to choose one photo from my big pile to represent each significant family member ("that photo would be the one to stand for my father, because ____"). If we have been doing a lot of work around expressing feelings, I might ask the client to find five angry photos and five happy ones or some that communicate other feelings we've been working on. If I have been focusing on self-issues and using self-portrait tools like instant photos in session or photos of the client found in albums, I may ask the person to select a photograph from my large collection that goes with the self-portrait photo. I might even ask the client to affix the self-portrait to a photocopy we make of the projective photo that fits with theirs, so that we have a collage of self-in-context.

Sometimes I have clients make their selections in silence, while other times I ask them to tell what is happening inside them as they consider the alternatives, because even their reasons for rejecting images can be useful clues to their inner maps and values. Sometimes we go on to be quite active and have a conversation with the image or pose ourselves as if we were part of it, as a temporary sculpture, and explore what that brings forth. Other times I may have the client look at all the photographs with me and instead of asking questions about what the person sees, I may suggest that he or she question me about those images.

Questions, Answers, and Discourses on the Photos

Once we probe initial general reactions to a photograph, I will ask the client questions based on where I wish to guide the therapy. I may ask about the overall image, its component parts, portions not visible (beyond the physical borders), imagined related images, or how the subject or emotional content fits with other images the client has discussed in previous sessions. The questions are open-ended and can be infinitely creative: I may suggest clients speak as if they were that river, ask that window what it can see, or what story that shoe might be able to tell if it could speak. If their chosen photos contain people, I might ask them what that person seems to be feeling or thinking about, why this person is in this place (and where he or she would rather be), or perhaps what that person was in the middle of doing or saying when the photo interrupted. If the stimulus for projecting on is one of their own family snapshots, I may have them "become" their own grandmother or "be" their father's hands to talk about what that feels like or what story could be told from that viewpoint. I might even ask them to become objects in a photo, pretending to be the dining room table, parental bed, or living room ceiling light, and ask them what as objects they've "seen" and "heard" of the family they have served throughout all these years.

I may have them physically assume the pose of a certain component of a photo's subject matter as if they actually were the table or those people and talk about what is going on in the surrounding room. I may ask them to become part of that photograph metaphorically by stepping over the edges of its frame into its scene, perhaps, or by walking on over to the ocean and wading in to then be able to tell me what that feels like, or becoming the chair and telling me what it has seen and heard before. "I am the field of flowers; I feel or remember ____"; "I am your bedside light; when you turn me on, I can see ____ and when you turn me off, it's because ____"; and so forth. I may have them *be* an entire photograph itself and talk about what *it* can see, hear, feel, or note about the client's life. Or I may have a photograph serve as a mask or puppet to talk to me *for* the client or to dialogue with yet another photo.

Whatever clients offer reflects information about themselves. When they are intensely involved in interaction with the photograph and fully attending to it with their face, body, or memories, I may check with them to see if their kinesthetic existence at that moment of "being with" the photograph reminds them of anyone in particular. Or I might ask them to become the pose of a component of the photo and hold that pose for a minute to know more about how it might feel to really be that person or object.

I might ask them to even project upon the probable intentions or feelings of the photographer, asking who they think took this photo and why, what they think the photographer was originally hoping to get and whether she or he did, who they think the photo might have been taken for, who posed in it and how that person felt, and so forth. Because we both know it is just fantasizing, it doesn't matter if they know I originally took most of the images. Creating the persona of the supposed photographer can be simply another level of imagining.

I am curious to know if the client feels that the image is incomplete in any way, if something is missing, or if anything would make its meaning or message clearer to viewers. I ask about which portions could be removed without any significance being lost, and how they might have taken the photo differently if they were themselves the photographer. I sometimes explore the parts that are not the central focus for the client, as the empty ("negative") space has its own reality, its own weight and potential significance.

I believe that the opposite of something is not always just "nothing"; there cannot be any opposite to something that is part of a whole, encompassing the entire image. Things only exist in relationship with everything else; they do not exist in complete isolation, even in a photograph. If there is sunshine, there is shadow. If there is a subject, there is also potential significance in its absence. Appearances signal not only what may exist, but also the potential of both its context and its opposite. In photos and in human emotions, whatever appears defines its context or "alter" possibility. For this reason I am also interested in the potential significance of even "empty" space, the area called "negative space" in artistic terms, meaning that which is not within the visual boundaries surrounding the actual subject matter of the photograph, as can be seen in a later example in this chapter about a brick wall and the shape of the "empty" sky that appears above and beyond it.

When clients first view a photograph, I usually ask them to try to be aware of any feelings, thoughts, memories, or ideas that come to mind. Sometimes it helps if I start a sentence and leave a blank to fill in; for example, "When I see this photograph, I find myself feeling ____, wanting to say ____, remembering ____, having the reaction that ____, wanting to ask ____." Or "When I explore this photograph, I think its message for me is ____, it makes me think about ____, or my response to it is ____ and I think this is probably because ____." These and other sentence completions can be spontaneous during therapeutic dialogue or can be given as assignments to be finished later in writing (or by using other photographs for answers).

I sometimes ask clients to continue sentences I have started, such as "If this photo could speak, it would likely say ____"; "If I were to title this photo, I would call it ____"; "If this photo were to be able to teach me a lesson, it would be ____"; "If my mother were to know this is the picture I chose, her response would be ____"; "If I could give this photo as a gift to someone, I would give it to ____, because of ____." This sort of nonverbal, nonthreatening activity can draw emotionally laden material from the client's unconscious. A useful follow-up is to go back over these statements, finishing them the way the client's parent, lover, spouse, or child might. Another approach is to return to the large collection of photos and ask the client to pick an image one of those other people might have selected as "calling" to them ("Which photo do you think your mother would have chosen as a metaphoric self-portrait? Why that one?")

These exercises provide insight for both therapist and client as to how fully the client knows the mother (or other significant persons). If therapy has been initiated because of the client's difficulties with a particular person, and if it seems useful to explore that person's life beyond the usual surface roles, this can be a very good way to begin. Even better would be to actually involve the other person in the exercise to see which image he or she actually picks and how the person completes the sentences.

If the other person does participate, it will be useful to ask him or her to hypothesize about which image they think the client might have picked as a self-portrait image, how the client might have completed the statements, and perhaps, which photo the client might have thought this person would pick, and why. The result is an encompassing multivectored "self-other projective analysis," which can provide considerable data about how the two people perceive themselves and each other. The ideal would be for each to observe the other's process, both in choosing a self-image and in picking the image the other one might choose. If each listens to how the other completes the statements, both will learn a lot about how the other thinks, evaluates, and projects personal and emotional meaning.

As a therapist firmly rooted in the systems approach to therapy, I often find it valuable to involve more people in the actual counseling session than just my particular client (if not physically, then at least conceptually). Therefore I try whenever possible to use overlapping techniques, such as those just described, to help people communicate by using photographs as a focus; this reduces people's fear of being wrong or losing face. Nothing a person says in explaining his or her reasons for choosing a certain photograph and in speculating as to why another person might choose a different one is disputable because it is clearly only their version and is true for them. In this way, projective techniques can be used in family or couples therapy as dialogue starters and values clarifiers, even if the other significant people only "participate" in the client's imagination. Alternatively, if direct confrontation is too risky, a video can be made of each person's session for the other person to view (with permission).

Another layer of complexity can be explored by asking the client to pick three to five images that seem to call or appeal to the person, lay these photos out on the table or floor, and tell a story that connects them together. Begin with "once upon a time" if this helps the person get started. Art therapists might prefer to have the client draw the story and/or collage the snapshots together, perhaps laying the photos on newsprint and drawing in the connecting images. The client may then tell the story to the therapist or let it evolve silently during guided hypnosis or visualization. In group or family counseling, clients can work in pairs. The important thing is that almost always, the story that emerges without prior rehearsal will be synchronistically more significant than would normally be expected from a random spontaneously-initiated tale, as working with visual and metaphoric images can evoke personal and emotional information from the unconscious if the process isn't too self-conscious and thus guarded. The story thus told often produces catharsis in the listener as well, as that person finds personal meaning in it. Finally, if several people are involved, they can hand their own few images to people who have not heard their stories so that those people can make up new stories. When they are compared with the original ones, clients will discover how differently meaning can be constructed from the same visual stimulus.

As mentioned earlier, "snapshots" used as projective tools don't have to be emulsion-covered photographic paper. They can be taken from magazine pages, newspaper clippings, calendars, posters, greeting cards, album covers, or advertising flyers. They can even be blank paper upon which one "sees" the image in one's mind. I have often recommended that therapists ask their photo lab to produce standard-sized 3-by-5-inch or 4-by-6-inch blank prints. They can even be ink-stamped on the back with the manufacturer's mark or date, just like regular photos, if desired. Viewed from the back, such prints would be indistinguishable from any other photos, and they will feel just like other snapshots in the client's hands. I use these blanks one or two at a time, to fill in for missing images that I wish existed in the client's hands at particular moments of discussion.

For example, when a man told me that he no longer had any photographs showing his recently deceased lover in happier moments before he got sick, I grabbed one of these blanks, put it in his hand with the shiny side facing him, and said, "Well, OK, now you have one such snapshot to look at. You're holding it and I can't see it anyway, so I don't have to know it's blank. Pretend it's the missing one, and tell me about it. Talk with it, look at it, and share with me what happens." He stared for a moment, and then an inner picture "came up" on the blank. The client "saw" an image as if it were actually photographically fixed on the paper in his hands. We continued to "work" this image as if it were really there. Because I couldn't see it, he became even more personally invested in it by trying to make it real for me.

I often use imaginary photos in this way, saying something like, "Pretend for a moment that you are looking at a photo inside your mind that I cannot see and tell me more about it". It works. They try to help me see what they are seeing in their "inner eye," and we discuss and explore something that does not exist and yet can stimulate hours of work. Other chapters in this book go into more detail about such applications. For example, one of the brief transcripts accompanying the next chapter describes using a blank piece of cardboard to "stand in" for both real and imagined snapshots interchangeably. It is always the photograph inside the mind that is being worked anyway, even when there is a "real" image in the hand.

For therapists who have clients do visualization work while in hypnosis or deep relaxation, or who work with dream re-creation processes, photographic blanks can be used to fix an image that was encountered inside the mind. While encountering internal images, the client can be asked to remember certain ones by "taking a quick photo of them" inside their minds. Later, they can be asked to recall these inner snapshots and to project them mentally onto the blank "prints," or even to sketch simple representations of them, to "see" them better. Similar image-activating work can be implemented with clients involved in self-healing work through visualization (people with cancer, AIDS, and other serious illnesses) and self-image improvement through mental imaging. Their visualizations can be made more real if they mentally place them on photographic blanks, which can *be* those images for them, even if no one else can see them.

Seeing the actual photograph that a client is viewing is useful in projective work. One woman perceived an image of a twig poking through a snowbank (perhaps 6 inches long in real life) as a sandstone cliff with an old tree growing at its edge (discussed later in Chapter Five). Another never could see the phallic shape in the silhouette of a person's arm and clenched fist that her son thought was obvious (and was giggling about).

Clarifying perceptions through speculations about photographs also can be useful in exploring gender-based issues such as sex-role expectations, family conditioning, tolerance of homosexuality, and so forth. For example, I photographed a man close-dancing in dim light with a partner who has a medium-length ponytail and whose back is to the camera. When most heterosexual clients have viewed this photo, they have usually responded to the image based on their "natural" assumption that the man's partner is female. Such assumptions have not been so quickly forthcoming from my nonheterosexual clients when discussing the photo, and often they have commented on the nonspecificity of the ponytailed partner's gender as something that originally attracted them to the photo.

ILLUSTRATIVE EXAMPLES

The preceding examples have generally illustrated a specific therapeutic topic being discussed. The vignettes that follow have been arranged according to the best structure I could formulate for mapping projective technique possibilities. This framework differentiates among categories of "one person with one image," "one person with several images," "several people with one image," as well as "one person with an image over more than one session." This is not the only framework for examining projective work, but I have found it useful in teaching this technique.

One Person with One Image

Several examples in this chapter have illustrated one person working with one image, so I provide just three brief additional anecdotes here. The transcript at the end of this section, however, deals at length with the exploration of one image by one person over many months.

Asked to select a photo that particularly grabbed her attention, a woman chose the image of a sad baby standing in a crib, holding onto the railing. "This is a photo of my oldest sister," she explained. "Not the baby—the railing! My oldest sister was always there for me, always a stability that I could lean on, hold onto, sometimes just lightly touch when things were becoming a little scary or crazy. I could always let go, and she wouldn't mind, but she'd still be there, solid and dependable, to protect me and hold me up if I became unsteady."

One woman in her mid-fifties chose a photo of a young pregnant woman as her self-portrait, "not literally, because I couldn't have a baby now at my age, but figuratively, because I'm just about to give birth to my thesis. What gift might I give this picture? For some reason my mother just came to mind, I guess because of her strength. She would be able to give me that help which would free me up to have more time to finish it."

A fellow chose a rather abstract photo of a wall completely covered with ivy. The photo was taken close up, so that it simply showed leaves overlapping, all turned toward the source of light, and looking almost like a blanket. "At first I imagined all the leaves as individual pieces laid on a table in straight lines, and wondered how someone could get them done so orderly. Then I also thought of a breeze blowing up and showing their undersides. Then, when I turned it around, upside down, it seemed to become a cover, like a quilt, that someone could hide behind or hide under and see out without others seeing in."

I asked, "Could it be you hiding under there?" and he nodded in silent assent. I asked him, "How old might you be when you're doing that?" "Six or seven," he responded. "I used to hide there because underneath I couldn't hear my parents screaming and I didn't want to tell them to shut up, or they'd just come turn on me instead." From one position, this was only a harmless hedge; from the other, a hiding place for a crouching child.

When I asked his "child" how he was feeling there hiding and crouching, and what he might say if he could speak out, he said, "Diminished, insignificant, unimportant, covering my mouth so I couldn't say anything. The words that come to mind are 'the less I'm seen, the better.'" When I asked the adult man if there was anything he might say now to that child of long ago, he said, "Stay put." Why? "Because as long as no one can see you, you're safe." He added that he could say much more from under the leaves than he ever could if exposed. Later, when exploring his family and his deep love for his protective grandmother, he revealed that it was she who always made his bedquilts.

One Person with Several Images

Some of my images seem to attract more responses than others. Photos 3.7, 3.8, and 3.9 are examples of landscape, still life, and building images that have served in many therapeutic discussions as metaphors for the self.

The triangular rooftop (3.7) has appealed to many people for very different reasons. One woman was at first strongly attracted to a photograph of a round table in front of a window. The table was covered with knickknacks resting on its crocheted cover. She explained her choice: "I would probably like to know the person whose room this was. I can imagine the stories those treasures and trinkets on the table could tell and would love to handle them myself. The darkness around the window probably hid many secrets and you'd have to be patient to really get to know the rest of the room's insides. But if this were my room, I would soon be bored with staying inside. The window draws me to look through it, to see what else is out there, what else might be going on. I'd want to go out there, walk among the trees and flowers, and see what is happening beyond the narrow view the window provides."

For her second image, she chose the triangle roof, as a contrast to the first picture. "I chose it probably because I didn't like it, but the negative feelings were so strong that they also needed to be recognized and honored! I'm bothered by things that block my view, so even though it's a nice old building, and perhaps full of interesting things inside, there's

Photo 3.7

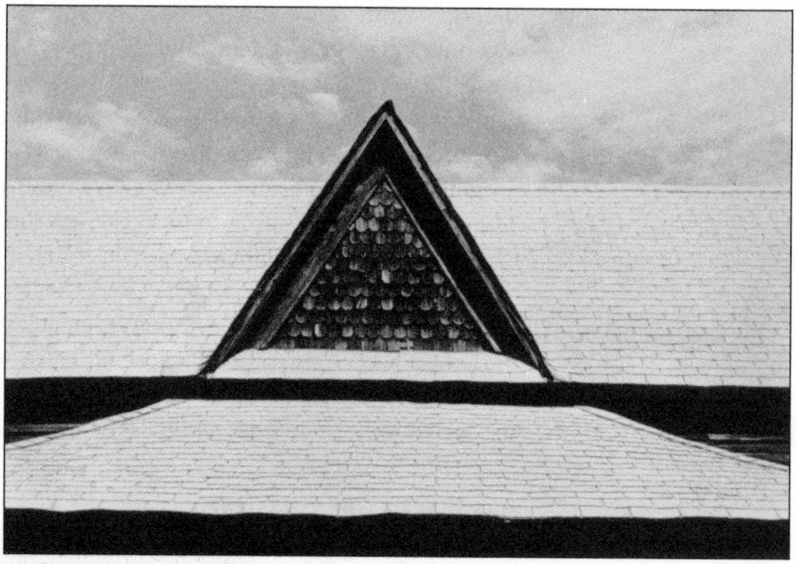

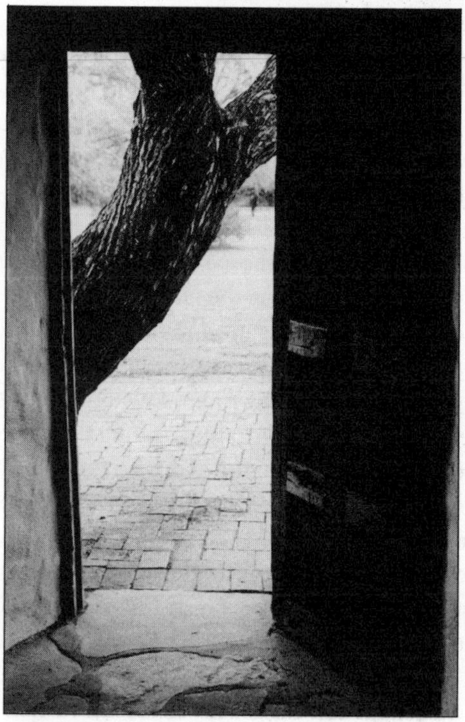

Photo 3.8

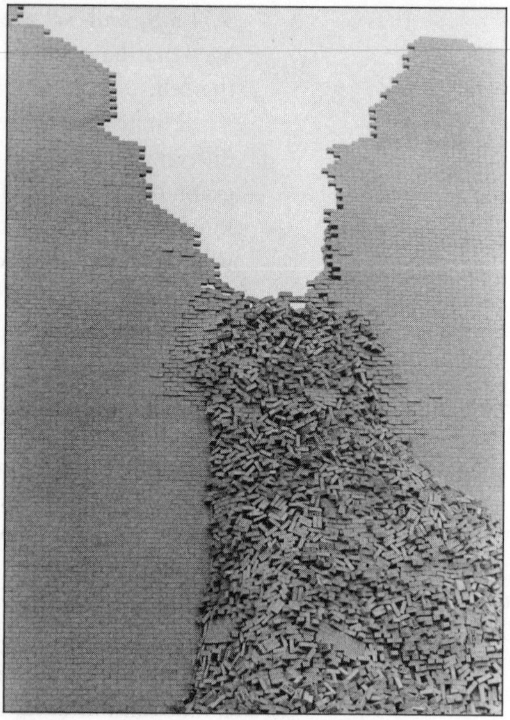

Photo 3.9

no way I can see to be able to get in there. It's a trap. It will never go anywhere, and it obliterates the background. It's just there, blocking out the rest of the sky, and hiding whatever might be behind it. I'd name it "the hanging one." I'd want to get over the top, or around the side, or move it out of my way somehow, so that I could explore all the possibilities beyond it! I really don't like it trying to keep me from seeing what else could be there."

This woman was a therapist. She was always welcoming changes and exploring the full range of possibilities she believed were available to anyone willing to open up to their potential. She was always looking on the bright side of things and finding something of worth in everyone she met, but she was intolerant of blocks to discovery. Her explanations of her responses to the liked and disliked photographs well illustrates these tendencies.

The very same rooftop was selected by another woman because it felt extremely spiritual to her. She said its triangularity signified the Trinity and thus Christianity and God. She commended me on being able to see this and capture its symbolism photographically. Although I was pleased she got such strength from it, I had to honestly share with her that I was not at all religious myself, and being ethnically and culturally Jewish, I would have been extremely surprised to think I might have accidently used this kind of symbolism on purpose, even if only subconsciously!

A third woman found the closed quality of the roof to be very comforting, yet simultaneously almost claustrophobic. She had chosen this rooftop image, along with one of a house interior that reminded her of her grandparents' farmhouse, as the two that most strongly "called" to her. Coincidentally, she mentioned that photo 3.8 (the tree) terrified and threatened her. Her comments, which follow, reveal some of the issues underlying her reactions.

In some of our initial work, this woman had been assigned to bring in some photos of herself as she wanted to be. She told the person helping her that she wanted to be photographed "hiding in the trees"; later she included several such images in a self-portrait collage about the part of her no one knows. These showed her roots being in nature, and her 'tree' of personal growth becoming stronger and fuller. This collage also included several pictures showing only her eyes.

She said that the farmhouse photograph (not shown here) "appealed to me the most because I would explore the second and third storey levels, and because I could run up and hide in the attic and just play. It's a memory of a staircase, childhood play, playing by myself in all of these rooms upstairs—I don't want to be up here long though because it's lonely." When describing her reaction to the rooftop photo (3.7), she explained, "The image that first flashed through my mind when I looked at that was that it was a hiding place [and her voice became very soft and low at this point], and somebody was scrunched in there and was hiding—a person, yeah, a child."

Whereas a man had selected the tree and doorway photo (3.8) as being quite an enjoyable, humorous image because "the tree seemed to be leaning in like a giraffe, playfully peering in, asking to be invited in for dinner," the woman above found it so negative that she could not bear to look at it for more than a few seconds. Where the man saw it as "a surprise, a pleasant surprise! I open the door and here's this tree come to visit me," the woman perceived that image as full of danger. She expressed wanting to be "anywhere but there" and to "escape by any means, including becoming invisible, flying up to the ceiling to remove myself."

She said, "When I saw that photo, I just gasped. The tree felt like it was keeping me in this room. I couldn't get out, and it really frightened me. I couldn't get past it." When I suggested that she might instead think about being outside the door, looking at the image from its other side (as a way to give her some power over its intensity and signal that she did have some choices), she replied that if she were outside, she would wander far enough away that she could see the doorway from a distance, with the tree no longer in front of it, and fully open. But her feelings were still so intense that she was not willing to even physically hold the photograph in her own hands, and in fact she later decided its title should be "The Golem," which she said meant "monster" to her.

Several People with One Image

Elaborating upon the discussion in the first topic (one person with one image) this topic illustrates the wide range of varying responses a single image may evoke in different people at different times. The tree seen through the doorway looked to one man like "my dark side, my fear and my shadow parts. The tree blocks my movement, even after I managed to get the door open after much struggle. It's threatening. It's open, yet still blocked." Yet a different man had a contrasting view of the same photo:

"I like the open quality and the 'through' quality of air going through openness. It's inviting because all that fresh air is coming into the room. At a more symbolic level, it's me going through into my life, going forward, leaving part of my life. I am right now, today, walking out into the world, over the threshold, not knowing where I'm going or where I'll end up. The tree is strong. I think it's an oak tree, and it has two branches. I see myself as two different things, like sometimes serious and other times light and easygoing. Sometimes I forget I'm connected."

One woman could not explain why the photograph appealed to her. Once she began to describe it and what she would do if she were inside that photograph, she recognized previously unrecognized parts of her personality: "If I were in that room, I'd have to duck under the tree to get out. I would go out and then come back in. I could be photographed outside it or inside it, but if I were inside, I'd be wanting to go out into the sun, and if I were outside, I'd go off to the horizon. And then? Then I'd come back into the room again. The most important component of this photograph for me is the doorknob on the door. Without that, I wouldn't want to be in there. I could be in the room with the door closed, but only if I knew there was a knob on the other side, too. If not, no way. But if I were in the room with the door closed, I couldn't see the tree, and I need that tree to be there, even though it's in the way. Actually it looks like a crutch. Is it some kind of excuse? Oh, dear, I've been ducking in and out all my life—relationships, work, commitments. . . ."

A still life of a wall of bricks "frozen" in apparent collapse (3.9) has caught the eye of many viewers for a variety of reasons. For some people it relates to archetypal walls or barriers being broken through to achieve goals, while for others walls are protective defenses against other people or disappointments. Thus walls may be perceived as emotional buffers that may need to be chiseled away or permitted to crumble by themselves so their isolating and disconnecting qualities can be dissolved. The following examples illustrate how diversely one photograph can signal meaning within several different people's perceptual realities.

One man chose the wall as his favorite because "it could also be ice climbing, pure clear air, blue sky, my last ascent before reaching the top of the world, a frozen waterfall to climb, peaks on either side. Perhaps I'll find Shangri-la on the other side, once I get to the top. It's exhilarating, with short breaths but mind clear. I'm almost there. My quest is almost done!" In contrast, another fellow picked this photo "as a story to tell about myself because I have cancer. Although I don't plan to die, it has obviously been on my mind a lot. I used to see death as a wall, a finality, and I couldn't imagine passing through it or going beyond it. But the wall is cracking open and it's like a doorway to all that is beyond. Now I can see beyond it. This wall is my heart. It's opening now, as it cracks in two, letting my inner self come out. It's a window in for other people to finally be able to see me, and a window to let me come out. I'm losing my fear—which kept it all stitched tightly together—and I'm no longer having to control everything permanently in stone. It's suddenly OK now."

I've also heard it described as "a collapse that's in perfect order, like how I'm going to feel when I finally have that nervous breakdown"; "so much time wasted, just like my life—whenever I get something started, it never can get finished"; "a picture of war and all its damage"; "a picture of 'The Awkward Age,' like coming out of my own shy adolescence"; "a detail of the perfect wall being broken down and the possibility of something much more beautiful being built in its place—I would title it 'Rebuilding.'" More recently, there have been many comments relating it to the collapse of the Berlin Wall and the hope this concept conveys. Several people have likened it to computer symbology: "Oops, sorry, systems error. Start again"; "Putting a whole day's work into a word processor and forgetting to save it—look at all those words falling, rushing, spilling out"; and "Oh, no, the power went out and I hadn't saved my term paper."

One woman saw the wall as crumbling: "It fell down by itself. I really think that some big wrecking ball knocked it down from the other side, and I think that probably what is on the other side is expansive, is green, maybe a field, is quite open with lots of space. I'm drawn to the part that's crumbled, falling away. I'm interested in how it happened and what's on the other side." When I asked how that wall might be feeling, she replied, "Impatient, because it wants more knocked down, more faster, like 'get on with it.'" When I asked her what else the wall might say, she continued, "Help me! Push me over!" and when I asked her to name the wall, she said, "The wrecking ball in my life would be anybody who would help me begin to break down my own barriers. It could be my therapist, friends, even myself. The wall itself would be named 'Expectations.'"

When I asked her to "peek around" the back side of the photo, she discovered a path there (which we later metaphorically traveled down), and when I asked her how the bricks felt being part of the still-standing wall, she replied, "Oppressed, squashed, secure yet anxious about becoming one of those already-fallen bricks." When I suggested she try out being one of those types instead, she said, "It means I would be less attached, more on my own, more independent, more self-contained. It was painful pulling away from that wall, where I had my place, but the old patterns are broken now."

One family was having difficulty recognizing their interrelated roles and responsibilities in the events leading up to the emotional breakdown and suicide attempt of the sixteen-year-old son. I wanted them to realize their different understandings and expectations of what their life together should be and how this presented an inconsistent reality and conflicting messages to the boy. I believed that until they could begin to respect each other's positions and share communication, they wouldn't be able to leave their extreme positions and make progress. I asked each of them to write responses to five photos I selected from my collection, and then share these with each other. When it was clear that no one could be wrong (in an absolute sense), they began to acknowledge that each saw the same thing differently and began to explore the feelings underlying their different perceptions, as well as what would have to change for each to perceive what another saw.

As one of the five photos, this one of the brick wall produced a range of perceptions and responses: "Looks like somebody forgot to set the brakes," the father laughed, "It's obviously a brick wall tumbling down, a breaking of a wall, a destruction, possibly an accident—but it's a collapse that's in perfect order somehow, almost looking like it was etched out and looks and feels quite comfortable." The mother saw it as "a high mountain valley of stone, a thin river cutting through and down. If it were to mean a person, then I'd find it sort of vulnerable, a breaking out of something private, not meant to be seen, but sort of an awkward 'oops' feeling of something that wasn't supposed to happen." The daughter said it felt like her "stabbed" ears being subjected to her brother's incessant, loud stereo music, but softly added that "it was *too* quiet when he was away in the hospital." The son, the original focus of the therapy, described the image as "like a wall of frozen anger—and you have to take it apart slowly, brick by brick by brick—starting to trust people again, starting to believe what they say. It's the wall between me and other people, the wall I've built myself, by choice. I was aware I'd put it there, to keep people at a safe distance, and that way nobody could hurt me again 'cause they couldn't get close enough. I wonder how many more bricks there are to go—and how high it really is."

The following final set of comments about the image of the wall of bricks demonstrates how one picture can hold several meanings, without these producing any dissonant push for closure. In this case, a woman had selected the photo as being the one that "called" to her the most. "The bricks could be falling down or being built up. They remind me of change, the constant process of growth, learning, movement, and shaping my life. The lack of stability in a brick wall reminded me that obstacles can be overcome. It also meant that the things I tend to feel secure in, like a house, job, ownership of something, all the things our lives so constantly revolve around, are superficial structures prone to collapsing. This doesn't mean lack of control in my life, just lack of permanence. Life is change and movement for me. Permanence is coping with change, inner strengths, and striving to learn and understand the world around me. On the other side of the wall a living, thriving world exists. I want to be able to see beyond the structures we build around ourselves and allow myself to experience more of my life. To see beyond the wall of our consciousness would enable us to see horizons beyond our immediate selves. We could see an entire universe. For me that is what the brick wall crumbling down meant; seeing beyond the structures we build around ourselves, allowing the light of other experiences to shine through.

"Within the wall I also saw a woman's body, which didn't surprise me, as I have lived happily with a woman for over six years now. During my earlier years, I was afraid of my forming sexual identity and couldn't accept being lesbian. I built my life according to the blueprints of society, a false structure for me, and a painful time. An inner pressure built up until one day my real self just blew a hole in the carefully contrived image I had created. A shaken person emerged from the rubble, but one truer to herself. The photo of the wall spoke clearly to me about this aspect of my life. And if that weren't enough, I looked at the empty space itself for a moment and it became an essence itself; the shape in the wall that the falling bricks had created [was] an outline of southern Africa. This just blew me away, because I had lived in Zimbabwe for two years, and it had an intense impact on my life in changing how I perceived the world and myself. It is quite amazing, especially when you realize that the literal English translation of *Zimbabwe* is 'house of stone'! Wow!!"

In making a self-portrait about a year later, this woman chose to pose herself on some steps, with a sign reading Public Relations on the wall behind her (see photo 3.10). She had not viewed the brick wall photo in many months, but upon viewing her snapshot, I saw a striking

Photo 3.10

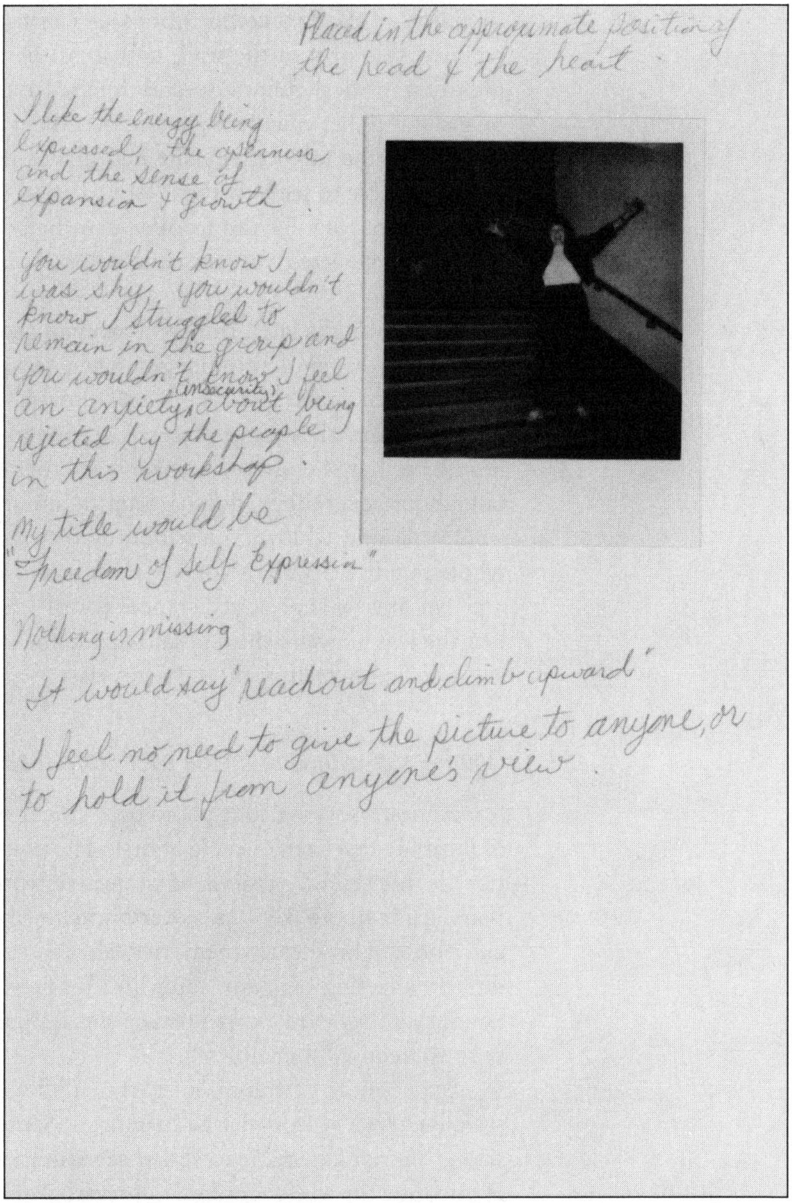

Placed in the approximate position of the head & the heart.

I like the energy being expressed, the openness and the sense of expansion & growth.

You wouldn't know I was shy, you wouldn't know I struggled to remain in the group and you wouldn't know I feel an anxiety (insecurity) about being rejected by the people in this workshop.

My title would be "Freedom of Self Expression"

Nothing is missing

It would say "reach out and climb upward"

I feel no need to give the picture to anyone, or to hold it from anyone's view.

similarity in the two compositions: her arms and legs seemed to me to replicate the form of the wall, and so at the next session I put the wall photo on my desk among several others. Passing by the group of photos on her way to her chair, she glanced over them and grabbed the wall photo to bring to the table where she had placed her self-portrait. She called me to the table to see how they "looked alike" (so my perception was validated without my having to offer it verbally). She said she wasn't sure how they connected but was certain "both photos were saying the same thing!"

Many months later, this same woman again unconsciously returned to wall imagery in describing her sister, "who has cancer and has been battling it for years. Now the X-rays show it's all through her body, riddling her liver, all sorts of places. I've tried to talk with her about it, tell her I care, but she always keeps me at arm's length. She never wants to talk about her feelings, doesn't want to admit she has any. She's a damn solid wall, and I'd love to just put my fist right through it. Actually, my whole family are walls. Nobody talks to me about what they're feeling, and I'm always kept at a distance." Until I repeated her words back to her, she was unaware she had said them, and upon playing the videotape, she watched herself with great surprise.

One Person with One Image over More than One Session

Sometimes, "working" one photo over several sessions can peel back layers of meaning that aren't visible at first. The illustrative example in this section details several sessions of projective work, spaced over nearly two years, using photo 3.8 to uncover buried memories of childhood trauma and abuse. Those early memories, alive in the man's unconscious, were directly affecting his daily adult life. Yet he was initially completely unaware that they even existed (except for a vague feeling that parts of him were somehow "shut down").

Experiences of trauma in early childhood are often absorbed and stored as deep sensory-based memories. Some of these are vaguely conscious but not amenable to verbal searching, while others remain buried at unconscious levels. Trauma in preverbal years can strongly affect people in ways they can feel but find difficult to describe. They know something is bothering them deep inside, but do not know how to open up those secrets. People who are urgently trying to reconnect with memories of early trauma, such as abuse, fear, or extreme anger, so that they can consciously examine them in the hopes of escaping their constraints, often find that they are simply unable to make contact with these things through verbal or inner-thought dialogue.

The layers must be lifted slowly, sometimes over several years, and there are sometimes "slips" that send us back again—usually because we have gone too fast, and the unconscious defends by, for example, "forgetting" the discoveries made at previous sessions. This was the case with the man I will call Matthew, who returned many times to the image of the tree in the doorway, each time almost as if it were new. Although he remembered it as being very powerful for him, he kept having to rediscover its contents' meaning for him. This was useful because not only did he recover information from previous sessions consistently enough that he knew them to be true perceptions for him, but also each reencounter with the photograph permitted new memories and even deeper discoveries to emerge.

Much has been written lately about therapeutic work with clients who experienced childhood abuse. Most of this work has aimed at helping these "victims" become "survivors" through various processes of self-empowerment, self-informing, and redistributing the power balance between the event and the person experiencing that event. The various approaches involve confronting the perpetrator for direct communication of anger, hurt, validation, and/or retribution, or confronting the issues in order to reexperience them cathartically and finally drain off some of their overall control on the person's present life.

Such buried memories inevitably affect a person's emotional expression or experience; they cannot be left unconscious without there being some vague gnawing anxiety that something is wrong, that the person is somehow different from others. Often people who have experienced early abuse cope with it through various dissociative disorders or even multiple personality disorders, and there is a rapidly growing body of psychological literature about consequences of abuse and treatment options that is far beyond the scope of this chapter. In any case, to defuse these feelings, clients must do more than just think about them; they must actually try to re-experience them again, "live," and understand them with the body as well as the brain. The example that follows illustrates how projective

PhotoTherapy techniques helped one person regain unconscious information and begin to heal.*

I conducted a workshop for therapists on PhotoTherapy techniques, attended by a colleague who enjoyed the various experiential exercises and found that he had serendipitously learned a bit about himself in the process. In the first exercise with projectives, the group gathered around a table covered with nearly a hundred of my photos. Each person selected the image that most "called" to him or her.

I then handed out a list of questions for participants to eask each other as, working in pairs, they began to explore each other's inner realities and feelings using projective PhotoTherapy techniques. I had noticed that Matthew and his workshop partner were deeply engrossed in the exercise, and also that after the exercise, he was very quiet and seemingly self-absorbed. Sometime later, he contacted me and said, "You know that picture of yours that I saw last week at the workshop? Well, I can't get it out of my mind, and I want to know if we can set up some time to work on it some more. I think there's something in there that holds some clues about my past that I just haven't been able to find, though I know something's there. Do you think we could get into it that way?" And so began one of the most interesting journeys I have ever undertaken with PhotoTherapy.

When we got together to work with that photograph, I began by asking him to remember what had happened the day of the workshop. I wanted to hear his memories of the image and its impact before handing him the actual photograph (in case there was additional information residing in any dissonance between real and remembered contents). He began, "In the workshop, my first reaction [to the photo] was simply 'I don't like that.' I had a negative reaction to it, but it wasn't all that intense. I was very engaged with looking at it and feeling more and more strongly about how much I disliked it. I found that the door itself seemed to be the focus, rather than the doorway, and my reaction was all to the door itself. The reaction became stronger and stronger. I really hated this photo.

*There are over seven hours of videotaped sessions with "Matthew," spread over two and a half years of reencounters with this one image. The very sparse transcriptions selected for inclusion in this chapter are those most salient for illustrating the points made in context of projective PhotoTherapy work. However, "Matthew" has fully 'released' the remainder of these tapes for viewing by therapists and other mental health professionals or students in training. Arrangements to view them can be made through the PhotoTherapy Centre (on-site only; no duplicate copies available).

I wanted to kick it down—kick through it, get it out of the way. And that had something to do with the difficulty of actually going through the doorway—I would have tremendous difficulty simply walking through that doorway with that whole door there." He said that since the workshop, that photo had stayed in his mind, he had come to believe that there was something about the door that reminded him of his mother, and he could not just bypass the door. ("Bypassing my mother is what I've done all my life—being something that she manipulated, being someone who is afraid to be himself with her.")

When I handed him the photograph, he said it was much as he remembered. "The door itself is still exerting something of a pull, not as strongly this time as before, but—what is it about this door? Something to do with those flagstones [on the ground]. It's almost an image of blood. I guess it's the concrete that's flowing between the large flagstones, so that image of blood is there. [He paused and sighed and then continued.] I don't know what it is. I guess there's an air of menace from that tree outside. It's looming, kind of looming in, or peering into the room. It's really a feeling of being trapped inside this space, of maybe there being more than one thing that's keeping me in there. Not just the door but also the tree—the fear of passing by either one of them. I still don't like it. What can I do with that door? I still have this image of me just putting my foot through it."

I suggested he imagine being in a situation where he could perhaps do that, and he replied, "It's a very strong door. It's not a door that would easily yield to my foot. I think what it would do would be to bang against the wall and then come back and strike me. There's also the sense of imagining myself walking out from this place and seeing this door swing to on me and trap me between the frame and the door." When I probed at a bit more metaphorical level about the fear and who or what it might connect with deep inside him, he said, "There's something there in the sense of perhaps having been afraid all these years of someone who might not respond, might not react, might just be a door." I asked what it might be like for him and the door to have a conversation, if that door could speak, and he replied, "It would whine at me, like creaky old hinges." When encouraged to get into the actual dialogue, he continued in a whiny, voice, "It's a whining, bitching, complaining kind of a door. One that you could never satisfy, no matter what you did. It would whine, 'You don't love me. You never come and see me,' and things like that." He said he felt like he needed at this moment to distance himself from the door, but that was a problem because "I see this as a very small cell rather than as a large room, so I feel backed up against a wall already, with no room to move in relationship to the door, and I'm too close to it. I'm uncomfortable in this relationship with the door. I'm too close. I'd like to get farther away, but I can't within these confines."

I had him change positions by suggesting that he consider the possibility of being the door, and he spoke of the door remembering and feeling the past as a live tree. It felt used and dead now just being a door with no life of its own, something no one takes any notice of, in comparison with the person in the room (himself), who is at least alive and able to go where he wants. He said the door itself would feel stuck, being tied down to one place, and being something it never wanted to be and alien to its basic nature. I found all this material very interesting in terms of his earlier comments about his feeling that the door connected inside him with his relationship with his mother. I wasn't certain where we were heading, but found his tightly focused attention wasn't examining much else in the photo besides that door!

As it happened, he was planning a trip to the country of his birth (and his adoption), and although he wasn't on very good terms with his adoptive mother, he was expecting to go visit her. He was also going to try to find his birth mother and find out more about both her and the reasons he was given up for adoption a week after he was born.

He had mentioned blood on the flagstones earlier and this had piqued my curiosity, so I asked a bit more about this. "It seems to be coming from the door, or behind the door. It's spread out across, underneath the whole of the door, and then it runs away like a river, away from the door and down." I asked if it was flowing toward him or away from him, and he replied, "Away from me. In fact it's sort of across in front of my body." Somewhat surprised by his answer (because I had heard him incorrectly), I slowly repeated in a puzzled tone, "It's a cross in front of your body?" He laughed and corrected me: "Not a cross [making a plus sign with his fingers], but across. I'm standing inside, facing out so [it runs] across my body. My sense is that the door has bled, either in the past or over the years. My suspicion is that it was one occasion where there's been a lot of blood because there's a real sense of flow there—some traumatic experience." We continued along this track, considering what may have happened to the door that it would bleed so much. For a while it was real blood we were discussing and then we shifted to seeing it as a metaphor for a psychological trauma, "an emotional pain, something that happened at some point in time that drained the life blood out of the door—when the door was quite young." At this point, he suddenly grew quieter and seemed almost hypnotized by the photo.

When he became a bit more "present" with me in the room, he said he had experienced, or rather felt he had reexperienced, something very intense, "some experience that happened early on, to me, [because] I can't know about my mother's early traumatic experiences." At that point, he seemed lost again inside himself, mentioned that the tree suddenly was becoming more menacing and there was a sense of something about to come up, "a sense of abuse—a physical abuse here, that's where it's leading." As he proceeded with this journey, I asked him to just throw out any words he could while it was going on and that we would then return to process it after it seemed over (assuring him he was safe to let it unravel inside him).

In summary, what he said happened was that he felt movement, as if he had moved closer to the door, the doorway frame, and the tree, while feeling "I'm the focus of hostility and that sense of physical abuse or some sort of abuse about to happen." It was only then that he noticed the figure in the background, "a very tiny figure walking away, and the sense I got there, [although] I don't know how much of this is just a cognitive rationalization, was of my birth mother walking away and leaving me in the hands of these two strangers that I feel terribly threatened by."

We then spent quite a lot of time discussing what his early years of life were like and what he thought might have happened to instill such fears in him. In the first part of the session he had been responding to the photo and then speaking for various parts of the image. I next asked him to talk *to* it: "If you could tell the door, the tree, or the stones anything, what would you tell them?" After a long pause and a heavy sigh, he said, "I would tell them that I, too, am tired of being trapped in the same place for all these years, but that, unlike them, I am human and I do have the potential to move out."

From this more positive shift, and knowing that the hour was soon to end, I tried some more focused reframing to give him a sense of being able to negotiate this process to a positive end point. He, in turn, discovered that "one thing I would do is thank the door for telling me its perspective, to thank the door for letting me share its views and insight about what it is like to be 'just' a door, and to feel some heart connection with that door that I hadn't had any of before." He expressed sympathy for the door, which he said surprised him, as well as disassociating from the door a bit by telling it that he couldn't set it free and couldn't change it (nor could it change itself, although it could change how it felt about itself).

He then concluded, "I've hugged trees before, but I've never hugged doors before—and I give this door a hug." I asked, "Have you ever wanted to hug the door before?" (speaking on both levels simultaneously), and he responded, "Not this door. Oh, yeah, I've got it now." I asked, "What have you got?" and he said, "You meant, have I ever wanted to hug my mother before? Have I ever had any insight into what it feels like to be her? No [shaking head], no. But even then, I proceed out there, but only as far as the door, but then I still have this tree there, that feels—"

As he seemed lost in thought, I waited a while and then prompted, "The tree there, that feels ____. It says 'I am a tree, and I ____.'" He contributed, "I am a tree, and I don't want to let you out [because] I want to keep you stuck where you are the same way I'm rooted where I am." I prompted, "Because, if you got out, ____," and he said [still speaking for the tree], "If you got out, who would I have to look at? Who would I have to talk to?" When I asked why the tree couldn't talk to the door, he answered, "No. Talk to that dead old thing? No, I don't think the tree and the door talked for years." I then asked how the tree might be feeling, and he replied, "Sad. Sad, sad, sad—for two. Yeah. That lack of communication between the tree and the door hadn't even occurred to me. It hadn't even crossed my mind that the tree might want to speak to the door or the door to the tree. The tree is facing the door, but the door is facing in, away from the street and not looking."

To summarize what I noticed from this session involves detailing a multilayered and multifaceted set of possibilities, in that the door and tree seemed to serve dual, or even triple, roles, often simultaneously. At one level, Matthew and the door interacted from a position of son and adoptive mother, and the original feelings of anger or fear of being trapped seem to be involved in that relationship. At another, especially if using a context from archetypal imagery about lighted openings surrounded by dark walls resembling a cave or womblike area, rivers of blood, being moved forward unwillingly or struggling to emerge from restricted dark places, and so forth, I couldn't help but wonder if we were uncovering some sort of very deep early memory about either his birth process (was it bloody and difficult? unwanted or resisted? traumatic?) or his adoption (was he battered? unloved? abandoned? abused?).

If this session was also about memories of his own birth process, then all his comments about what the door and doorway would do or say become a lot more communicative (wanting to kick through the door and get it out of the way, feeling trapped and being unable to bypass it, having no room to move, being too close to the door and being unable to get further away, blood running across him while he faced the opening blocked by a forked tree, and so on), especially as he connected all these feelings so closely with the idea of "mother," which he assumed to be adoptive mother (but I wasn't so sure).

If instead we were uncovering early abuse, then the same comments were equally important, but from a different perspective altogether. The point is, at this stage of the dialogue, neither of us knew any answers. If the door was his mother, was it too easy to assume the tree was his father? He said at the end of this first session that his early very strong negative reaction was to the door, not so much to the tree; yet earlier he feared the tree's "looming." He said, "The menace of the tree I've seen today, that was really not there, or was below the threshold [when first viewing the photo earlier]. The anger toward the door's gone—there's a sense of empathy, of heart connection with the door, coupled with a sense of sadness. Earlier I didn't understand the nature of the door. I didn't understand its point of view, and I felt threatened, locked in, trapped by it—trapped by my own expectations of how that door would respond—or should." All these layers of meanings were potentially available, and all options had to remain open until the discussion of the imagery developed into a tighter focus. This is the way projective PhotoTherapy works: all the threads of a weaving keep moving along in parallel until the larger pattern begins to emerge.

I asked him what he might say now to the door, and he began, "I'm talking to my mother. The reason that I haven't spent time with you, haven't enjoyed being with you in the past, has been my feeling that you're always trying to push your feelings onto me, to get me to do or be the way you want me to be, rather than the way I really am." I asked what the door has always wanted to tell him that it feels he's never heard, and he said, "That it loves me. That's the message. That it loves me and wants what it sees to be the best for me. And the message back from me is, what you see as being best for me is not usually best for me from my point of view. [I must] be myself, and not pretend to you that I am the person that you want me to be. The door still loves me anyway. And I never understood that. I never understood that she would still love me even if I was, even if I went my own way, even if I insist on being me. I thought that would lead to the loss of her, that she would somehow withdraw, that it was always like a conditional love."

In response to my earlier question about what he might have titled this photo if he could, he now said, "The first title that came to mind was 'Exits.' [But] that didn't really capture my sense of what was going on; what has come up through our talking about this photograph is more than exits. So now the door is benign. The doorway is approachable, but I still have that tree to get past, and that's probably a whole other session on its own. The tree is still looming. The door is no longer threatening. And so the next stage for me is to work with that tree image. But at least I'm now standing in the doorway. It's a real step forward. [But] there's a lot of work left in this one photograph!"

We ended the session with the usual summarizing and reflecting and then discussed some ideas for his upcoming trip abroad to visit his adoptive parents. He mentioned that he felt a more neutral and comfortable relationship with his adoptive father since their lines of communication had improved due to his adoptive mother's no longer being able to do the letter-writing as a result of her several strokes. She was not well, and Matthew expressed regrets that her memory was no longer dependable; thus his chances for gaining additional information about his birth family and early childhood might be slipping away."

I recommended some photo-taking assignments as well as that he copy any family album photos he thought might be significant. I also asked him, if he did find his birth mother, to try to get someone to take a photograph of the two of them together, as well as find out any details available about his actual birth. I had not intruded with my own hunch about the photograph relating to a difficult birth process, because at this point it was truly only a wild guess on my part. If it were true, it would be better if he made the connection between early event and later unconscious perception for himself. I did a final checking in to find out how he felt, and then ended the session; his response assured me it was all right to end: "I feel not bad, sort of warm inside, no anger—[and] a sense of completion up to this point."

Several months later, Matthew rebooked to continue working this image. Since our last session, he had been to visit his adoptive parents. He described his encounter with his adoptive mother: "I had been told that her mind was going, that her memory was going, that she was dementing. So I went back with some trepidation, but when I got there, I found that in fact what was left of her was the good side of her—the warmth and enthusiasm of her life was left, and all the manipulative side of her was gone. And so that made it very easy just to open up to her and deal with her as she is now. And all the other stuff, which began with the first tape we made, had been so well diffused by the work that came before, that I was just able to be with her and enjoy her and she enjoy me for the first time, instead of having to protect myself all the time."

He quite joyously informed me that during that trip he had also found his birth mother, who welcomed his reappearance and shared information as well as good times. "That was exciting. The process of finding her, of looking for her, spending the first ten days of my trip searching for her was frustrating but interesting." They spent a lot of time together, and he was able to find out about his birth: "I found out that she had a terrible time with me. She had toxemia for four months prior to my birth. When I met her this summer and asked her about the circumstances at the birth, she told me she remembered nothing of it; she doesn't remember [because] she was so out of things.

"I went and read the hospital records, and found that I was lying transverse [breech birth], so I had to be rotated, and they used forceps to deliver me. So clearly it was a very difficult birth. My mother was in hospital for a full month after I was born and was still very sick during that time." So Matthew had found out that he was born to a sick mother; his body was manipulated by sharp instruments into a different position for delivery, and then he was grabbed by branched forceps and pulled out. This might well have something to do with the power my photo held for him. Then again, it might not—and although there is no way to know with complete certainty, a perceived reality that makes sense and feels valid for the client can be worked with therapeutically.

Matthew also brought to this session several photographs from his holiday. The compositional qualities of one of these were strikingly similar to the image we'd been working with, though he was not conscious of this when he took the photograph. I know this because he showed me all the photos together, like a pile of souvenirs, and it was only when I paused over the one that caught my attention and asked him about its composition that he suddenly saw the pattern repeated.

That snapshot (3.11) was of a special place where he had enjoyed spending time in his youth and that he had pleasantly anticipated visiting

Photo 3.11 ***(left)***
Photo 3.12 ***(right)***

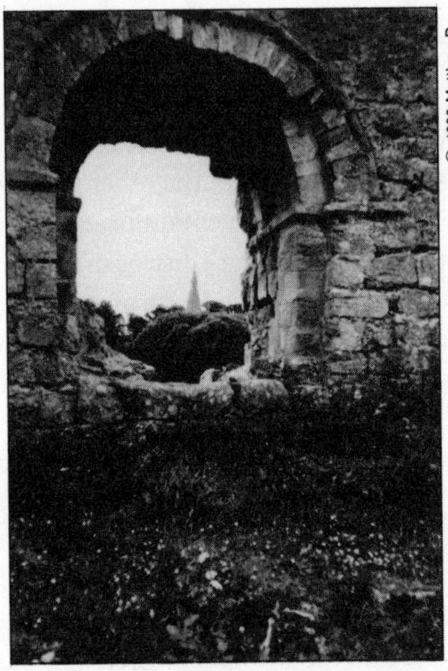

© 1990 Matthew D.

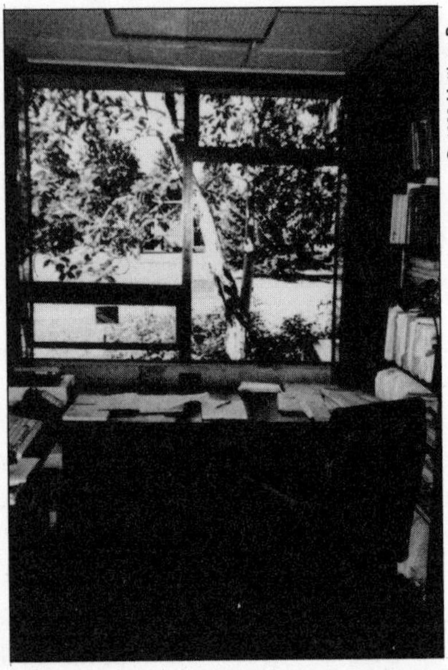

© 1990 Matthew D.

on his trip. "There's an old church close to where I lived as a child and it kept pulling me back to its grounds. I felt very much drawn to the old castle across the road from the church, and so in climbing around the ruins I took this photograph, which shows the spire of the church. I think I spent a fair amount of time composing [the photo], getting what felt like just the right shot so [that] I had the church spire."

I asked him about the amount of forethought he had put into composing the scene because, to me, it strongly repeated elements of the photograph—heavy black, the heavy door and wall, the flagstones leading up, all surrounding the lighter opening. The only difference was that there was no looming tree; there was just the small spire in the background (similar to the distant figure in my photo).

When I presented these perceptions to Matthew, clearly owning them as being only my particular ideas and not absolute truth, he replied, "You know, I hadn't seen that until you saw it. I had not seen the echo of that other photograph until you pointed it out to me." I replied, "But that was *my* perception. Did it fit for *you?*" He responded, "It fitted perfectly for me, once you raised it up to that level for me, but I hadn't seen it before that. I certainly hadn't thought about that when I was framing the photograph. But considering the second photograph I brought, it sure makes sense. The other photo is [even] more evocative of the part of that original photo that I still have work to do on." This second snapshot, photo 3.12, was taken from the doorway of his office toward the window.

"I had one frame of film left and had the camera at work with me and thought I'd just shoot the last one. For some reason I didn't want to go outside to look for a subject. So I thought, well I'll just take it through my office window, because I'd never taken a photo in my office, and I'm leaving the university, so it would in a sense be a way of getting a memento of where I've been. I had a lot of difficulty working in that office. It's never been a comfortable atmosphere for me. It was improved by bringing in plants and putting a rug on the floor, but it always had sort of an oppressive feel to it. When I got the photos back and looked through them, there wasn't a sort of 'aha!' experience, so it's hard to reconstruct just when I realized. I looked through them and put that one aside—and then, I'm not sure whether that was after I'd gotten a copy of the transcript [videotape transcription of our first session], but something twigged about that photograph and I pulled it out again and looked at it, and realized that there was the forked tree through the lit doorway [window opening]. There's something in the configuration of doorway and tree that is particularly powerful in the original photograph I saw at your workshop. I think that the evocative power of that photo is something that comes from intrapsychic causes; that is, *something* happened in childhood [that relates]!"

However, this was not to be the final encounter with my original photo. When Matthew compared his own two snapshots with mine, he again had a strong emotional reaction to viewing it again, particularly in response to the tree trunk: "Now that tree trunk is just looming in at me, coming right in to get me. That's amazing. The door no longer has any power, the door is a door. The power of this picture is really incredible. I didn't think it would have done anything this time, because—I had a good connection with my father this time, so I thought that if this does represent my father, then this picture may be defused, but it's not. That tree trunk is just looming at me [he snarled half jokingly at the photo] Arrgghh!"

However, it has been my experience that such things, at least in PhotoTherapy work, are rarely so simple as to convey a one-to-one correlation, and thus the image could easily still carry additional power and impact for Matthew. He also felt that it still triggered other memories for him, particularly abusive ones such as the possibility of seeing someone being flayed, witnessing someone else's bloody birth, even torture or crucifixion.

"The nasty, gnarly black tree that is looming out at me [reinforces] my suspicion that there's some abuse here. And I have no memory of any abuse in my childhood. But that's the feeling I'm getting around this tree," he sighed deeply.

Matthew remembered his father being rather passive and quiet and though not openly affectionate toward him, still conveying good caring for his son, so he found it difficult to search there for the suspected abuse. Yet he had strong feelings that something nevertheless might have happened, so we scheduled another session to work with my original photo again, and planned to concentrate on the tree trunk specifically. Because he now lived several hours away, it was several months before we met again.

Matthew began our next session by saying, "We ended up the last time with me just about to go out of that door, go past the door in the photo, and confront that tree." Although he feared that in this latest viewing the photo would have lost its power for him, it had not. Even after two years of working with it, the original photo still inspired an uneasiness that he described as "spooky—real scary." He expressed fear and sadness about getting into the image again, as well as worries about unpleasant consequences of finding out what was in there. He said that if the tree "found" him, it would be physically dangerous—as if he were being beaten.

I tried a deeper form of hypnosis with him than I had used before, including some basic age-regression techniques, and had him "be" the child in that room for a while. His reaction was immediate; he emphatically threw the photo down onto the table with such force that it veered off onto the floor. "It's going to hit me," he quickly exclaimed through gritted teeth, "That's what it is, it's going to nail me [and indicated a slapping type blow]." I said simply, "Because?" and he answered that someone was "very angry, very angry with me. I don't know why." He was encountering his self of approximately two years of age, on the floor near a crib in a bare room, "sort of down—like I'm squatting down or being knocked down." When I asked him to describe the hand that was coming toward him, he sighed deeply and perplexedly said, "It's sort of moving backward and forward between being a woman's hand and a man's hand."

We continued this for several minutes, exploring the room and his bodily sensations. As he was unable to identify whose hand it was, I suggested he approach a mirror in that room to see what he looked like and who might be approaching behind him. These explorations located the probable abuse in his baby years, not later, and Matthew continued to express feelings that neither of his parents had hurt him. He also was certain that the hitting was unexpected, happened many times, and that he was fearful because he couldn't connect it with being 'bad' in any way, so it was always without warning and thus irrational. He said later, "That's why it gets in the way of all sorts of things like intimacy—in the way mainly of dealing with other people and their anger, because my child part of me [still] gets frightened and triggered so damn easily that I have great difficulty staying in my adult self and dealing with that angry person as the adult." This connected for him to his fear of being vulnerable or trusting others with his emotions, that getting in touch with real emotions would find him going crazy, as well as his fear of rage or anger in himself or others.

Still in trance but looking now at the photo again, Matthew found it was taking on a three-dimensional quality and beginning to move through the doorway toward him. He grew frightened, and to help him regain some control over it, I asked him to describe in minute detail what he was seeing. After giving specific details about white glistening patches and dark gnarly textures, he added, "For a moment there, there were features of the tree trunk—that reminded me of my paternal grandmother, who was a foul-natured woman. She had so much hatred and anger inside of her—my father said she was just terrible [as a mother to him]. She was very dark-skinned. She looked like a gypsy, very black hair and very piercing eyes, very dark eyes, and tended to wear kind of gypsy-type earrings and scarves. I have the sense of her sort of jangling, so maybe bracelets and bangles. Dark and aging hands, so the skin was starting to wrinkle." I was beginning to have another hunch about these dark, wrinkled, and occasionally sparkling hands, but again did not want to intrude on Matthew's perceptions, so I went at it a bit sideways: "Were they big or small hands?" "They were big." "Were they particularly male or female looking?" (This was what I really wanted to know.) "Really it could have been either. They weren't women's hands, but they were a little on the small side for a man's hands."

As we continued, Matthew described his grandmother further. As he thought of her and her home, he actually, right in front of me, crouched over in a protective manner. He traced this memory to an old horsehair couch in her living room where he feared unpredictable violent action—unexpected and unjustified—inflicted by a hand that was neither totally male nor female, connected in his mind to his father, and yet a woman. And he remained totally powerless in front of that constellation of explosive danger. If the door was his mother, he'd been expecting the tree to turn out to have deeply hidden secrets about the father he knew to be quite gentle, but now he said that the tree had been "a female tree" all along.

Regardless, it still remained in his way, blocking him from emotional freedom, so I proceeded with another hypnotic exercise, having him find a way by himself to neutralize the tree's power over him. He had earlier said he was afraid to kick it down, because that might not work and then the tree would know how much he hated it. Now, within the safe context of our session, he decided to risk going back and reexperiencing the original terror, with all its intensities, to find a path to where that hold on him would be released.

The first step, similar to his becoming the door in the first session, was to have him find, to his surprise, that he had become the tree itself. In searching the tree's life and feelings, he discovered that the tree had grown up bent and gnarled, unbalanced and off-center, because of abuse to it as a young sapling (or baby). "I was twisted out of shape. Grew up full of anger, full of spite, just hating, just really hating." When asked what it was doing there in that doorway, the "tree" replied, "Not much, just standing here, but I can see that my appearance is very frightening to the child inside the doorway, and I take some savage pleasure in that." Why? "Because then I have some power, while I know I really have little power to change things or be different, but I'm capable of scaring this young being."

I then asked the tree why it had so much anger in that relationship with that child, and "it" (Matthew) immediately answered, "Because he's not family. He's not blood. He was adopted; he's an outsider. He doesn't belong." I asked, "Does he know that?" and the tree/grandmother replied, "Not yet, but I'll make sure he does." It/she explained further that a hint or two, dropped just right, would suffice, and that this gave her "a perverse pleasure, [which] seems like the only kind of pleasure I can get. If he found this out, it would hurt him the most, and it also might put a bit of distance between him and his mother." Matthew continued to connect things, explaining that the grandmother and her own son (his adoptive father) had a terrible relationship, and that putting strain on this baby's relationship with her son's wife seemed to please the woman. When asked how her son would feel if he knew she was harming his son, "she" replied, "I'll make sure he never knows. I'll do it when he's not around." And the child would grow up feeling hatred, anger, and fear.

That summary made a lot of sense. Matthew, still deep in trance, was apparently stuck with this new discovery. I wanted to move him into a more active position and into neutralizing her power over him, so I asked what the tree was afraid the child might do in return, once it was grown. "I hadn't thought about him doing anything to me in return" (and the voice seemed genuinely surprised). I added, "He's not going to stay a child forever. He's going to remember the anger. He may not know where it came from, but if he ever figures it out, and you're still around—what would you be afraid would happen?" I wanted him to consider that the old lady's power over him could be stopped as soon as he decided it didn't succeed any more, that he could seize the power back.

He sighed deeply and then, with voice slowly rising, began, "You bitch. You little bitch. This tree is rotten through and through. It's just an outer shell. The inner core is dead and dying, so the least push will send it crashing to the ground. I just have to be careful that I'm not standing underneath it when it falls." He looked at something in front of him, invisible to me, but which was clearly the now life-size tree. "It's starting to fall, and at the same time the image is changing [speaking now in a very thin, shaky, and emotional voice]. The tree, the image of the tree, is now the image of a man coming out of the shards, and he's flying. [Matthew began to sob.] He's taking off!" Matthew removed his glasses, wiped his eyes, continued to cry for a while, blew his nose, put his glasses back on, picked up the photo again, studied it, and then looking at me, said, "Thank you."

I, somewhat transfixed by what just had occurred, asked him if he could fill me in on the details. He said, "In talking through as the tree, realizing that it was an embittered and twisted old tree, the realization came to me that it was a facade that I was seeing, just an outer shell, just a husk was left. The whole inside of the tree was rotten, crumbling, and powerless and dying, and the tree went from looming in to falling back, reeling away, and falling down. All I needed to do, I didn't need the drop-kick; I could just simply push it. Although I didn't say so [out loud], I kicked it, and then realized that I didn't need to kick it; it just needed a gentle push, and that my directing its fall could help insure that I wasn't caught. In my mind's eye I didn't see it actually fall to the ground and disintegrate;

rather it metamorphosed into this figure of an angel, a male figure, with wings coming out of his shoulders, who was taking off, moving away out of that doorway completely. I feel that figure symbolizes myself. Growing, dealing with the past, and being free of these things that do drag me down; the fears of dealing with other people's anger; the fear of dealing with something else that didn't come up before: the fear of being passionate in my life, about my work, my interactions, and commitment, committing myself to any course of action wholeheartedly."

He appeared so refreshed and cleansed that I felt it unnecessary to continue any further deep work at that time, especially as he had brought himself out of his hypnotic state naturally. I headed toward closure of the session, asking him to review and summarize with me what had happened, and he mentioned finding some extra connection in discovering that the two prominent figures throughout this whole process that were most directly connected with unexpressed anger were both female.

He suggested that this might have been part of his difficulty maintaining emotionally intense relationships with women in the past and that it might not be so much of a problem in the future. He might be able to become angry with a person and yet know that they still loved him, even if they were angry in return.

I found this last experience quite different from the door work, in that with the door, I probed for information, while in this session, I simply set the stage and let the material do its own emergent and evocative work. He said he felt quite comfortable ending at that time, and that having knocked down the tree, he no longer felt it necessary to go find the exact abuse. I agreed to stop on the condition that we could always do another session in the future if he wished.

For Matthew, the forked tree trunk blocking a doorway had carried multiple meanings simultaneously: possibly unremembered birth trauma, perhaps later abuse as an infant, and certainly some intense memories of childhood terror, along with symbolic representations of his life being blocked by those restraints (and his acceptance of them). His goal throughout these sessions was to work the image until there was no more psychological tension in it when he looked at it. Using PhotoTherapy techniques as often as I do, it was not surprising that one photograph encountered in a workshop could initiate such powerful and informative results. However, Matthew, who was previously rather skeptical about synchronicity, now enthusiastically uses these techniques in his own work.

SAMPLE EXERCISES

Begin with a large collection of many photographs of all varieties of subject matter and contents. If no real photos are available, create a collection from old magazine pages.

1. Sort the images into groupings that seem to you to go together, while reflecting about how you are making these choices.
2. Find those that evoke the strongest emotions in you or best express how you are feeling today, noting those images that are particularly attractive or repulsive.
3. Find those you would like to keep for yourself or give to someone else as a gift.
4. Find those that most interest you—that most call to you, make you smile, make you want to know more about them—or that you find yourself continually returning to.
5. Find those that repel or frighten you or that you would never tell a secret to.
6. Find those that could serve as metaphorical self-portraits of you, even if the photos are not actually of people at all, that you feel most (or least) represent you, and/or those that might remind someone else of you.
7. If you could travel through time or space and put yourself inside any of these pictures anywhere that you'd like, find the ones you would choose to be in.
8. Try to find those images you think your spouse, lover, mother, father (boss, friend, child, next-door neighbor, or anyone else) might pick in response to any of these questions.
9. Find images that you think any of the persons suggested in question 8 would guess that you would have picked out in answer to those same questions listed above. Consider whether the choices are similar or different from those you selected and explore the possible reasons.

Examine the photo or photos you selected.

1. Consider the thoughts, feelings, memories, and fantasies that you have become aware of, even if they are not expressible in words.

How does each photo make you feel? What do you think about when viewing it?

2. Explore the photo's highlights and shadows, its subject matter and the less obvious background. What is it of, and what is it about? How do you know that from looking at the picture? Are you absolutely certain? If not, what other details might you need to see to be completely sure?
3. What are the most obvious things noticeable in this photo? What parts do you think you may have missed in your first glance that are now emerging to your eyes? What are the obvious and not so obvious, intangible (nonverbal) elements, such as its tone, the relationships expressed within it, feelings conveyed from it (and to what degree), any noticeable symbols, apparent metaphors, and the like? Turn it around, get close, and step back from it to see it from other perspectives and notice if anything else becomes evident. What, if anything, seems to be missing? If anything is, what would be needed to make it more complete?
4. Ask the photo its name, its identity, what it means, and whether it has anything to tell you, any message for you. How well does it know you? Are there any other questions you would like to ask it? If you did ask, what might that reply be? How would that feel? What question would the photo like to ask you if it could? Who or what does it remind you of?
5. Is there anyone you know of who would like to have this photo? Why? Would you like to give this photo to anyone? (If you did, what do you think or hope they'd interpret this gesture to mean?) Is there anyone who you definitely wouldn't or couldn't give it to? If so, who? And why wouldn't or couldn't you?
6. Try to title or name the photo. See if it seems to belong with any others in the original collection, in a group or collage? (Does it miss any other photos that should be accompanying it?) Does it have a sound, a movement, a color, a pose, a feeling, or a secret to share with you?
7. Try mentally pulling and stretching the edges of the photo outward/upward/downward, exposing more than was originally in the image. What else is brought to light that was left out of the original image? How does this additional visual field affect the contents of the image, its meaning, its feelings? If you were to make

the photo smaller by removing part of it, where would you choose to focus it down to (and why)?

8. Try stepping into that photograph, to become part of it. Where would you go in it? What would you do there? What else might you then be able to see, do, know about, or feel? From in there, imagine yourself turning now to face the camera. What can you see of the photographer (who is that person, why is this photo being taken, and so forth)? What can you see of the scene the photographer is participating in?
9. If you could time-travel to be in this photo, where would you go? What would it be like to actually do that? (What might be your perceptions and thoughts and feelings?) Would you like it there? Would you stay there? Would you want to stay?
10. If you could change anything about the photo, what might that be? How would that alter things? What about changing something in the original scene itself? What do you think would happen then, and would there still be a photograph worth taking?
11. Pretend that you *are* the photo (or particular parts of it). Try imagining how it feels to be that photo (or part of it) and then try acting, feeling, and talking as if you were actually it. Speak with "I" statements about the whole photo, its various parts and/or the relationships expressed within it, such as, "I am the tree (the chair, the child, the sidewalk), and I am thinking ____, seeing ____, feeling ____, imagining ____, remembering ____," and so forth. What do you think that photo (or part of that photo) would say if it could speak, hear if it could listen, see if it could look, feel if it could sense? Who would it like to have with it for company? Where might it go; what might it do next; what might it dream or want? Experience being that photograph or a part of it, and explore these things.
12. What kind of relationship do you think the photographer had with the subject of the photo? Why do you think the photographer took this photo in this way, at this time? Would you have taken it? Why or why not?
13. How does what you noticed in the photo fit for yourself? Is it like your own life in some way? If so, how? If it reminds you of something or someone, what is the connection or association about?
14. As you think over your answers, consider both what you knew and

how you knew it. Why did each answer come to mind at this particular time? What in the photo—what visual data or clues—did you base your answer on? *How* would the image have to change for you to have a different feeling or thought? How might your answer be different at some other time?

If the photo in front of you is of a person:

1. Who do you think this is a photograph of (who is this person)? What does he or she do? Where does this person live? Does the person remind you of anyone you know? If so, who, and what kinds of memories are recalled?
2. Do you think this person is happy? sad? bored? anxious? proud? shy? fearful? friendly? hard to get to know? possibly abused? nice? homosexual? an orphan? a cat lover? perhaps depressed? generous? dangerous? alcoholic? trustworthy? unstable? deaf? a musician? a teacher? a politician? a therapist? a truck driver? a grocer? illiterate? How can you tell?
3. Tell some of this person's story. How might you title it? What is the person's past, present, or future like? Does the person have friends? What is the person's family like? What are the person's parents like? If the person were to give you a gift or tell you a secret, what might that be?
4. What is going on in the photograph? What has happened in the person's life that has brought her or him to this very moment of being photographed? Where was the person when it was taken, and what was he or she doing right then? How was the person feeling at the time the photo was taken? What happened just before or after the shutter was snapped? Where might the person have been going? Would you go with him or her (and if so, what would happen)? Where and who is this person now?
5. Could this person be having the same sorts of problems (dreams? experiences? feelings?) as you are today? Did she or he have the same kind of childhood as you, or the same sorts of family difficulties you experienced? How can you tell these things? How does the photo communicate this information to you?
6. What does this person's background seem to be like? What do you think is his or her cultural, ethnic, or racial group? What do you

think her or his religion, family values or traditions might be? Is this person heterosexual or not? What is this person's home environment like? Imagine what his or her neighborhood, work, job, interests, or hobbies might be like. What do you think is his or her favorite food or movie? Does this person have pets? What does this person like to do for leisure activities?

7. Why might the photographer have wanted to take a picture of this person in this place? Did this person know the photographer? Was the person aware that the photographer took this picture? Was that all right with him or her or would the person have preferred not to be photographed? What does she or he think of this picture? What would he or she change in it if it could be changed? Who might the person want to give it to? How do you know these answers?
8. Would this person have let you take this photo? Would you have wanted to? If you did, how might you do it differently? Would you let this person photograph you? If so, on what conditions?
9. Imagine that the person in this photograph is now looking at you and then speaking to you. If this photo could speak, what do you think it would say? What is the message that you think might be behind the words? What might your dialogue be like? What does this person see when looking at you? What might that person say to you, remind you about, say about his or her feelings? What questions might this person want to ask you, or what secrets about yourself might he or she want you to reveal? What questions would you want to ask her or him (and if you got back the answers, what might they be?).
10. If you could climb into this photograph to be with this person, how would you pose the two of you together?
11. Which of the other photos does this one seem to fit with or belong with? Try placing it next to these and imagine a story that connects them. Imagine a dialogue between the two (or more) photos. What might they discuss, share, argue about, or need to ask each other? What could they tell each other about you and your life?
12. Pretend that you could cut this person out of the photograph and place him or her on another background (either inside your mind or within another photograph). What would this new context be like for the person? How might it change your reaction to him or her?

If the photo in front of you is of a place:

1. When you look at this photo, what thoughts, memories, or feelings come to mind? Does this place interest you, make you feel uncomfortable? safe? happy? threatened? worried? excited? or any other feelings?
2. What kind of place is this, and what does this photo seem to be about? What was going on there, and why might the photographer have wanted to take (and keep) a picture of this place? Where is it, and what else is nearby? What sorts of things happen here? What will occur there after the photographer has finished?
3. Would you *want* to be there or live there? Why or why not? If so, would you want to live there yourself? If so, would you prefer to be there alone or with someone else (and under what conditions)? If not, what would have to change for you to want to go there?
4. Does this place remind you of anywhere you have been before? Does it remind you of a place someone told you about? Does it match fantasy places you've imagined? Why do you think these connections come to mind?
5. Are there any people who belong here? Who are they, and what might they be like? Would you want to know them? Why or why not? Where were they while the photo was being taken (and what were they doing at that time)? What would they think if they found out that someone photographed "their" place while they weren't there? Would they want a copy of the photo? Why or why not? Can you describe a conversation you might have with them, and what they might tell you about this place and what it is for them?
6. Think of people you know and consider whether they would like this place or being there, either alone or with you. Who would and who wouldn't, and why might that be?
7. Could you have taken this photo? Would you? If so, what would you have wanted to capture? If you had taken this photo, what might you do with it, and who might you give it to?
8. If this place (or parts of it) could speak to you, what do you think it would say? What might it remember? What is the message that you think might be behind its words? What would you reply? What secret might it share with you? If you could ask this place a question, and then get the answer back, what might that be like?

9. Try to become the place (or its parts) or the photo of it for a moment, and speak as if you are it. How are you feeling? What are you hearing, seeing, touching, smelling, thinking about, hoping for, dreaming about, wanting to say, remembering, or perhaps wanting to tell the photographer?
10. If you were able to put yourself anywhere you'd like inside the image itself, where would you be? If you were there right now, would you want to share that moment with someone else? If so, whom would you like to be there with you, and why? Could this place be yours (would you want it to be)? If not, what would have to change to make it yours if you'd want?
11. Which of the people photos does this one seem to fit best with or belong with? Try placing it next to these and imagine a story that connects them. Imagine a dialogue between the two (or more) photos; what might this be like? What might they discuss, share, argue about, or need to ask each other? What could they tell each other about you and your life?

If the photo in front of you is of an abstract image:

1. Did this photo call to you visually, or was your response more from your body or your feelings? What was this visceral response, and how does this photo make you feel? What is different about the photographic choices your eye is drawn to from those your body or feelings selected? Why might that be?
2. What sorts of other images, or people or places you've known, come to mind when you view this? What thoughts, ideas, or memories does it evoke?
3. Turn the photo around several times and explore whether this difference in perspective brings forth any change in the thoughts, feelings, memories, and so forth, that it has stirred in you. Move away from it and then closer in to view it in detail; do these differences change how the image feels or communicates?
4. What do you think is the real subject matter of this photo? What is it of, and what is it about? Where is it? What is its size or scale? Are you sure? If not, what else might you need to know to be sure?
5. What would you title this photo? Try speaking for it, or express how it feels by posing, dancing, or moving as it would or should

if it could. Consider how it might smell, taste, sound. What are its colors? textures? What else is beyond its borders?

6. If you were able to put yourself inside the image, where would you go? How would it feel? What would be your perceptions, thoughts, feelings, and perhaps memories?
7. If you could speak with this image, what might it say and what might you say back? What is the message that you think might be behind these words? Would you want to ask it any questions, and if so, what? If it were to give you a gift or tell you a secret, what might that be?
8. Which of the other places or people photos does this one seem to fit with or belong with? Try placing it next to these and imagine a story that connects them. Imagine a dialogue between two or more of the photos; what might this be like? What might they discuss, share, argue about, or need to ask each other? What could they tell each other about you and your life?

If time is too short for lengthy explorations, try the following quick version of the exercises.

Pick one photograph that really catches your attention, that you are strongly drawn to, or that inexplicably just seems to "call your name." Place it in front of you and consider, both for the photograph as a whole, and for each individual part of it (person, object, place, and so forth) the answers to the following questions:

1. What is the story that goes with this photo?
2. Has the photo a name? If so, what would its name be, and why? What about a title? Why would this be its title?
3. Has it a 'home'? If so, where, and what would that home be like? Why?
4. Has it a question to ask? If so, what question, to whom, and why? What would happen if it asked that question? Is the question to you? What might the answer be? What would happen if the answer were given? Is there a question you would like to ask it, and if so, what and why?
5. Has it a message to give? If so, what message, to whom, and why? What effect would that message have, and would it be truly understood? Is there a message you would like to tell it, and if so, what and why?

6. Has it a need to express or a hurt to share? If so, what need or hurt, to whom, and why? What would happen if it risked doing this? How would this feel? Do you need something from this photo or perceive a pain? If so, what and why?
7. Has it a wish to make or a gift to give? If so, what wish or gift? Who would this be made to, and why? What would happen if this wish were actually granted or gift actually given? Do you have a wish for it?
8. Has it a hope or dream? If so, what is this and what would happen if these were fulfilled? Is there anything the photo is hoping you don't tell or ask it? What might that be? What would happen if you did?
9. Is there anything you need to find out from this photo or that you hope it doesn't tell or ask you? What might that be? What would happen if it were expressed? Is there anything the photo needs to find out from you? What and why?

If, in any of these exercises you are using the same image as another person has chosen, it could be very useful to compare answers to find out how differently one snapshot can affect individuals. Try to examine those differences without worrying about being "right" or "wrong" (or getting trapped by esthetics) and talk with each other about why you might have had such differing perceptions and what your responses say about each of you.

4 Working with Self-Portraits

Understanding the Images Clients Make of Themselves

The clown paints on a new face and suddenly those watching find themselves in disbelief, suspended between knowing what they have just observed and the fact that this magical character standing in front of them has quickly become a different entity from the person who had just moments before been maskless.

The mask takes on its own identity, talks for itself, and covers up the "real" person underneath it. Sometimes there are so many different masks available for use that we grow confused about which one to choose to put on. Sometimes they are so convincing that they even can mask us from ourselves. Occasionally we look in the mirror only to find one of our many masks instead of ourselves. Sometimes we cannot locate the key to unlock their hold on us and despair of ever being able to find our true self again (or worse, we don't recognize it when we do manage to uncover it).

For many clients, getting to know themselves better is often a major presenting goal for therapy. This is often joined with the desire to clarify the separation between who they are individually and who they are in their many relationships with others in their lives. There may be dissonance between what they want to do or be and what other people are demanding or expecting of them. Thus they want and need to improve their understanding of themselves, and increase their awareness of all the underlying and unconscious factors that bind them to others. I have found that most of my clients' difficulties seem to lie in areas where their self-knowledge is weak, confused, distorted, outdated, or simply unexplored, and thus they find it hard to know just who they really are and what they really feel or want.

As a result, working with them to help enhance and enlarge their abilities to perceive and recognize themselves becomes foregrounded for me as a therapeutic goal. I believe that increasing their understanding of who they are and how they came to be is an extremely important part of our work. Therefore I design a lot of my interventions to activate self-esteem, self-confidence, and self-acceptance and to help clients find the boundaries between themselves and others (not to perceive these as barriers but to clarify their effects so that choices open up).

I believe that as clients get to know themselves better, they can become more assertive and confident about making their own decisions and less emotionally reactive to the whims and expectations of others. If they know better who they are, they won't be as dependent on others for self-definition. They won't need others' approval or validation in order to be who they wish to be and can risk exploring life more fully. If their self-image strengthens, there will be less dissonance between how others see them and how they view themselves. If people have to wear fewer masks in order to relate to other people, then their own faces are freer for not having to grow into them. If people's self-representation to others isn't so cognitively controlled, then they are freer to act spontaneously and unconditionally.

How we see ourselves is how we define ourselves; how we choose to represent our identity is how we hope it will be known by others. Basically, how we *believe* ourselves to be is the only reality we can truly operate from, because our perceptual filters, values, expectations, and so forth, get in the way of our ever objectively observing ourselves just as much as they prevent us from doing this with other people. In this sense, beauty (or any other attribute) is not just in the eye of the beholder but also in the mind of the beheld. People may present different opinions in giving us feedback, but we will not internalize these as being true unless they resonate with our own internalized picture of ourselves.

Similarly, when people expect us to do new things, especially things we are certain we cannot do, we encounter not only their expectations as potentially limiting factors because we view them as unrealistic, but just as often we run into our own assumptions about our abilities and limitations. It is very difficult to do what you don't think is possible or what you truly believe yourself incapable of doing. Yet therapy is based on the premise that people can indeed change or grow in ways that they themselves may not believe possible or have failed at before. One of the most difficult tasks for a therapist is to let clients discover for themselves their own abilities to grow and change, because if we take on the role of enabler or animator, there will always be the component of dependence on us as the ones who "made it happen." If we are integrally attached to a client's process of self-discovery, then that client has not learned that he or she can do the process even when we are not around.

Therapeutic movement can begin with a client's simple shift from "I can't" to "I can; it's just that I won't." This is a shift from giving others the power to define and limit the self to recognizing the choices in life. In such ways it becomes clearer how self-concept and self-awareness are at the heart of much individuation and differentiation work.

Most therapists work from the proposition that in order to change, a person must first be able to cognitively conceive of him- or herself as a distinct individual and reflect on the consequences—for that person and for others—of any changes being contemplated. For any therapist for whom the client's perception and awareness of self is central, PhotoTherapy techniques that permit clients to get better internal and mental pictures of themselves can greatly enhance their potential and process of self-knowing. Self-portrait images give clients a means of symbolizing themselves to themselves in their own privately coded language and of seeing themselves from an external position much as another would see them. Self-portraits provide external representations of inner symbolization of self that can be held, visually examined, and used to bridge into others' knowledge about oneself. For clients to be able to examine their images at their own pace and probe them with questions (even if silent ones) allows for reflective self-observation that no input from another person can match.

Visual information about the self that has not been filtered by others is difficult to ascribe to them. Negative information about oneself that is obtained through self-perception is more likely to be accepted as true and internalized. Positive information obtained in the same way can hardly be disputed either, for many of the same reasons. If self sees self in positive self-regard, and no one else has been there to interfere, it is possible that such revised self-perception may well pass through the barriers of defenses and rationalizations that usually block such information. Self-confrontation that produces positive reactions can strengthen self-esteem in ways no other process can. As with photos described earlier, it is not the appearance of the self-portrait that is so important, but rather the meaning of that appearance to the creator, subject, and viewer of the image—in this case all the same person. Therapy with self-portrait images is based on what the client thinks of him- or herself as presented in the photo, regardless of the image's effects on others.

For example, if a client brought you photo 4.1 in response to a self-portrait assignment and you had to therapeutically "work" the image with him, you would first encounter your own reactions to it, how it makes sense to you, how it makes you feel, and what you think was happening for the client for him to have chosen to pose this way. Then you would have to put your ideas aside to also explore how the image made sense to him, both during the photo-taking process and upon later reflection.

The surface contents of the photograph are only our beginning point, and our immediate assumptions about it are often incorrect because they are based more on our own reactions than the client's intentions. We cannot

Photo 4.1

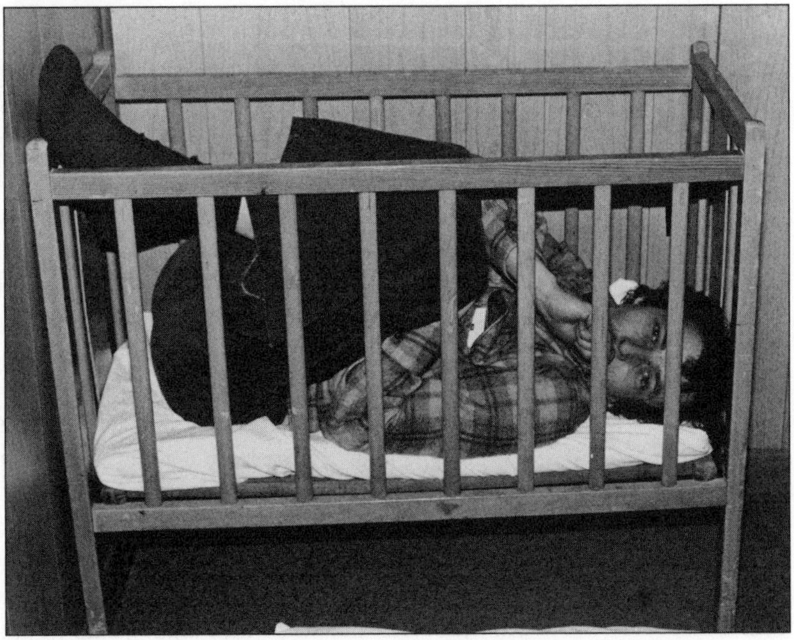

objectively decode this image to find the intentions and communications consciously and unconsciously embedded in it. We must involve the person who appears in it, who took it, who is looking at it now, and so forth. Interpreting snapshots is always a collaborative effort between the therapist and client; there is no way to look at this or any photo and know definitively what it is about. Keeping in mind the list of questions recommended in the preceding chapter for using photos as projective stimuli, readers might want to consider what questions would be helpful in "working" this self-portrait with the client.

Disempowered people are those whose voices have been silenced and whose existence is given little recognition, even in silence. As they have had no influence on how the world runs, they are seen to make no difference in society, and thus are not seen to be there. The consequences of this are central issues, though often unconscious ones, for marginalized or devalued individuals, and they frequently prompt people to seek therapists for help in taking more charge of their lives.

This can be true for races, for cultures, and for groups based on disability, gender, or economic status, but it can also be true inside the minisociety of a family, where "emotional orphans" live side by side with other family members who knowingly or unknowingly oppress them, usually while they are children. Often the consequences are that not only have their voice and feelings become silenced, but they often no longer recognize that they have a voice at all (or have the right to have it back). PhotoTherapy techniques, especially those involving self-portrait work, have proven to be powerful adjuncts to therapy with abuse survivors and other societal "victims," precisely because these techniques depend on nonverbal information, which the words of others (or even the self) cannot devalue or disempower.

There is no doubt that seeing photographs of oneself taken *by* oneself, without contributions from any other person, cannot help but document the identity of that self. When such images show change, they help the person pictured perceive and accept responsibility for that change. The "proof" is in the image and is thus less arguable and more impervious to outside criticism. Making self-portraits (even if only in imagination) is the first stage; therapeutically "working" them is the necessary second one that allows clients to better integrate and synthesize the picture of who they are and what they want to do about it.

HOW THIS TECHNIQUE WORKS

Pretend for a moment that you have won a free portrait sitting at the best place in town. You may pose as you wish, with whomever or whatever you want, including pets, as your props. The picture can be taken anywhere you wish, and you may order any clothing, adornments, and assistance in your visual preparation (such as hair stylists) that you might feel you require. You may even be nude if you choose to. It is your picture, and the photographer will follow your instructions. This will be a self-portrait in the ultimate sense, as you get to do this repeatedly until you get exactly the photograph that you want. Picture this perfect photo portrait of yourself in your mind; get it very clearly arranged, and examine it thoroughly for its messages and secrets (that no one else need ever know). Once you have done this as fully as you desire and achieved the ideal you for yourself, the next step in this fantasy exercise is to give this very special portrait to your father or mother (or employer, or ex-spouse, or . . .).

Did your image change once you found out you had to give your special portrait to that person? What sorts of revisions, limitations, censorship, protections, and so forth suddenly got imposed? If it didn't make any difference, then I would risk a guess that you and the imagined recipient are in a fairly comfortable and unconditional relationship. If you are resistant to showing that recipient what you really are like when you are being who you want to be, it is likely that you would feel hesitant or even threatened to give that person your freely created image. If you repeated this exercise knowing that you were to end up giving away your portrait to that person, what kind of a picture of yourself would you create? Is it different?

This is what "working" self-portraits can lead to: not only the physical/visual elements of self-presentation, but also those more unconscious, nonverbal, subtle and psychologically loaded facets of self-communication that ride along with these images of ourselves. And, as readers who participated in this fantasy discovered, it hardly matters whether or not the self-portrait actually exists!

As the fantasy exercise illustrates, there is more to self-portrait PhotoTherapy than the images. Among the important elements are what is going on inside clients' minds and feelings when they are planning such snapshots; how they think about what they have been "assigned" to take, make, or find; and the entire constellation of both cognitive and emotional processes that take place around their encounter with the idea and the task.

Photos of the client taken by others may well suffice as stand-in's for self-portraits as long as the client feels they are truly representative. However, usually the influence and selective needs or expectations of the photographer get in the way, especially if such snapshots are posed rather than candid. Photos that we have posed for may be more acceptable as realistic than candid ones, as we believe that by constructing our pose we have somehow contributed more of ourselves. Candid shots that catch us unaware, and thus more naturally, often end up being less resonant with our inner picture of ourselves, so we may reject them as being only someone else's accident. If actual self-portraits are unavailable or insufficient for therapeutic purposes, then these other kinds may of course be substituted, but their inherent limitations, plus the photographer's agenda, must be recognized and considered.

In self-portrait PhotoTherapy I may initially use as our focus something as simple as a client's photo identification picture on a driver's license, security pass, or student library card, and have the client tell me her or his reactions to it. We may discuss more metaphorical self-portraits or photo-album images, or I may ask the client to proceed through structured assignments and exercises whose components are specifically focused for definite reasons, based on what I hope to precipitate in the encounter with the photo.

Very often these later kinds of self-portrait artifacts are created during the session with a Polaroid camera. Some therapists even provide a room where clients may try on clothes, masks, makeup, body paint, and so forth, in private, taking photos on their own by using a self-timer or cable release mechanism. (I do not have such a room, but it would be wonderful.) Whether the client does the self-portrait work during our session, or before or after it, or whether I lend a client one of my simple office cameras all depends on the client's particular needs and situation.

Like all other photographs brought from home or created in the therapist's office, self-portraits are original photographs and should remain undamaged, but all extra copies may be useful for various reworkings. Photographic copies can be made by most commercial labs, but photocopying machines are much cheaper and usually easier. With them clients can enlarge, reduce, crop, and build collages. It doesn't matter whether the copies are in color or black and white. The self-portrait can be reworked as many times as the client wishes to make changes to it. Copies of self-portraits can be attached to cardboard or paper and a variety of art materials can be used to detail or enhance them.

Ideas for combinations with various art therapy media were presented elsewhere, so I will not repeat them. Readers will note that many of the creations made by PhotoTherapy clients and workshop participants shown throughout this book are enhanced with art materials and thus have import from art therapy debriefing perspectives as well.

Self-initiated Self-Portraits

I recently received a snapshot from a childhood friend I had not seen in over twenty years. She looked nice and was being lovingly hugged by her husband and children. It seemed an ideal family portrait, and I quite liked it. However, she wrote on the accompanying card, "I hate this picture because I am still too fat." I honestly had not noticed her figure. It wasn't part of the criteria I was using to evaluate how she appeared to be doing, who she had become as the years had passed, what her life seemed to be, or whether her friendly, enthusiastic self that I remembered from high school was still alive twenty-four years later. Her spontaneous, self-critical comment signaled an apology for her appearance and reminded me how often we measure ourselves by an internal standard. We condition our own acceptability to ourselves on that standard and assume that everyone else uses it too when deciding whether or not we are worth knowing: "I won't be acceptable *until* I lose more weight"; "I am not OK *because* my body is too heavy."

However, had my friend been my client, I could have asked a number of questions about that snapshot that would have precipitated deeper therapeutic discussion, such as, "Who is this person when not being part of this photograph?" "If this picture were sent to strangers, what might they be able to learn about that person from it?" "What will be different about this person's picture in a month, a year, ten years, or forty years, and how would that change the meaning of the photo or your answers to these questions?" "Who might the person in this photo want to give this picture to?" "What would that person in the photo like to change about the picture?" "Does this picture remind you of someone?" "If so, who and why?" These kinds of questions may be asked about any photograph a client offers for discussion, even those made long before therapy began. It is not the questions or the image itself that are important, but rather the process initiated inside the client's mind and feelings, and what the image means to the client.

I would ask any of these or other questions from a two-part, and often interchangeable, framework. One viewpoint would be more from an "outside, looking in" position, as if the client and I were jointly observing a photograph of a third person, and the other from the closer level of asking the client directly about him- or herself. This would be the difference between asking, "What does the person in the photo like about the picture?" or "What would the person in the photo like to change about the picture?" and asking the client what he or she personally likes or would wish to change in themselves. Frequently, the answers from the two viewpoints are radically different, and this can be therapeutically useful in establishing personal perceptual boundaries, enhancing self-reflective explorations, and helping with separation between the client's and others' expectations of themselves.

People generally understand the power of self-portraits to ground us in more realistic perspectives on ourselves. For example, dieters often place photographs of their past thinner selves on refrigerator doors to remind them of their goal—and of its achievability. One woman told me, "I am an alcoholic, and I have four pictures of myself that remind me of how I was when I was drinking. I keep those four photos in my wallet all the time for my own special reasons." Another client once told me that on business trips he carried photographs of himself with his children as reminders of why he was working so hard. He didn't choose photos of the children alone, but rather pictures of him playing with them, as it was his own involved commitment that the images signaled to him, along with the children's identities.

One client brought in his self-posed holiday photos of himself. I noticed that in several he was standing in front of directional markers and road signs, some appearing to be growing out of the top of his head, and so I gently asked him if there might be some sense to be made of this repeated imagery. At first he joked about how often this accidental theme appeared. Then he paused to stare seriously at one "?" sign (indicating a nearby tourist information center) and commented with unexpected insight that suddenly this made sense. He had taken the vacation after quitting his job, and now at age fifty he was trying to decide what to do next. The "accidental" poses showed what may have been unconsciously affecting his choices of self-imaging.

To start clients in self-portrait work you may want to ask how well photographs of them by other people have represented their real selves. Are there things people seem to never really get right? Are there things that seem to always be in these kinds of photos that the client wishes were different? And are there absent components or qualities that they wish would someday finally manage to be captured and seen? Asking clients about such things in photos they already have of themselves can often yield important clues about how they see, or wish to see, themselves in external representation of what they already know to be their inner identity.

If you then ask them to consider helping these changes along by taking the photo themselves, or allowing someone to push the shutter when they are ready, they may be willing to give it a try, especially when they know that there is no wrong way to create the image and thus no way they can fail in attempting to create it.

From this position, self-portrait exercises can actually be a great deal of fun, and if the client is at all hesitant, the therapist can model the freedom and flexibility offered by doing some self pictures first. If the client gets to observe the therapist planning, creating, and then viewing a self-portrait, this can serve as a good model of how expectations and reality can sometimes be surprisingly different, and that this is all right. The client can even be asked to look at the self-portrait of the therapist or of themselves, pretend for a moment that to be the therapist of the person in the photo, and imagine what questions they might want to ask "their" client.

Most self-portrait PhotoTherapy techniques involve (1) discussing and exploring what happens when clients plan and then pose for snapshots of themselves and (2) further interactive debriefing of the image that was created. Sometimes the "heaviest" therapy may take place in the earliest stages of thinking about what the photograph might look like, or would need to look like, if it were to really be made. Sometimes these imagined or fantasized images, which are quite real and viewable inside the client's mind, are sources for hours of therapy. An instance that comes to mind is a long discussion a client precipitated when simply trying to decide whether or not to smile in her photo ("If I smile, it's for other people to see; smiling covers up the real me!"). Other times, the "meat" of the insightful or cathartic work is in the live process of making the image.

In yet other instances, the most valuable progress comes with looking at the finished self-portrait and responding to it through the therapist's questions.

Self-Portraits Made in the Therapist's Office

If people have grown up with only conditional approval or love, their sense of self becomes primarily other-defined. Such clients need to find out who they are when none of the definers are around. Self-portrait PhotoTherapy work can help clients clarify their self-images and raise their self-esteem and self-confidence through making, viewing, and accepting images of themselves and owning their positive perceptions.

One sign that this process is starting to succeed is that people begin to comment favorably on photos of themselves; they begin to keep them or ask to have copies of them, and when criticizing themselves, they begin to identify certain family members as the sources of such devaluing. If we wish clients to start taking responsibility for their own lives and begin to initiate action rather than just react to others' constructions of them, we can design self-portrait work to correlate their inner perceptions with outer documentation. In this process they can self-validate their feelings and let go of introjections from others that are irrelevant to true self-awareness.

I asked one adult client to pose for two instant photos while we were talking about her current difficulties with her parents. I asked her to pose as "Daddy's ideal little girl" and then as "Mommy's ideal little girl." I wanted to make concrete for her some of the hidden "scripts" she still, at age twenty-two, seemed to be perpetuating from childhood messages about how she should behave. In the first, she looked cute and smiled coyly; the second picture showed a depressed passive version of herself with her arms drooped at her side. Her family's standards of behavior were based on gender expectations, and she appeared to still be trapped by them, fearing to assert her independence and choice of career for fear of what they would say. I then had her pose as her own "perfect little girl," then as the adult version of that little girl, then the little girl she had been all along inside herself, and last, as the adult self who she was keeping secret from her family. The different body language and posing behaviors communicated to her much more than she could explain to me in words, but she later told me that it wasn't until she saw all those different selves together that she realized how much they conflicted and made excessive demands on her store of psychic energy.

Self-portraits can also be very useful when working with issues involving goal-setting, assertiveness, and other self-esteem issues. They are important aids for clients who need to cognitively accept that they can actually do or become something that they previously thought impossible or beyond their abilities. As discussed earlier, snapshots can be posed to permit people to see themselves doing what they "know" (think) they cannot actually do in real life. But, there they are in the picture doing it, looking as if it is really happening, and it *is* real because the photo shows it as proof of that moment's true existence. If they recognize that they were photographically documented looking like they were actually doing the activity or being a certain way, then it is only a very small reframing of perceptions to comprehend that they *could* actually do or be this way, or else there couldn't have been a photograph made of it. Thus it has moved into the realm of at least being possible.

In a somewhat similar vein, PhotoTherapy can be useful in work with clients who claim that they cannot feel anything or who state that they cannot comfortably express their emotions. One productive approach is to ask them to pose looking *as if* they were feeling, for example, angry, happy, sad, confident, or worried. If photographed *pretending* to be expressing a feeling, "as if" they were actually experiencing it, several things happen simultaneously (and can be even further enhanced with various psychodrama or video techniques if wished):

If a person tells me he or she cannot express a certain feeling, then poses pretending to show that emotion, the photographic evidence shows the person expressing the feeling. And there is the chance that the person actually will experience the feeling. When we use our bodies to try to communicate a feeling, we will often connect with that emotion, and sometimes even physically precipitate or cathect it, unexpectedly.

The power of the photograph to serve as a form of proof or truth sometimes precipitates in the client the perception that what they are looking at has actually occurred, rather than just been posed for. Sometimes seeing themselves looking sad, angry, in tears, happy, or whatever, will allow them to temporarily see themselves *actually experiencing* that feeling. It has all moved into the realm of being a definite possibility, and suddenly the choice to act or not becomes clearly theirs—"can't" has become "won't"!

Scrutinizing the frozen moment as long as they wish, clients can contemplate consequences, communication of affect, stirred memories, and voices from the past. It is a way to see the self unlike any other in therapeutic process. Techniques such as these are based on theories of cognitive dissonance, objective self-awareness, and internalization of locus of control, to name just a few, and they work well in visually activating such theories, as the examples in this chapter well illustrate.

Another way to work with such inner dissonance, or with polarized extremes inside clients' perceptions of themselves is to have them show the therapist the oppositional qualities or stances and photograph each new pair of opposites separately, such as "me when I'm good," and "me when I'm bad," or "happy" and "sad." The client then has in hand two photographs of the same self expressing contrasting realities, which can then "face" each other and "talk" with each other through role-play, like puppets. Or each can address the client and have dialogues, or the two can be end poles of a continuum and the client can pose for and photograph new in-between steps to better understand them as metaphorical stepping-stones. This resembles the concept of "polar splits" familiar to Gestalt therapists and helps activate some of their "empty chair" techniques. I call this the Polarized Polaroids exercise, and it is the basis for the two transcripts that end this chapter.)

Photographing the two poles of a current dilemma, such as particularly complex feelings or inner conflicts, can be expanded by having the client make a context for them to coexist on a sheet of paper large enough to physically and philosophically encompass both. If the images are attached to the same sheet of paper, the client can use art materials to create a joint "reality" or narratively establish their connection, no matter how tenuous. Such visual synthesizing on one piece of paper permits the understanding that dissonant parts are still encompassable within the self of one single person.

Additional techniques can be implemented to create metaphorical intermediary stages to bridge or join the extreme positions of any bipolar continuum, such as creating additional self-portraits to fit between the two extremes. These in-between images would symbolically represent middle-ground solutions, less polarized feelings, resolutions of expressed conflicts, and achievable stages in goal setting. Examples might be "my life now" and "my ideal goal" or "me at work" and "me at play". This provides a way for the client to work in syntheses apart from (or in conjunction with) therapeutic dialogue.

Another way this technique of visually precipitating perceived extremes can be used is in working with underlying dualities that the client feels exist inside him- or herself (or is unaware of the full dimensions of, but wishes to explore anyway). Examples of this are the male/female (and/or androgyne blending), which can be worked with as gender issues; representative components of anima/animus or ego/shadow parts of the self, such as various archetypes postulated by Jung and others; commonly described dualistic aspects of the self like good/bad, outer/inner, known/secret, liked/disliked, carnal/spiritual, and real/ideal aspects of the self, or the human/animal self components associated with the belief structures of many ancient cultures. All present the self as comprising two "alternatives," or poles, which are actually part of each other, or two sides of one thing.

Dualities may surface when clients are directed to create one self-portrait for one assignment and another for an assignment that contrasts or extends that first one. For example, I have asked clients to use photographs to show how they are feeling at this particular moment in contrast to how they usually feel, how they think they will look when therapy has finished (successfully) and their problems are solved, the person they are now in contrast with the person they would like to be (or the person that their mother or father wanted them to be), how they see themselves as compared with how they think others see them, their inner secret self versus their outer public self, the self that no one knows, the parts of themselves which they don't like or want to change (sometimes in conjunction with the parts they like or want to keep), how they see themselves and how they would like to see themselves, and on a more affirmative and empowering note (which can be a very positive goal-forming image), their self in a place they would most like to be (or most like to be seen), with things and people around them they would most like to have. If useful to the therapy process, they can even be asked to make pictures of themselves "when I'm dead," "at my funeral," "when I'm in heaven," "when all this pain is over," and numerous other possibilities.

Some very exciting work has happened with this sort of dualistic imagery worked jointly, including dualities of time and space (such as past/present self or present/future self, before/after frameworks, and so forth). I also have found it exciting to use the paper itself as a plane of reality by suggesting that clients put their face, profile, or frontal view on one side of a piece of paper or stiff cardboard, clay figure, or other movable object and their back view or back of head, shadow, or alternate profile (the other eye) on its other side, as in "me" and "another side of me"—in this case quite literally. These sorts of expressive creations can assist the client's recognition that, although these parts of them are sometimes very different, they are still expressible and thus conceivable as being part of the same reality.

Sometimes creating self-portraits allows a person to confront fearful possibilities directly, such as death, divorce, suicide, disability, or loss of identity (through bereavement, retirement, and so forth). These are also useful for permitting clients to play out the final steps of processes they are about to begin. If they can photograph themselves "being" in those future situations, they can often more directly address them. An example of this was work with a woman dying of cancer who was emotionally unable to confront her own death. Cognitively she knew she had to, but emotionally she always resisted. Finally, she decided to photograph herself in a coffin-shaped cardboard box and then look at the photos as if at her own funeral and observe what people were saying or emotionally revealing in response to her death. She said it was very important that she take the picture herself (using a timed shutter-release), because if anyone else did it, she thought she would still not believe it.

I have used this technique with adolescents contemplating suicide and people exploring their own imminent deaths, such as people in late stages of AIDS-related illnesses. Helping them place their inner sensory-based images outside themselves provides a bit of added control over the vague unknown. Goals can range from acceptance of death, to creating photographs as remembrances to keep your memory alive to others, to making photos (and elaborate art-enhanced "frames" for them, even if only on paper) to serve as "wellness" pictures for health-imaging work.

Exploring the ultimate consequences of something provides a framework for bringing it into more realistic perspective, even if that "something" is one's own death. When people have not been able to discuss death openly or contemplate it directly, it forces itself out through less concrete means, as in photo 4.2. This child's spontaneously posed self-portrait led to serious concern on my part about his possibly suicidal tendencies.

I took this snapshot at a group home where I was the therapist for several First Nations children who were attending the local school for the hearing impaired. The children were familiar with my using the camera in activities with them and often playfully posed for me even when not

Photo 4.2

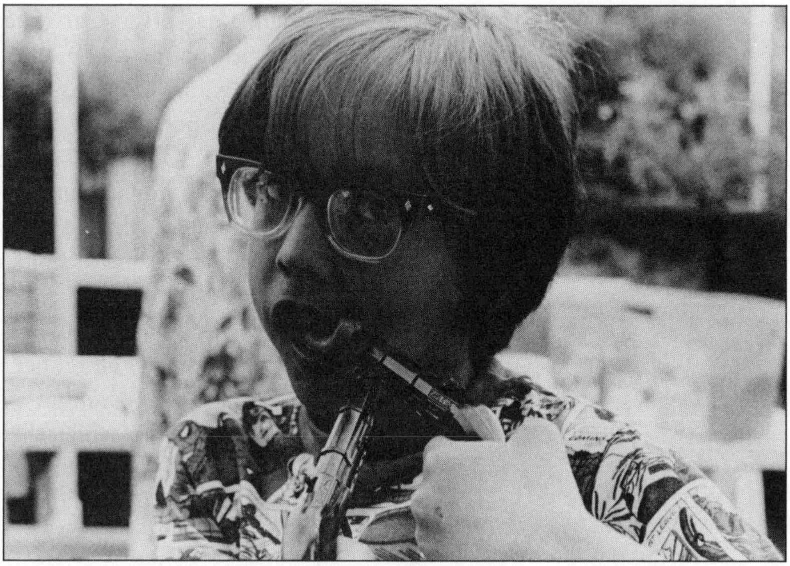

doing PhotoTherapy exercises. (Readers can find further discussion of these activities in Weiser, 1975, 1983a, 1983b, 1984c, 1988a, and 1988b.) In this situation, we were making portraits to send with Christmas cards to the children's families in distant coastal villages, and this particular boy, usually quiet but friendly, chose this pose and directed me to press the shutter. The other children had posed themselves in playful and even clowning activities, but this boy, who had been playing alone as a "cowboy," took his time and carefully arranged himself, even checking his pose in a window reflection before signaling me to go ahead. After finishing all the photos, and sending the other children out to play, I sat down with him for a while to check things out.

Of course, this one photo by itself did not necessarily mean anything conclusive; he could have been reenacting something he had seen on television. But the pose was so striking that it bothered me. Rather than challenge him, I owned my concern as mine and asked him if I should take his picture seriously, or if it had just been a moment of pretending. He wasn't willing to talk directly, but got some photos I had taken earlier of him in "emotional affect" expression exercises, demonstrating various feelings for the camera. He showed me the sad and depressed faces of himself as a way of telling me how he was feeling. We talked further about his sadness of missing his parents at Christmas, his low self-regard, and his recent suicidal feelings. But he had been otherwise unable to initiate this conversation and, unwilling to discuss it directly with me in sign language, he used various self-portraits to speak through.

In the following example, I activated my concerns about a client's wellbeing PhotoTherapeutically. A woman whose parents were both alcoholic brought in several photos of herself that she said she liked a lot. In all of them she appeared only from the armpits up. As she was extremely thin, I suspected she might be anorexic, and I noted aloud my observation about the rest of her body being missing in those snapshots. Also, in all of them, although she was smiling, her mouth was tightly closed. I asked her to try to repeat these poses, but with one or two differences. I wanted photos of her entire body (which she refused to do, because she was "too fat"), and I wanted photos of her smiling with her mouth open, which she agreed to, but found awkward to actually pose for, so appeared strained in the final print.

To get around this impasse, I got her permission to make photocopies of the images she had brought in, affixed them to large sheets of paper, and requested that she draw in her body and a social context for each image. Next, I asked her to use crayons or pens to draw open her visibly closed mouth. As she "opened" the mouth on one photo, she began to clench and relax her own jaw. I asked her to speak for that now-opening mouth, and she began to let out anger that had long been held in, anger toward her parents and the shame she had felt. I drew numerous speech balloons on the big page, each coming from her now open mouth on the photocopied image, and asked her to fill them with words. I sat quietly as she filled the space with torrents of words and then continued out along the border of the paper. After we processed all of these discoveries, I suggested an additional self-portrait closure for her whereby she posed holding the paper covered with all her words and images in order to synthesize the overall event and ground it in reality by means of a tangible photograph. In this pose, she requested that I include her whole body, because she said it was time she finally looked at it.

As mentioned earlier, another way to explore the self is through masks or decorated faces, costumes, hats, and other metaphorical equivalents of self, such as one's possessions. Masks are particularly useful for showing personas and the various roles or facets of the self they represent. A client can be asked to pose with a mask of their own finding or creation, such as art on cardboard, magazine people with eye-holes cut out, drawings that cover the whole body, other photographs in collage with those of the client, and so forth.

Any mask can be addressed by the self in face-to-face dialogue, or the mask can be applied and the person photographed actually wearing it. The resulting photograph can then say or do things that the client might not be able or willing to. This can be further "worked" by using two photographs of the same client in the same session, one masked and one not, so that the client can make the two images confront, converse, and compare with each other (or interact with the client in three-way dialogue). The client can ask the mask (or the masked self) questions and then respond from the mask's perspective, or the therapist can establish the process by directing what each should do next. Masks can be interrelated with album photos, collages, or even selected projectives with which they "fit" for the client.

One of the most important facets of self-portrait PhotoTherapy techniques is their ability to provide validation for the client far superior to self-evaluation based on the opinions of others. In a true self-portrait, if there is anything positive seen by the subject, it is indisputably there only because the subject put it there (by virtue of it being already a part of that person when photographed). Photos of a client taken by that client over the course of therapy can give the client proof of improvements that have occurred that might be discounted as flattery if spoken by the therapist. I often have clients make self-portraits in my office at one of their initial sessions and again at their final one—and sometimes several in between so that they can see for themselves how their presentation of self is changing. This sort of demonstration can be powerful therapy in itself.

Following are examples of the kinds of homework assignments that help clients explore whatever problem, feeling, or issue may be the current focus of therapy. Self-portrait assignments, especially if another person is involved as a neutral shutter-pressing assistant, can blur a bit into the kinds of techniques addressed in the next two chapters. The difference of course is that as maker of a self-portrait, the client is the director and animator of the entire process and the true creator of the results—not the object of someone else's construction.

Self-Portraits Assigned as Homework

Self-portrait assignments can help clients learn more about who their selves are, what constitutes the self apart from its construction by others, and metaphorically where the self is (where its boundaries are, where it leaves off and others begin). Most such assignments are given so that the client will not only see the results but also carry out the planning and creating, which may be especially important when personal emotional risk-taking is needed to achieve the pose or final print. Self-portrait assignments that require clients to spend time alone addressing their inner concerns, or where the photo making requires them to go somewhere new or be somehow different than usual, are sometimes their first experience of taking time to reflect in any detail on their private lives, indulging their own needs instead of others', or even acknowledging that they have their own internal feelings, apart from what others have told them.

An example of this is an assignment I gave a client who was trying to differentiate from her parents' strong demands for her attention and involvement in their lives and their beliefs that, even though she was in her late twenties, she should not have a life of her own because they needed her to stay with them. I requested her to photograph herself with them (which pleased them) and then the following week I asked her to spend twice as much film photographing who she was when she was not busy being their daughter. With very mixed emotions (and ambiguous messages from her parents, with whom she shared these instructions so as to have "permission" to do something on her own), she tried very hard to find things about herself to photograph.

It was a slow climb into her own identity, but it did progress. To begin to form an external image of herself, she initially needed her parents' assent. She presented it to her parents as "her psychologist's homework requirement," which she must complete, and they cooperated by supporting her involvement in the activity. Before she could begin to separate from them, we had to find ways for her to see that this was actually possible, initially without risking their disapproval until she was strong enough to counter it. For her to even consider individuation and liberation from their control and authority without rejecting the love that was also there, she had to recognize for herself that a life of her own could be seen and acknowledged by others.

Self-portrait work can be an "accidental" component of other techniques. It can surface in album-review work (where one imagines, remembers, or recreates one's own self-image) or it can emerge out of photo-taking assignments. It can even be part of projective work in which clients find images that seem to reflect their selves in some way, or in which they bring in photos from albums, magazines, or whatever, that best describe them, their lives, and their relationships with others.

An example of this kind of technique-blending occurred when a thirty-six-year-old client told me she was offered a promotion into her company's public relations department, but surprisingly found herself somewhat resistant to accepting. She was delighted with the honor, but for some reason disturbed by it at the same time. When conscious probing failed to come up with any answers, I asked her to have herself photographed in two ways: what she is like at her current work and then as she would be in the new position. She discovered that posing for her current job was easy; she just took pictures of herself as she already was. But she found that when preparing for photos of herself in the new job, she ran into all sorts of inner turmoil and kept putting off the photo-taking task.

The following week we discussed what had happened, and she shared her photo results. We discovered some significant differences. In the "now" photos she was in casual slacks, informal shirts, and comfortable-looking shoes. In the "new job," she was wearing dresses, high heels, makeup, and earrings, to fit the image she believed the company expected of its representatives. No, they had not "required" this; she had simply "known" that this would be necessary. When she saw the differences, she began to understand her resistance to making the change. It turned out that the problem was not in having to change her appearance (to her surprise, she liked how she looked dressed up), but in what the change meant to her. She was the only daughter in a family with five brothers, and throughout her childhood, her mother had made her wear ruffles and frills. The day she left home she switched to jeans and slacks and "comfort clothes." It was the 1960s, hippie styles were in vogue, and she could finally be herself.

She had long maintained this "independent" image of herself, but now to advance her professional career, she had to go back to a look her mother had forced upon her as a child. It turned out that the change of clothing meant that her mother had "won" after all. The therapy was therefore geared to helping her see that even in opposing her mother's position, she was still being controlled by it. In her determination to be the opposite of what her mother had wanted, she was not free to appear however she wanted. And "dressing up" didn't have to mean that she'd lost a power struggle, unless she wanted it to mean this.

We reviewed family album snapshots the following week, and she showed me numerous images that supported her claim about being forced into what she termed the "pretty-girl" mold. But surprisingly, there were more than a few images that refuted that claim. In several pictures of her as an adolescent she looked fairly sloppy and not at all girlish—she was in jeans, up trees, even hammering a dog house. These had been erased from her selective memory of her adolescent power struggles with her mother. The album review, combined with the self-portrait work, led to the client being able to let go of some of an old agenda and explore what her mother might have been going through at that time. She began to explore in therapy why it was that, nearing forty, she still seemed to need to remain invested in adolescent issues. She began to realize that the emotional distance she perceived as coming from her mother may actually have been created by herself, and that she could simply end it if she wished.

Some therapists have directed clients to find published photographs in magazines and books that demonstrate aspects of themselves that words alone could not express. I have even told clients to "shoot" pictures with cameras that have no film inside, to "take" their self-portraits—and have then asked them to draw what the camera would have got *if* there had been film in it. This is particularly useful for correlating expected with real body images and in cases where the client is too fragile for direct confrontation with the real image. Metaphorical responses to self-portrait assignments can also be useful. One client brought in an entire roll of pictures she had taken of her shadow. Another, assigned "to describe himself photographically," brought in snapshots of objects personally associated with him (his desk, glasses, hat, slippers, special coffee mug, car, and so forth), but none in which his own body appeared.

Applying projective PhotoTherapy techniques to "found" images can result in self-portrait work. Clients can create collages that represent them, take photos to show parts of themselves not usually perceived, and find album images that unexpectedly share secrets, even when they are not in the photos themselves. They look in my large collection of photographs (discussed previously) for images to serve as metaphorical self-portraits of themselves or that seem to fit with their just-taken instant self-portrait. These can be worked as if they were photos of the clients, or they can be processed visually by the client posing for an instant photo with their chosen image in a way which makes sense to them.

Such indirect approaches can reach buried or repressed material, as the following example demonstrates. Joanne was asked to select a photograph from my "projective pile" that seemed to her a metaphorical self-portrait of herself, even if it didn't picture a person. She selected one showing a woman lying on her back with her eyes closed and her hair spread out around her head (see photo 4.3). She said, "I was originally drawn to 'my' self-portrait for both personal and esthetic reasons. I am very much enamored of dreamlike images, which this one appeared to me to be. The

Photo 4.3

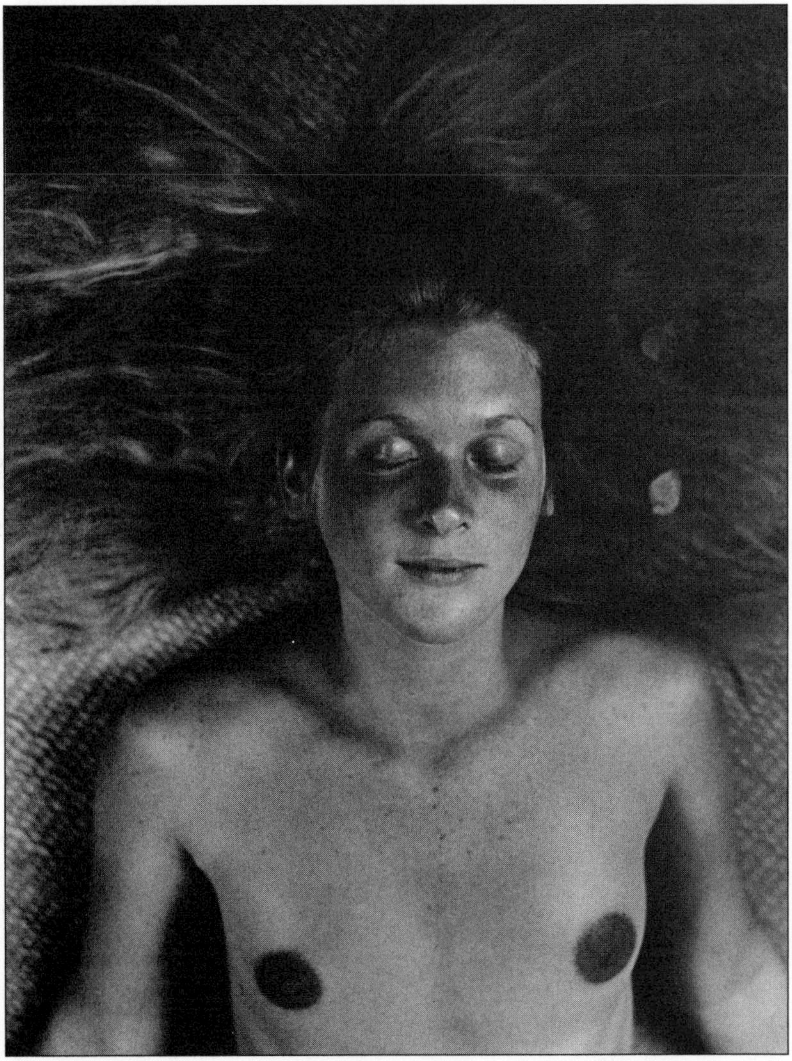

girl looks very relaxed, content, totally trusting, and as if she is being dreamed or is imagining something, and it appears that this something is giving her much pleasure. She seems very relaxed with herself and her self-image. Put succinctly, she is my ideal, what I would like to become."

To further "work" this image, I assigned Joanne to pose herself with this photograph in any way she wished, and she chose to mimic the pose of the person in the picture. In it, Joanne is lying down, eyes closed, with the other photograph resting on her chest. She shared these results and her assignment with a few of her close friends, and told me that they refused to believe that it wasn't her in the original photograph, as they found the resemblance strikingly similar.

Examining both photos closely, Joanne talked with me not only about the images, but also about how she felt making the second photo. We focused on them when our discussions touched on stressful topics. Joanne kept returning to how they suggested "a feeling of comfort and happiness, of being loved, secure, and out of harm's way." She commented that the original photograph seemed to touch something deep inside her, resonating somehow in ways she couldn't put to words, and she mentioned the hair resembling straw or hay (which I thought might have been suggested by the tatami mat the woman in the photo was lying on). A few weeks later, after a visit to her mother, when she had spent time exploring her family's photo album as I had assigned her to do, she returned to my office clutching a small faded snapshot (photo 4.4). She gleefully placed it next to the other two, and we found the similarities uncanny.

This photo was of her own mother about twenty years earlier, when she was about Joanne's current age. Her mother had liked the photo a great deal herself and had told Joanne that she kept it in her wallet for several years, even though she had felt a bit strange carrying around her own picture. When it became too fragile, it was placed in the album. Her mother also mentioned that when Joanne and her sister were young and bored with adult socializing, she would let them look through the wallet photos for entertainment. So this image had long been resting in my client's memory as a nonverbally-coded and unconscious trace of childhood. The photo she found later in my collection connected with it in ways neither conscious nor verbally explainable, and not traceable until the combined self-portrait and album-review assignments.

As Joanne's story illustrates, people frequently carry around mental images that they may not be aware of but that serve them as touchstones

Photo 4.4

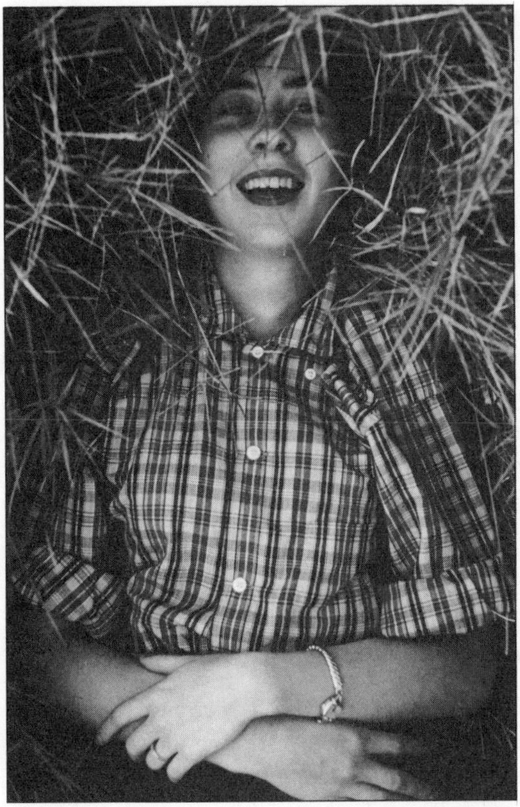

© 1960 Joanne's Mom's First Husband

for determining meaning about events and people in their lives. It is not infrequent that we find we have been carrying around images in our minds that turn out to have been actual photographs rather than our own intangible memories. The above example illustrates how common it can be for such unconsciously remembered images to have such emotional importance without our even being aware of their existence, and later examples in other chapters will further demonstrate this truth.

Another component to self-portrait work that can be extremely significant for some clients is that, if they wish, they may destroy, mutilate, alter, or actively distort their self-images. Of course it is preferable for their stability if this is done in the company of the therapist, or at least that such events be shared with one. There are times when this sort of metaphorical destruction of undesired parts can be especially constructive or cathartic, but it can also be dangerous. In the safety of privacy, if necessary, clients can also literally try alternative ways of being, such as cross-dressing and experimenting with makeup, transcending class or race limitations by up-dressing or role reversals, using their bodies as paper-doll templates for a variety of identities by means of clothing changes, and so forth. Identity can be explored as creatively as client and therapist can find ways to do so. Clients may even be assigned to photograph their "self-equivalents" for themselves (inanimate objects or those from nature; appropriated images from media, such as magazines; surroundings; whatever represents them to themselves).

As most of these assignments involve clients going out with the express purpose of taking or making photographs, even when they are of themselves, these can be considered as relevant to Chapter Six, on snapshots taken by the client. So as not to repeat this material, many of the assignment-related PhotoTherapy techniques appear in that chapter. Readers may want to cross-reference these two (and the exercises recommended in both) for future consideration of either set of techniques.

Additional Aspects of Therapeutic Focus

Numerous innovative self-portrait techniques and interventions have been documented as demonstrating the power of self-encounter for all clients, especially those who are members of traditionally devalued or marginalized groups who have taken up the camera as an active agent of change. It becomes obvious from a survey of the existing literature on PhotoTherapy, most of which is listed in the references or the recommended readings at the end of this book, that a high proportion of written documentation of the field has concentrated on self-portrait techniques (even if only as part of a multitechnique application matrix)—a fact that probably mirrors the natural interest most people have in themselves.

Particularly worthy of attention is the work of Wolf (1976, 1977, 1978, 1982, 1983), who has used instant-film self-portrait techniques in combination with art therapy and psychoanalysis, particularly with children and adolescents. Another pioneer is Ziller (1989, 1990; Ziller and Lewis, 1981; Ziller, Rorer, Combs, and Lewis, 1983; Ziller, Vera, and Camacho de Santoya, 1981), who has clients do what he calls "auto-photography," whereby clients take self-representative photos even if not appearing in them directly. Readers may turn to the list of recommended readings to learn how he uses auto-photography to find people's "psychological niche," a term he uses for what is individually and socioculturally important to them.

WORKING WITH CLIENTS' SELF-PORTRAITS

The process of asking questions about the image and having the client interact with it (based on the therapist's guidance) actually probes the same aspects of self, regardless of the particular object of original photographic attention or its size or visual format (album page, collage, hand-held image, fingerpuppet, face photo stuck on sand tray object, photo in the middle of painted or sketched scene on a larger piece of paper, hand-drawn self-portrait, and so forth). Later in this section, readers will find a list of in-depth questions useful for beginning therapeutic dialogue with any self-portrait images.

To try to see oneself from the perspective of an outside observer—objectively—is rather like the quandary, expressed to me in a personal communication by Shaun McNiff in 1990, of trying to separate the wind from the sky. It is not possible to view an image of oneself, knowing that it is oneself, and see it as if it were of a stranger. There is always privileged knowledge that cannot be removed from the perceptual process. Yet this is what I ask clients to do, even though I know that it is impossible. Clients must confront what is defining and thus binding them, to free themselves to experience life more fully. But therapists need to assess clients' readiness for such work carefully, and work up to it slowly. Clients' confrontations with their self-images are among the most intense, raw, and risky of therapeutic encounters. As such, they should be handled very carefully (or not at all) with clients whose self-image is fragile or whose self-esteem is very low; damage to such clients may be severe.

In light of these concerns, one of the strongest benefits of real or imaginary self-portrait techniques is that they allow therapists to ask clients self-oriented questions in indirect ways. The snapshot can serve as a stand-in for the person, and occasionally as a mask for the client to speak through. It can also serve as a safe focus, an attention deflector when the topic is stressful. People are usually more comfortable talking about how they feel about their own photo, or even how "that person" in the photo is feeling, than about themselves directly. In the move from a third-person perspective to a first-person one, using a self-portrait as a transitional object to join the client to themselves can be empowering to a client who may have been initially hesitant to "own" their own feelings or image if asked to do so directly. The procedures for doing this begin with general queries and then, as the client permits closer work, move slowly into the client's more intimate boundaries.

To establish partnership and a relatively equal power balance, I often begin self-portrait work by asking things such as, "Who is this person and what is she doing there?" "Tell me a story about this person." "What do you think this person would say if he could talk?" "Is there anything you might want to ask this person?" This general, impersonal approach keeps the image distinct from the client's self so that the client can risk saying things for, or about, that person that they are unable to say directly. This serves as a model for the client to get an external perspective on him- or herself without feeling attacked.

Implementing more flexible, less-structured dialogues regarding client self-portraits can be done fairly easily with the use of specific questioning techniques. These can be used with virtually any self-portrait images, even nonphotographic ones. Therefore I will direct readers through this "nuts and bolts" section about how to really get started by illustrating the kinds of questions that can be asked about self-portraits and how to use the information each evokes.

Making the Self-Portrait

Either the client is directed to bring to the session a self-portrait that they controlled the making of, or I work with the client to make one in my office as a prelude to the following exercise. If someone assisted the client by pushing the shutter, the client is to have made certain that the other person gave no critical advice, no esthetic suggestions, and made no attempt to make the client look "better" or "different." This image is supposed to be as true to the definition of a pure self-portrait as the client could make it, and the client is required to accept the very first image he or she creates as the one and only snapshot to be used for the exercise. No conditional judgments are permitted, such as, "this one didn't work out right so I want to try again." That first and only attempt may not be the one the client wanted, but it is the one that was made. This can be a good beginning lesson about self-acceptance and actual limitations versus unrealistic expectations.

What the client is to do with this snapshot (usually a standard 3-by-5-inch size or one about 3 inches square), depends on how the therapist wants to proceed. The image can be processed using the questions that follow, on its own, without further elaboration, or it can be affixed to a background and/or joined with art media for more complex expression. To use additional media, the client would be asked to place the photo anywhere they wish on a large sheet of paper (or shirt cardboard, or manilla folder, if the bigger size is a problem). The client is then invited to use art materials (on a nearby table) to "decorate" or enhance it, if that feels right. (I prefer folders or cardboard to the lighter newsprint traditionally used by art therapists; they can be held up in one hand and moved about and used as masks or puppets in dialogue.)

Some people choose to center their image on the paper's surface and some place it at the top left, as if starting to write a page. Others can't decide on a location and move it around during the remainder of the exercise. A parallel often emerges between where the client places his or her photo on the larger paper background and the positioning of his or her own body inside the frame of the snapshot. Some choose to cut out their body outline from the scene and place only it on the paper (sometimes they put in their own preferred background), though most keep the entire image to work with. Some people later use the empty space from the cut-out as a shadow aspect or use the negative space, perhaps as an alter ego. Some clients use the art materials to fill in every bit of space on the page or cardboard, while others are very sparing in their artistic expressions or use the space specifically, for example, for bordering the image to the point of producing highly-bounded enclosures, frames, or mazes that have special meaning for them.

Some people draw or paint "themselves" into becoming part of a yet larger scene whose edges now become the borders of the larger "picture" from which the photograph was "cropped" when created. Some actually "finish" their bodies or surrounding environment by providing the remainder of missing parts which the photograph had excluded (bottoms of legs or tops of heads that had been photographically "cut off," legs of chairs, remainders of window frames, continuing perspective views outside windows, and so forth). Some are comfortable with the photograph remaining incomplete, whereas others artistically express a strong need to finish the "not closed" or unboundaried portions of themselves or their setting.

Some use the snapshot as the very center of a mandala; others show a strong urge to further contain the snapshot's borders within even more boxes, circles, constraints or restraints. Some choose to use their image as a starting point for expressive movement opening outward from themselves, and others place themselves at the end-point of a series of progressing steps, directional signals, or other forms of sequential evolutions of time or space (like an unfolding narrative). Some people prefer to do none of the above, which is fine. Just as people are unique, so will their self-portrait creative expressions be. Photos 4.5 through 4.8 show some of the creativity that clients bring to self-portrait assignments.

All the above is still a prelude to the actual live therapeutic process, which I am most interested in probing with carefully conceived questions. I use the self-portrait and its larger constructed form, if the client chose to enhance it, as our focus, and I ask the client questions based on answers he or she gives to "explain" that image. I keep referring to "the picture" or "the person in the picture" because I want the client to tell me what she or he sees and what it means, as if the subject of the self-portrait and the viewer were two different individuals. I may also want to know more about what it was like to plan this photo, whether it came out "right," how it felt to pose and have to choose exactly the right shutter moment, and what, where, when, and how the client chose the final image. These questions are more general approaches than those discussed below, and processing them involves not only the information given here but also suggestions given in the next two chapters. Thus, I will not address these further here.

But for now, I will return to discussing how to begin working with only one image, possibly attached to one piece of paper, decorated or not, and one fairly consistently used set of questions with which to explore one single self-portrait of one client. The questions that follow are some of my favorite ones, but they are by no means the only ones that will succeed in connecting clients with emotional information. Readers may devise better ones, and I welcome your writing to me about additional questions that you would recommend for PhotoTherapeutic uses.

Photo 4.5 ***(left)***
Photo 4.6 ***(right)***

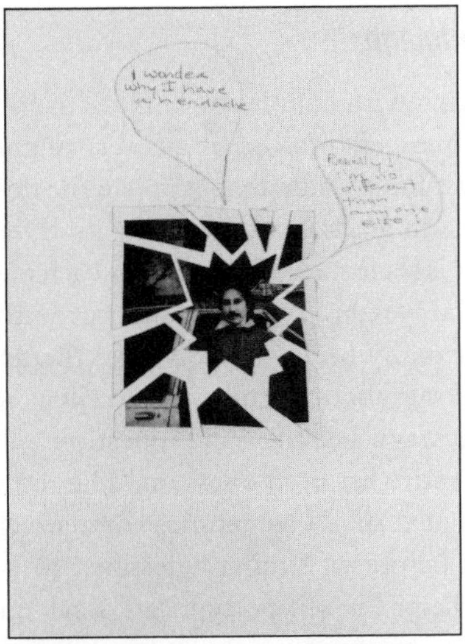

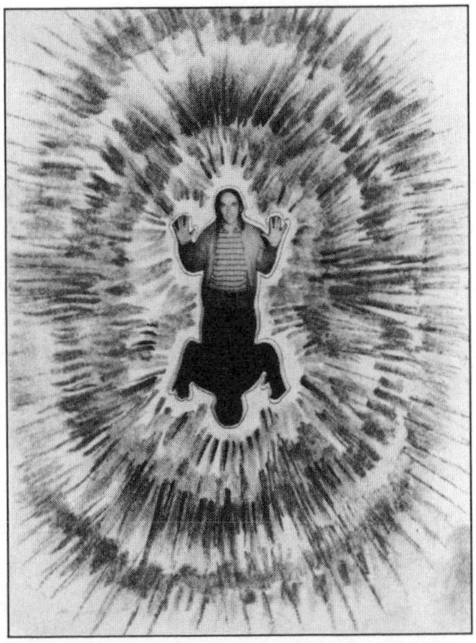

Photo 4.7 ***(left)***
Photo 4.8 ***(right)***

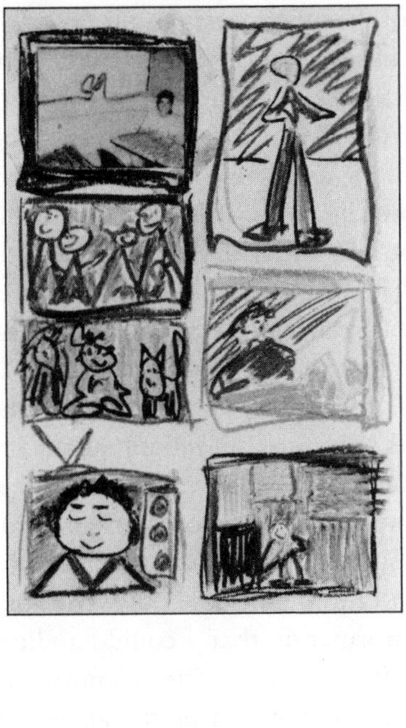

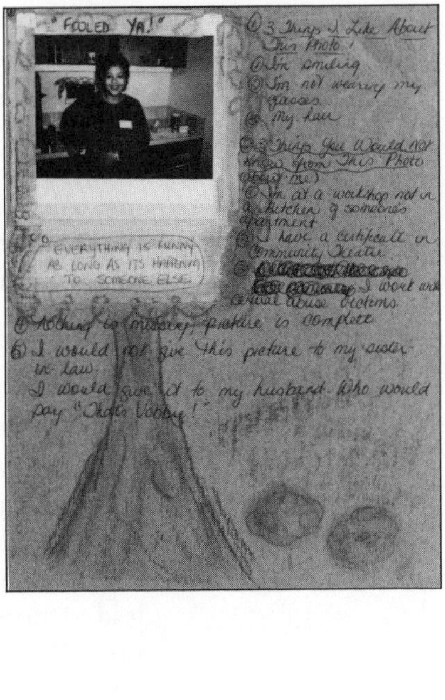

Working the Image

If I am working with couples or families or in a group or workshop setting, where one person's verbal answers might influence what the next one would say, I make sure that people write down their answers and then have each person read from the writing itself, rather than reply spontaneously when it is their turn. This protects each person's comments and gives them all equal weight. Writing responses onto a self-portrait construction can be equally useful in individual therapy. Writing down answers and then talking about them gives excellent results too.

I don't always ask the same questions, and I frequently don't go through the entire list in one session. The response to one question will influence the next one. I sometimes compare clients' answers with those made weeks before to similar questions to see how their therapeutic progress is reflected in self-perceptions. Each question that follows is useful by itself, but becomes even more helpful when connected with answers given to some of the other questions on the list. There are no formal directions for combining questions. This will be situationally unique for each therapist and client.

What Do You Like About the Picture? I often try to begin on a relatively positive note, as so much of therapy concentrates on the problems and pains of the client. So I usually begin by asking the client, "Tell me three things you like about this picture," or even better, "Please complete this sentence: "Three things I like about this picture are: ____, ____, and ____." This can be an interesting kind of question, as most people are much more willing to share what they don't like about a picture (and metaphorically, themselves) than to give compliments. (In our society, we aren't supposed to go around talking about how wonderful we are; it's considered rather rude. We are taught to criticize ourselves, to always be trying to improve our appearance to others, and to seek to better our lives and the impressions we give.) I ask for three observations to avoid excessive fixation on one single "best" answer. (Four or five would probably lead to more information than I could handle within the debriefing session.) Once a client has made three comments, I sometimes go back and ask which of the three would be the answer if only one were allowed.

Many people find it difficult to respond positively to questions about what they like about themselves. Such people often find it easier to compliment the picture of themselves because it is outside their own physical borders. What people like in their photo strongly reflects their feelings about themselves, and their choices indicate something about underlying values, usually buried too deeply to be easily verbalized in direct reflection. Sometimes they give answers, such as, "I like that I don't look too short," or "I like that I don't have that dumb smile on my face, like I usually do." These are not really purely positive statements, but they provide clues about what sorts of components make up their internal critical maps and what expectations mold their lives.

If clients find it particularly difficult to come up with answers to the "what do you like" question, or if all their replies focus on the background or details, I might ask if it would be better if I had asked for three things that they didn't like about it. And, not surprisingly, they frequently have a long litany of self-criticisms and deprecations and usually find it difficult to narrow those down to only three. It can be useful therapeutically to move off that particular image and on to imagined ones, by asking, "What would have to change in this photo for you to not have that particular criticism of it?" Or "Here's a photo of you that you *do* like" (pretending to hand them a photograph, fingers pinched as if holding a print, though there is nothing really there). "If this is one that really pleases you [injecting this possible reality where they may not even believe it could be true], in what ways is this 'new' image different from the first?" In this way we can work backward to find those physical characteristics that signal the most information to them about themselves.

The hidden message in all this is that many people think they are never good enough as they are. They are certain their self-perceived shortcomings are much more noticeable than they appear to others in reality, and often blame their troubles on their perceived physical attributes, or lack thereof. When answering this first kind of question, people begin to encounter those expectations and judgments long embedded in their silent conversations with themselves—those "ought's," "must's," and "should's," the internalized introjections that dictate expectations. I might explore this further by saying, in reference to what they liked, "Who in your family would say such complimentary things about you?" or, if there are negative aspects to the comments, "When you hear yourself talking about the things that keep you from liking yourself, the expectations about how you ought to be instead of how you are now, whose voices do you hear inside your head?" People know the answers to these sorts of questions, even though they are probably stored nonverbally and are hard to find using only words as the impetus.

Sometimes all three answers suggest a difference between how the person appears and how they actually felt when posing: "I like that I seem happy, I seem friendly, and I seem relaxed." These suggest that I may want to discuss with the client what would have to change in the photo or in the person's life for those statements to say "I like that I *am* happy, I *am* friendly, and I *am* relaxed." Other times their answers reflect surprise, such as "I look better than I thought I would" or "I like that you can't tell how uncomfortable I am in front of a camera." These sorts of responses indicate dissonance beginning to grow between clients' expectations and their actual self-perceptions; they cannot blame the talent of the photographer because they—the clients—were in charge of taking the snapshot. One man quickly posed his self-portrait at a desk in front of a blackboard. Though he later said he had not thought much about the significance of the pose, his "likes" included "I look alert and competent" and "I appear to be happy in my work." Later, when I asked him to tell me something a stranger wouldn't know about him from looking at that photo, he said, "I always wanted to be a teacher." These comments led to deeper discussions about career dissatisfaction, which had only begun to surface.

This opening question, plus the remaining ones discussed below, are designed to permit people to interact with themselves face-to-face. Seeing themselves as they are seen by the world (through the eyes of a camera) often provides direct, and often previously unrecognized, clues to how they construct themselves for presentation as well as how they expect to be perceived.

What Is Most Obvious About This Picture? At this point, I sometimes ask clients to fill in the blank in the sentence "The most obvious thing(s) about this picture is/are: ____." As mentioned earlier, what a photo seems to be of and what the client thinks it is about are usually two different things. One woman said the most obvious thing about the photo of her standing in front of a large old tree was that she appeared to be part of the tree, including its strength and gracefulness. I simply saw a person in front of a tree, and did not find myself perceiving them joined, yet for my client this union was obviously real and significant, particularly as later, speaking for the photo, she said, "To live is to grow; to grow is to be alive." Another person called his self-with-tree photo "growing up and taking root." Tree archetypes appear often in therapy and can be particularly striking in PhotoTherapy self-imaging work.

Another example that illustrates the difference between what a photo is of and what it is about involved a woman posing as if swimming in a gushing fountain's surrounding pond. "I didn't want to be my usual guarded self. I didn't want to pose like I usually would. I wanted to present myself as I am, not covered up, being careful. I am obviously having fun swimming. The fountain looks as if I'm throwing up the water [with her hands, playfully]. Water is nurturing for me, and I find it soothing." Her title for the photo was "Water Baby," and she described resting in water as a pleasant fantasy, as water was "calming and nurturing" for her. In a later session, however, she brought up her difficulties separating from the influence of her mother, even fifteen years after leaving home, and ten out of twelve photographs she showed me of her mother included lakes, rivers, water in numerous placid appearances. I went back to the self-portrait, which she had described as "throwing up the water," to see if perhaps the phrase was intended to mean purging, and whether "treading water" had ever gotten her anywhere. I wondered if she wanted (or planned) to do this the rest of her life.

Tell Three Things about You that This Picture Doesn't Show. The next question is to "tell three things you wouldn't know about me (the client) from this picture." This permits clients to go beyond the identities they use to introduce themselves ("Nice to meet you, too. What do I do? Oh, I'm a carpenter" "Who's my boyfriend? Oh, he's in the army." "Hello again! What have I been up to? Oh, the usual—work, family, kids.") The answers to this question help clients to flesh out who they are when they are not filling those usual roles that usually define a person's activities in relation to others. Their responses frequently reveal information that a stranger might not get upon first meeting them, details that are more personally revealing or significant, such as "I have a kayak," "I like dogs," "I'm part Swedish," "I'm a responsible person," "My feet hurt," "I don't want to be so shy," "I wheel a lot of manure," "I have four brothers," "I have fat legs," "I'm very religious," or as one man summed it up, "My history, my loves, and my intentions". One woman's list of three had "I'm originally from Brooklyn, I love horror movies, and I hate sailing"—not earth-shattering therapeutic material, and yet it gives me a larger idea of the parts of herself she feels have some importance.

One client listed "this is a new posture for me" as one of the things not knowable from his relaxed-on-the-grass pose; further discussion led to his sharing feelings of fear of being "caught" in this pleasurable pose, not being his usual workaholic self. We role-played the "getting caught" feeling to see who in his life would have something negative to say about his relaxing. The voice of his dead father loomed immediately, and gave us an indication of where some of the frustrations in his life might have originated. Another person said, "You wouldn't know from looking at this picture that my clasped hands are protecting me and keeping me safe inside their circle." This client later said the photo would say, "I don't like to feel OK. It's not safe to relax." In these sorts of responses, clients often share information that I don't believe I could have gotten through direct verbal queries.

This question also occasionally precipitates information that has been previously kept secret, sometimes repressed and sometimes protected because it is powerful privileged knowledge. Several times, clients have given one or two casual answers and then added a very "heavy" one. In a striking number of occasions, this has been either the death of a loved one or a secret about past abuse or sexual orientation. For example, one man listed, "You wouldn't know how I feel about my new glasses, that the birds were singing loudly right above my head, and that my father died last month." It has been my experience that intensely personal issues are frequently "squeezed" onto such lists, perhaps to partially neutralize, externalize, or control their power.

What Would You Title This Picture? Asking how a picture could be captioned lets the client summarize and frame the photo in a cognitive perspective. One person said the previous answers were about "heart things" and this one was more about mind and thoughts. Sometimes the answers to this one contrast with the other answers, while other times themes resonate consistently. One man titled his photo "Suspense," then had it "speak" impatiently, "Take the picture and be done!" He said later that this seemed to express his eternal inner tension over wanting excitement and mystery in his life while also wanting control, closure, and predictability. Another client chose to title hers simply, "Staring," and yet when asked what the photo might say if it could speak, was quite precise in adding, "My eyes see too much, but my mouth still half smiles." I myself felt like she, or the photo, was trying to let me in on some secret too raw to present to me directly. She later revealed her role in her father's sexual abuse of her sister—she had to lie silently in the other bed and pretend nothing was happening.

A woman had posed in a small boat that she realized later, answering the questions, was an old lifeboat with no oars. The irony of this seemed to catch her fancy; she said she liked that it was a boat unable to leave the safety of shore and face the rough seas. However, the boat could just as easily be seen as being "adrift and unsafe." She titled her photo "My Past Is Good Enough," which seemed a bit odd to me at first, but I figured I'd probe meanings after hearing her other responses. When she shared what her photo would say if it could speak, I began to have a hunch about her physical health: "The picture would say, 'I am moving on, and it's time to move on.'" She would be happy to give a copy of the image to anyone who wanted it, but wished to keep the original nearby "as a reminder of who's steering the course," and there wasn't anyone she would refuse giving it to, as she had recently "resolved all her outstanding family feuds." It wasn't difficult to conclude that some form of life-threatening illness might be happening to her, and I gently probed her situation, using my feedback of simply repeating all her answers together at once. Her tears flowed, as she told me she had been diagnosed with a fast-growing cancer and had not yet told anyone while she was still coming to terms with it. She was surprised to hear all those signals when reviewing all her answers, as she thought she had not been letting out any clues anywhere.

What Would This Photo Say? The questions "If it could speak, what would this picture say?" and "If the person could speak, what would the person say?" (which do not always yield the same answers) can give free rein to the imagination. I have heard answers as casually impersonal or deflecting as "How's my hair look?" "World, here I come" and "What now?" Others have larger potential significance, such as, "I should have listened to my Mom." One person posed under a no-smoking sign and listed a cigarette as what was missing from her photo. She had the photo say "Here she goes again!" and I found myself wondering what she saw herself as repeating—smoking habits or more global life issues. Both were correct hunches. She later explained that she had just begun smoking again after two smoke-free years and this had to do with the stress of again being laid off from work.

Another woman posed in front of a doorway opening onto an alley with a garbage container in it. She titled the photo "Doorway of Garbage," saying she hated portraits of herself and felt awful taking one. The words she said the photo would speak were "Which way do I go now?" She originally told me this was meant literally, as the door opened out into a messy world. We connected this to her issues of low self-esteem when she discussed her answers to a later question about who could have this photo of her—and who couldn't. She stated, "There is no one to give it to. I never give photos of myself away. I rarely allow photos [to be] taken. I never show the self-portraits I paint." This final reply was written onto the paper near her image in a continuous line forming a flat, oval-shaped, tight inward spiral (which to me resembled a barely open mouth, though I did not force this interpretation on her). The issues of opening up, taking risks, sharing and trusting others, beginning to accept her own feelings, and approaching others for social contact all arose from this quickly done exercise.

Deeper meanings may emerge when answers to various questions are connected. An example of interweaving themes representing underlying processes occurred when a woman told me that her photo of herself playfully pointing to a very large flower would say, "Funny, at first it wouldn't grow, and now I can't control it!" Later she mentioned that she could give photos of herself to her favorite teacher because "he's the first person who really took an interest in me, and I just blossomed." Even later she referred to beginning therapy at this point in her life as being the end of a long winter and said, "My seed is just now sprouting and reaching for the sun." A young teenage girl liked this question because "it [her self-portrait] gets to say things I've always wanted to say but couldn't get away with saying!"

One young woman responded to her poorly exposed (and thus extremely light-toned) self-portrait with the comment that it would say, "Oooh! I'm over-exposed," which soon took on additional layers of meaning. When I asked her how she felt being overexposed, she immediately answered, "Daddy," and then looked as if she would like to stuff that word back into her horrified mouth. It was a rather abrupt opening into childhood abuse issues; her father had continually pestered her into posing for borderline pornographic photographs.

How Might This Picture Be Feeling? I sometimes ask the client to tell "three things this picture might be feeling" or "three things this picture might want to be feeling." Questions I sometimes use to augment these are "How does this photo fit for your pose for the world: is this the real you? If so, in what way? If not, how not?" or sometimes, "What are three things this photo needs right now?" As these are relatively more specific, they often come later in the process.

What Is Missing from This Picture? The question "What, if anything is missing from this picture—if it is not complete 'as is,' what would be needed to complete it?" is another often successful catalyst. One woman's response, "Ugh! My mother would say she was missing next to me," is a good example of how clients' responses to all these questions add up to form a core theme. In another case, a woman who had said that the picture didn't show how alone and lonely she felt went on to say that what was missing from her was "another person beside me." Soon, however, she said she wouldn't let anyone else have this picture because she couldn't trust people not to emotionally wound her. As various answers combine to point to key issues, it can be useful to have the client consider how the photo might change if the missing component were suddenly magically supplied.

Another woman had decided to sketch her pose immediately after the camera documented it, because her son had recently dropped the camera and she wasn't sure her self-portrait would turn out. The photo did succeed though, and her sketch appeared to me to be quite similar to her snapshot. However, when answering the questions about the self-portrait, she chose to work with the hand-drawn image rather than the real photographic one, because, she said, 'I think it is a more honest portrait of myself"; and she liked it because "it fits my desired image of myself that I wish to present to the world, so part of me is satisfied." This reversal of usual validation of reality by snapshots versus drawings intrigued me, and yet some of her other answers provided signals about what might be underneath this comment: "You wouldn't know that . . . I am not whole, despite the fact that my circling arms are an attempt to create wholeness in the image, or that my feet [missing from both the photo and the drawing] don't always support me"; "The photo would say . . . 'bare with me while I grow.'" She did not notice or try to correct the possibly significant misspelling of the word *bear.* What she decided was missing from her portrait was "spontaneity"; to complete it fully "would require trust"; and "I wouldn't give this photo to anyone!"

Synchronicity and "accidental" errors of miscommunication, like the slips of the tongue or misspellings, can be useful factors in PhotoTherapeutic exercises. I spent one memorable session discussing with a client her feeling that "her son" was missing from her self-portrait, only to find out after much confusion that it was her "sun" that she missed (it had been raining heavily for several days). However, when I pointed out my error, she commented, "You know it's funny, but the two are connected for me as he's my only child and he lives down in Florida, and I do miss him a lot." Then we discussed her son and how the picture would change if he became part of it. Even therapist error can lead to useful process if acknowledged and worked through creatively.

One fellow said the most obvious thing in his self-portrait was that he was out of focus, and then added that what was missing in his photo was "everything." He also had chosen to cut the photo to the point where he only existed from the neck up, an observation that led us into deep discussions of body image and past abuse. Another client photographed herself on a ladder, but then noted that the bottom border of the photograph did not include the actual bottom rungs and legs of the ladder resting on the pavement below. She had already drawn in the missing "groundedness" (her word for it) before I got to the question about missing parts; she said she felt too tipsy without them drawn onto the cardboard. This led to discussion about who in her life provided this kind of support when she felt "tipsy" or ungrounded.

This brings up the connection between art therapy and PhotoTherapy in the use of archetypal symbology. For example, many art therapists have found consistent patterns of symbolic expression appearing in the art produced by previously abused clients, including phallic-shaped trees and other aggressive vertical shapes, zig-zags or wedged intrusive angular shapes, "floating" disassociated eyes, human figures drawn with no trunk (arms and legs descending directly from the neck), arms with no hands, hands with no fingers, legs with no feet, portraits of the self that show the head and body either not connected or "sliced" through with a disconnecting line or other markings, as well as other communications indicating possible emotional cutoffs or past witnessing of the unwitnessable. These patterns can also often be found repeating in clients' photographs, and therapists should be alert for such possible signals in ordinary photos that clients bring in, take, or pose for. Finding these clues doesn't automatically mean that abuse definitely happened, but when many of them appear repeatedly in the work of the same client, the therapist may want to inquire about that possibility.

In photo 4.9, a spontaneously posed self-portrait, the woman's arm separates her face from her body. This might signify little on its own, even though the woman once referred to "earlier portraits that reflect my detached self as being me." However, this person later took sixteen other photographs for my assignment to show "the me nobody knows," and in every picture that includes her body, the same sort of horizontal neckline separation appears. For example, in photo 4.10 the line is made with mirrors, and in photo 4.11, it is formed of a shadow "bending" up a wall. The pattern repeated so strongly that I decided to inquire about the possibility of past childhood abuse.

Photo 4.9

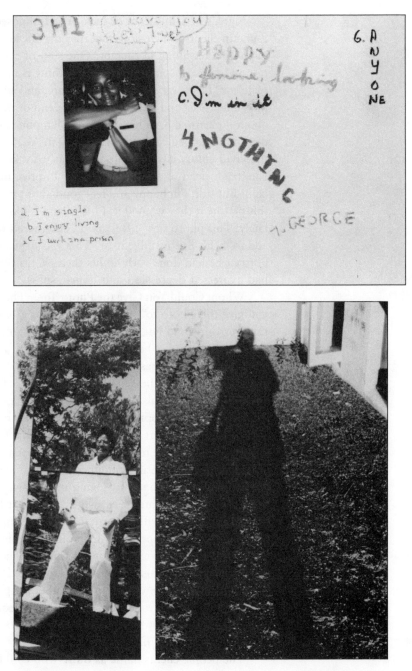

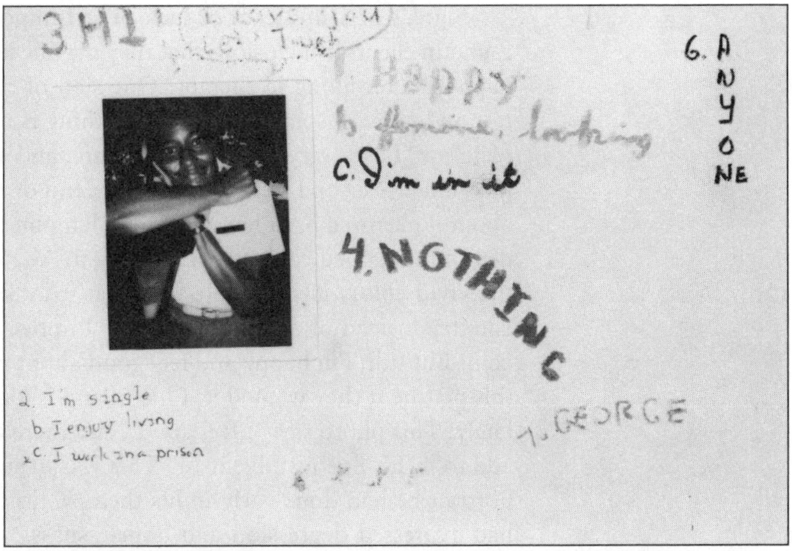

Photo 4.10 *(left)*
Photo 4.11 *(right)*

Signals of self-esteem or lack of self-imposed conditionality can be found in clients' conclusions that they are fine just as they are; this usually happens later along in therapy. One sign of this for me is to find them responding with something like, "Nothing is missing; the photo is complete" or "I like everything in this picture, and anyone could have it." One man made a second self-portrait at the end of therapy and his comments about it mirrored back his new-found happiness with himself, despite his deteriorating medical condition owing to AIDS-related illnesses: he liked the vivid colors in the photo and that it looked like he was out in the country instead of stuck in the city. "I notice that I'm getting a double chin! But still, I'm happy and feel good about myself. Anyone could have this picture if they wanted it. I like it and it looks like me and how I feel lately. This photo says 'I feel good!' and there's nothing I would want to add to it. It's fine just like it is!" This was in stark contrast with the self-portrait he had done early in his therapy, his observations about which had expressed depression and hopelessness.

Whom Could You Give the Photo To? The question "Whom might you give this photo to" (or "If you were to give this photo to someone, that person would be ____" or "A person who could have this photo if they wanted is ____") serves several purposes. First, the subtle nuances between the three phrasings often result in significantly different answers. People not only list the actual names or roles of such people (my mom, my best friend), but also frequently offer their explanations for why they would give these people the photo. One man responded that he would give his photo to a certain friend (but only that friend), because "he's the only one who would really understand why I'm in therapy." Conversely, another fellow haughtily announced, "I wouldn't give this photo to anyone. I'm not in the habit of giving myself away!"

A fellow in his late teens, who had at first liked his photo because he "looked 'macho' with his arm muscles bulging from his T-shirt," titled his photo "Mister Important." Later, however, he admitted that although he had appeared self-assured at the time, he had been fearful of the assignment and what his photo might look like. Now that he liked it, he still wasn't certain he wanted to hear other people's reactions to it, so he wouldn't give it to anyone. People of any age frequently signal unfinished childhood business by saying that they would be willing for friends, but not their parents, to have their picture.

The people clients name as those who could have their self-portrait are the people they trust or feel comfortable with "just as they are"— however they may be dressed or feeling. People you would give your self-portrait to, knowing it wouldn't be criticized or rejected, are probably people you'd give your real self to just as willingly. One client said she wouldn't give her photo to anyone who didn't care for her. Several others have lovingly and formally made gifts of their self-portraits to themselves to indicate their growing self-acceptance.

Acceptable recipients are often family members or close friends by whom one feels accepted unconditionally. Whether meaning family of origin or family of affiliation, *home* is one of those things best defined inside the heart; as one client told me, "that's where they have to love me even if they don't particularly like me right then". Similarly, the people to whom clients might give this self-photo are likely to be those people who accept them just as they are, without any significant preconditions or expectations. Therefore, this list also suggests who might comprise the client's natural support network—all those people who could be counted on in a crisis. This is a list of people with whom one feels emotionally safe and not having to act a role for acceptance. For example, in my work with people who have AIDS, I often need to know who will be able to help with caretaking needs without the client's rebelling at such undesired dependency. Their answers to the above question are usually a good beginning for constructing such a list.

Who Can Never Have This Photo? Clients' answers to the questions "Who definitely could not have this photo" and "Who I would not give this photo to, no matter what reason they gave for wanting it," and their often-offered explanations for those answers, can often trigger the most intense emotional processes of all the questions on this list. People usually aren't willing to risk giving themselves to others who they believe have power over them that they strongly resent. I have often found that the answers to the two questions "who could have it" and "who definitely couldn't" are paired when responses are given. For example, a client told me, "I could give this photo of myself to Sally and Judy, as it's a good way for them to remember me, but there's no way that Jane could have it, because she has lost the right to see how well I'm doing." Another client said, "My boyfriend could have it, but definitely not my ex-boyfriend!" A woman indicated her increasing acceptance of herself while also signaling some of her difficulties by answering, "I would not give this photo to someone who feels threatened by older middle-class women."

Exploring the emotional information underlying clients' answers to this final question can give them insight into what their unfinished business is and whom they perceive as having some degree of power over them. Note that these are not people who *actually* have power over the client; instead, the power imbalance exists because the client *believes they do.* The client is giving up power to that other person and assigning him or her responsibility for the imbalance. That yielding of control may be unconscious, but it is also voluntary. That is not to say that a person may not have been truly wronged, abused, or mistreated; however, if the wrongs remain unresolved or unfinished, the client has to recognize his or her part in maintaining the problem.

When clients have been abused or mistreated, I by no means suggest that they pretend it away (nor do I think they should always be able to "forgive," as so many books suggest is a necessary part of the cure). Rather, I encourage clients to acknowledge that the situation was indeed very real, explore it to clear away the emotional clutter remaining within it, analyze the situation consciously and examine what it means, and then, when able to see it all relatively externally, explore the feelings connected to it. Then the client has some choice as to what, if any, the ongoing significance of the problem might be. In the therapeutic processing of such events, it is not so much the factual details of an incident that we deal with as what its occurrence *means* to the victim (or perpetrator).

Often, just "naming" or even photographing unresolved vague anxieties or threatening relationships, which previously seemed too overwhelming to confront or consider changing, can give clients a modicum of power that allows them to come to terms with those problems at a conscious level. In the process of neutralizing what has appeared to be the problem's power over the client, it often becomes clear that, in fact, the client has been giving power to it. Chapter Six, on assigning clients to take photos, includes examples of how combinations of techniques can be used to "get a better picture" of the problem or the relationship that appears insurmountably difficult and ways clients can use these techniques to begin to reclaim some of their "lost" power.

From the perspective of systems theory (discussed further in Chapter Seven), cutoffs can exist in one person's view that the other person may not recognize, or one person's role can be fused with that of another to the point that the range of reality and emotion each independently experiences is severely limited. To keep people in our lives with whom we have conditional relationships, lack of trust, unwillingness to be vulnerable, or the need to maintain inflexible roles, is to remain impotent and helpless. It means seeing such situations as irresolvable, usually because we are blaming the other person for the problem's continuation.

One person, when asked who could not have her picture, said, "I hate him, and if I don't like him, then he's certainly not going to have my picture. I never let him take my picture either." Such strong feelings are clear indicators that work needs to be done, not because amends "should" be made, but rather because maintaining this kind of issue drains energy away from the client's mental health. If there are many of these sorts of conditional relationships in a client's life, so much attention is invested in protecting the self from them (or from expectations of related dangers) that there is little energy left for moving forward.

Therapeutically it would be very helpful for clients to consider the possibility that problems do not have to continue existing. Often when clients say they can accept such an idea, they mean only that the other person could easily end it all but that they themselves can do nothing about it. In such cases, I sometimes suggest exploring what it might take for the adversary, who could never have the client's picture, to become one of those who *could* have the photo. Clients often strongly resist this idea as an extremely undesirable possibility, but if pushed a bit to explore the necessary changes, they may be able to recognize how they themselves are controlled by their own need to sustain the adversarial role rather than risk establishing a more personal and intimate relationship.

I help clients explore such considerations in the following manner: I ask the client to keep in mind the person(s) who cannot have the picture; then I begin a process somewhat similar to peeling away layers of an onion, in that I hope the client will eventually see that she or he has some choice about remaining invested in the negative relationship. Making it clear that we are only pretending, I ask the client to temporarily consider what might happen if they actually *did* let that other person have the photo; what would be the worst thing or feeling that might happen? From this point, we go on to what would have to change in the other person for my client to be willing to really let them have the photo. Is this change possible or realistic? What might have to change in the client, if change in the other person is not possible, and would the client want to risk this move to improve the relationship? Is there a particular aspect of the photo that makes the client so vulnerable to this other person, and if so, what part is that? Is there anything that might make the client *want* to give the photo to the other person, and could any change happen that would result in that desire?

I push at these boundaries in order to find the resistances; I ask the client for alternate scenarios, to give insight into different, and perhaps new, contrasting viewpoints. What would be the worst thing that might happen if that person did somehow get this photo? If that worst thing actually happened, what would be the worst thing about that? Can the client imagine just for a moment that the other person has the photo after all, and what might transpire now that they do? If pushed gently through all these stages to explore what would take place if feared events happened, clients often discover that things are worse now than they would be if they tried to diminish the barriers.

In all of the above work resulting from such simple questions and their multiple combinations, "now" and "potential future" are compared through examining and discussing photographic metaphors for these states. Discussing difference and change, either at the tangible level of photographic evidence or in terms of inner mental pictures, engages the client's inner, unverbalized assumptions about what would need to change for things to be different. Future conditions, however desirable, are often perceived by clients as impossible to achieve. When they recognize that those conditions are indeed possible and approachable, they can begin to realize how much resistance has come from themselves and is thus within their power to change. Once aware that choices and consequences are within their own control, they can begin to take charge of their lives and start to differentiate out from their previous disempowered and undifferentiated position.

Whom Did You Unconsciously Intend This Photo For? Another question I sometimes include if I think it useful is "Now that you have done this self-portrait, does anyone come to mind whom you may have been unconsciously taking this picture for?" Although this is somewhat similar to asking who the client might be willing to give the photo to, it is not quite the same focus. What I am trying to access here is their mental picture of themselves. I would like to know if they made their image for themselves alone or perhaps also with an eye to pleasing someone important to them. This kind of question, particularly in combination with the question of who they would like to give this photo to, is useful for exploring differentiation and fusion issues. To encourage clients to consider who they are to themselves as compared with who they are to others, I might probe a bit by asking if they might have been unconsciously posing for someone. "Does anyone come to mind?" "Do you think that person would like the picture?" "Is there anything you can think of that might improve it even more for you or them?"

Similarly, I might ask, "If you took this picture mostly for yourself, and you like it (as the client has previously told me), tell me now, would your mother like it too? Would your father?" These responses could take us a number of places, depending on what issues we were focusing on. For example, if I wanted to explore triangulation in a client's family, this technique might well point to where the alliances might be. I might ask a client to imagine a self-portrait a parent might take and like and how that might differ from the internalized image that the client is carrying around as her or his "reality" of that parent. I might explore how the client's self-portrait might differ from a "good" photograph of that client taken by a parent, and try to find out more about how the client thinks she or he is different from the parent's expectations and perceptions.

This has occasionally led to assigning each member of a triangle to make a self-portrait, assisted by each of the other two, and then having each person photograph the others as he or she knows them to be. In a threesome, this would result in at least nine photographs (and sometimes more, when people are unable to make choices). Each person's photograph would have been taken by two others, plus one self-portrait. Combining the pictures for comparison and conversation can be a very good way to start therapeutic dialogue; differences can be kept at third-person distance, discussed as metaphors, and considered as visually frozen perceptions rather than treated as aspects of the people themselves.

I want to reiterate that the questions described here do not constitute a closed list of what must be asked in self-portrait explorations. Therapists should use the questions that most frequently produce the best results and should feel free to add others if they seem relevant to the situation, such as 'What else should I know about this picture?" "Who else in your family knows this?" "Does the photo hold any secrets?" "If so, who knows those secrets?" "Is there something you are hoping that I do *not* ask you about this photo?" or any others that come to mind. One client, who went through the full process involving all the questions given in this chapter, had this reaction:

It surprised me because it suddenly became much more serious once we began working on the photos. At first I found it playful, a self-portrait with absolutely no expectations. It was like a game, a masquerade, where I could do or be whatever I liked. So I went outside and posed myself. But once we started answering the questions, it became much harder and even mysterious to look into this image to find what else had become embedded in the lightness of the original moment. Was something missing? Could I have known this at the time? What was I feeling at that instant? If I gave the image permission to speak, would it leap into revealing some unknown or forbidden territory? And the questions—was it the photograph or actually me being discussed, and is there any difference? Would my answers about the photograph—if it could speak, if it were incomplete, things I like about it—be any different if I substituted "I" or "me" instead of "it" in the questions? Of course, that's why you asked them in the first place, to get us to recognize this!

Three things you wouldn't know about me from this picture? Should I be "nice" or tell you that the first thing that popped into my mind is that one wouldn't know from looking at this picture how obnoxious I'm capable of being. I look *too* nice in this photo. Now you're going to ask me the difference between "nice" and "too nice," I'll bet! Title the photograph? OK, but I don't want to think about whether the title could just as easily fit for me. It's "Here I am. Take it or leave it." Would I dare risk offering the same choice about myself?

I was fine when you asked me three things I liked about the photo or, really, about me, but when you asked about three things my mom would like about it, boy did my hackles go up! I don't want to ever be the kind of boy she wants me to be, so when you asked me to imagine letting her take a picture of me as she would want it to look, my immediate response was "No!" But my Dad could, because he and I are a lot alike, and I'd trust that his image of me would be very similar to how I see myself. Maybe that's why you weren't surprised when I told you he could have this photo—because I like it, but my Mom never could—probably for the same reason, don't you think? Wow, I didn't expect all this could come out of looking at one quick snapshot!

ILLUSTRATIVE EXAMPLES

The two illustrations in this section deal with two different people, each of whom made a general self-portrait (with no limitations in the assignment instructions), attached it to a piece of cardboard, and added decorations, including written answers to some of my questions.

Rita made only the first image—a Polaroid self-portrait of herself; the second image, which I handed to her midway through our dialogue, was actually a blank sheet of cardboard the same size and color as the one she had applied her photo and pastels to. Jenny also made an instant-print self-portrait, and on another day, she made a second one to illustrate "who she would be if she weren't being who she was in the first snapshot." Rita did not permit me to include her self-portrait construction in this book along with her transcript. Jenny, however, did allow the use of both of hers, and they appear farther on in this section.

I include Rita's example, even without photos, to illustrate how verbal exploration of self-portraits can quickly move into areas of deep feelings and nonverbally stored memories, and also to demonstrate how comparisons of real with imagined photos can be integrated into helpful therapeutic process.

Jenny's is a good example of several processes (often interwoven): we contrasted what she is usually like with what she would like to express or feel if she could; we made use of her previous encounter with a photograph of a woman that Jenny felt called strongly to her (on which we had already spent over an hour in projective work) and rewove that into the self-portrait discussion; we then used these to delve farther into family issues of which she was not aware in her initial photo-interactions. Both transcriptions are given in full, with brackets enclosing my clarifications and descriptive notes.

Case Example: Rita

Rita: Things I like about this photo [self-portrait taken a half-hour earlier]? I put down [wrote on the cardboard] "directness of look," "smile," and "colors."

Judy: What about a picture of you where you weren't having that direct look, that directness of look, what would be the meaning of that?

Rita: I might think I was hiding, or afraid, or shy, or had something to hide, yeah, not open.

Judy: And if you were hiding or afraid or shy, where would the difficulty be in that? Would that not be OK?

Rita: Well, I think I've done that a lot, and I'm happy that I'm not doing it very much anymore. But that doesn't answer your question. Um, I value openness, so the difficulty is that I'm not living up to what I value.

Judy: Hold that picture up in one of your hands and look at it. Now, this instead [handing her a blank piece of same-sized cardboard] is another picture where you're not having that direct look. Can you see that? I'm seeing a person here that's full-frontal, full-facing, and you're saying that if you weren't giving that direct look, you have some idea in your mind what that would look like if you weren't. Can you get that thing in your mind out there onto that page visually so that you can talk about it? [she nods] What are you seeing?

Rita: I'm looking down, I'm avoiding the person who's photographing me or talking to me. I'm more concerned with my fears than connecting with that person.

Judy: Can you think of a time in your life where you've seen a picture of yourself that looks like that?

Rita: I've taken many pictures of myself that look like that, self-portraits. I haven't allowed other people to photograph me very much. But I do have pictures like that. And I'm aware of that.

Judy: [noticing that her eyes are slightly unfocused and her gaze into the photograph is intensified] Something in there is stronger than just the words you are talking about. What did you go back to [inside your mind] when we were talking about those pictures?

Rita: I went back to family albums, from my own family. And to images [her voice began to break somewhat], particularly images of my mother, who was a big smiler. And I used to resent her smiles very much. They never showed anything about what was going on inside. So I may be reacting to wanting to show what's going on inside me.

Judy: So a picture where you would see her with a big smile would mean what to you?

Rita: It would mean that I was cut off, that this was a performance on her part that was the same for everybody, and that she was hiding and therefore inaccessible to me. And I'm hiding when I'm looking down.

Judy: And you said that you found, when you looked at the pictures you did of yourself, that you were doing a lot of that glancing down. Yet I hear you say that you like the direct look here.

Rita: Because I feel open. I'm not looking down.

Judy: I think I see a smile [on the visible one].

Rita: But that's *my* smile; it's not my mother's smile. It's interesting, I don't know how to put those two together. It's interesting that when you asked me to look at that, pictures in the album are what come to mind.

Judy: So it's not *her* smile; what's the difference?

Rita: It's an honest smile; it's not a performance.

Rita said that her smile was spontaneous because she was thinking about her children. My thought traveled on several paths simultaneously: she has children and when she thinks of them she spontaneously smiles. Yet when her mother was photographed smiling, even smiling at Rita, to Rita that signaled being cut off. I became curious to explore smiles and their contexts and meanings. I also wanted to know more about Rita's family, her mother's photographs, and whether there were any Rita liked. It turned out that there was at least one photo of her mother Rita liked. She said about that one, "Interestingly enough, she's looking down. Sort of the opposite, exactly the opposite of this photo." I continued:

Judy: Have you ever photographed your mother?

Rita: Yes. I've never made a picture I like of her.

Judy: Have you made pictures she's liked?

Rita: I don't think; I don't show them to her.

Judy: Does she know you're photographing her? [Rita nodded yes] Does she ask to see them? [Rita shook her head no] Would you show her this one? [another nod yes] What would she say if she saw this one?

Rita: Oh, probably nothing much.

She continued for a while with small talk, saying her mother would talk about the clothes or environment and what was going on. Her mother would not likely ask about Rita's feelings, and she described this as their usual style of communication. I asked her, if this was typical, how she would answer.

Rita: I would just respond.

Judy: If this picture [of you] could talk to her, what kinds of things would it ask?

Rita: It would ask [she didn't finish the sentence, but paused for a long time, lost in thoughts inside herself].

Judy: [matching what I perceived to be Rita's major change of tone and affect by speaking much more softly] Can you let me in on some of that?

Rita: I was kind of wandering around, questioning whether I wanted to ask her or not. Whether I wanted to ask her how she was feeling, or tell her how I was feeling. What I wanted to do, I don't know.

Judy: [still speaking very softly] Can you imagine doing that?

Rita: Yeah, but it's only happened a very few times. It's not normal or comfortable.

Judy: For whom?

Rita: For me. Or for her; it's getting more so.

Judy: This here is a picture of your mother [handing her a piece of blank cardboard for that imaginary photo to "be" on]. Have the two photos [Rita's self-portrait and the imaginary portrait of her mother] look at each other for a while. Can you share with me some of what their interaction would be like?

Rita: Again, I'm not clear. Do you mean about what I'd like to have happen, or what has happened? Do you want me to stick to reality? Or just let this be something that's happening right now?

Judy: Your choice [I wasn't sure if I was encountering resistance or just an attempt to regain some control over the strong feelings she was encountering, so I made sure she was in charge of where we went next].

Rita: OK, I'll let it happen now. I'll say to her that she's looking, I'll say that I see your lovingness in this picture of you [note the switch in pronouns]. I see your lovingness there. And it's been hard for me to see that, and I'm happy to see it now. And she's saying, "I thought you'd never say that" [Rita smiled]. So I see her laugh [Rita paused].

Rita turned the conversation then to more mundane discussion about their age differences and her mother's usual way of being and of her standard poses for photographs. I asked Rita to imagine that the cardboard "photo" of her mother showed her at the same age Rita is now (forty-four).

Judy: So here is your picture today at forty-four, and this [the blank cardboard] is her at forty-four. Get a good look at them, and hand them to me if you will. If I then turn them around, this is still you and this is still her [indicating the different ones, which she could no longer see, except for their identical backs], then I can see them now and you can't. Get a good "fix" on them both and tell me what you see.

Rita: You mean describe the two images to you?

Judy: No, let them both be clear together. Now, *what* do you see?

Rita: I see that we're both smiling. I see that we're both concerned about who's taking the picture, that we're both vulnerable people with a lot of fears. That we're not that different. I hadn't thought that before.

Judy: You hadn't *thought* it before. In *feeling* it now, how does that thought feel?

Rita: Feels right. Feels all right. Feels, feels all right not to have to separate myself from her. Not to have to protect myself, that she's no longer going to do things that hurt me a lot when I was young [and she began to cry, saying that she felt relieved by it all].

By moving her indirectly into accepting a consideration of a comparison with her mother, I helped Rita to discover some previously unacceptable similarities she found between them. She had indicated earlier that her mother had been "shelved" in her mind to a relatively safe "role only" existence, and usually that suggests to me some therapy might be helpful to try to lessen their distance (or at least the power of its meaning). The process I used was a visual-photographic form of "anchoring" and then "collapsing anchors" (described in several books on neuro-linguistic programming methodologies; for example Bandler and Grinder, 1975, 1979, or Lankton, 1980). By having her work each photo image and then discuss them together, she unconsciously synthesized the two polarities.

By accepting the two seemingly exclusive opposites in her mind at the same time, a third option opened up: Rita and her mother may also have a lot in common, including their feeling hurt by each other. With the blank piece of cardboard standing for both real and imagined snapshots interchangeably, it becomes clear that it is the photograph inside the mind that is always being worked with, even when there is a real snapshot being held and looked at.

Case Example: Jenny

Jenny, a counselor for women and girls in crisis, attended a PhotoTherapy training workshop. On the first evening, she selected as her favorite photo my portrait of a woman, chin on elbow, looking out a window. Jenny decided that this woman was likely an artist or at least a student of fine arts, and that "she paints delicately and finely." When asked what the woman was thinking about, Jenny replied that "she was thinking of the one she loved" and that if she could speak, the woman would say, "When I'm with you I feel love in my heart." When I asked Jenny to assume the woman's pose, she reported feeling rather sad; "I am looking at a sunset and [it] fills me with sadness, and I am reminded of endings." She mentioned a memory of being with a lover in Mexico as the orange ball of the sun sank into the ocean. With that memory fresh in her mind, she went home that evening and looked through albums to find a sunset photograph, which she brought to the workshop the next day. She later commented that "I looked at the sunset picture and remembered all the trials and struggles of this old romance in Mexico—love relationships, the complications of trying to understand a loved one and be understood in return, and endings, are very much on my mind right now although at this point in the workshop I am not sure why."*

*This selection of material about Jenny's encounter with PhotoTherapy deals only with the self-portrait component of her work. Readers interested in the other therapeutic explorations this led to, such as the connections of this projective stimulus with earlier images of her mother, or what evolved from her concentration on 'endings' might find it worth reading the additional material on (and by) Jenny in Weiser, 1990, in which some of her direct quotes above have been previously published, used here with the permission of Jossey-Bass Publishers.

The assignment the next morning was to pose in any way desired for an instant-print self-portrait to use in visually introducing oneself. Jenny decided to carry through the theme from the night before and posed herself in a chair "looking out" at a sunset. Then she combined the photo of herself with the one of the sunset she'd brought from home on a cardboard sheet and wrote answers to my questions on it (see photo 4.12). "I posed like the woman in the photograph and was pleased with it. I labeled myself 'The Philosopher' [in response to the request to title the image]." The next day there was another self-portrait assigned, this time to go photograph "the you that you would be if you were not being the you who you are now." Although she claims it wasn't conscious, Jenny chose to make the second photo of her feet and lower legs, saying she particularly wanted the flowers on her shoes to show up. "I was pleased with the second picture too and labeled myself 'The Fool.'" To this photo on cardboard she added more artistic elaboration in the form of what seemed to be a figure in a colorful net tutu, which seemed to me, but not to her, to be more of a dancer than a court jester (see photo 4.13).

We began to discuss both of these photo-constructions together.

Jenny: In my first picture, I didn't have any feet, and I didn't deliberately do feet in the second picture, except that when I chose to do my feet I realized, well now, I gave myself my feet. And, so, the 'things I like' [responses] are easy to do for me, both of them, but when I say what I am missing in this first picture, well I really feel like I'm missing my feet. So I really like in the second picture that I've put in my feet.

Judy: Now that you have feet, what can you do?

Jenny: [smiling and immediately responding] Dance! It's almost like they're opposites. The first picture is captioned 'The Philosopher' and the second one's 'The Fool,' and in a way, maybe they're the same, but it's like I've got two opposite parts of myself in a whole picture.

Judy: I don't want to assume that I know what that ["Fool"] means to you.

Jenny: OK. Well, the Fool to me is like a court jester—joking, dancing, laughing—a helping-people-to-laugh kind of figure, and laughs at themselves.

Judy: And that's the one that you shot to be the you you would be if you weren't being the you you are now?

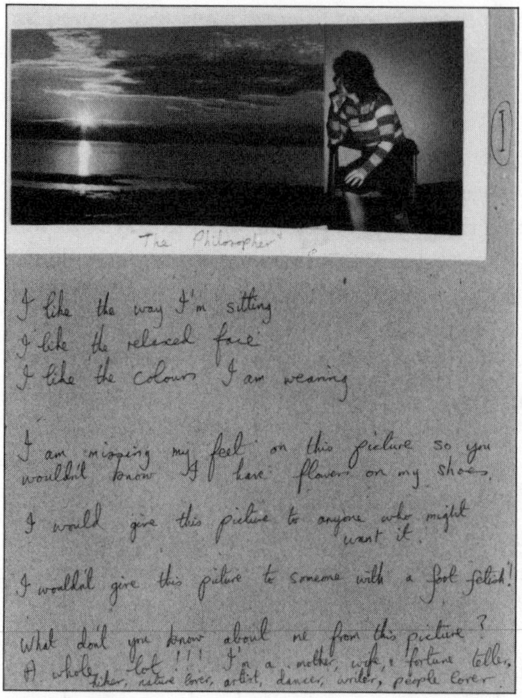
"The Philosopher"
I
I like the way I'm sitting
I like the relaxed face
I like the colours I am wearing
I am missing my feet on this picture so you wouldn't know I have flowers on my shoes.
I would give this picture to anyone who might want it.
I wouldn't give this picture to someone with a foot fetish!
What don't you know about me from this picture?
A whole lot!!! I'm a mother, wife, fortune teller, hiker, nature lover, artist, dancer, writer, people lover

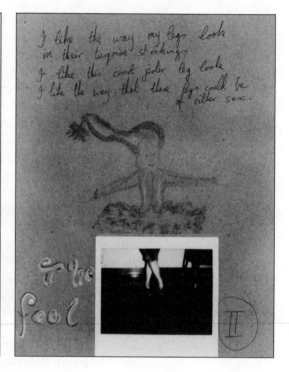

I like the way my legs look in their turquoise stockings
I like this court jester leg look
I like the way that these legs could be of either sex.
The Fool
II

Photo 4.12 *(left)*
Photo 4.13 *(right)*

Jenny: Uh-huh.

Judy: So the you you are now—

Jenny: Is a Philosopher.

Judy: What's the difference for you, Jenny?

Jenny: It's the lack of brain in the Fool that I like. It's the lack of having to use my brain, that seems to feel right.

Judy: The people around you, which are you to them?

Jenny: I think to my husband I'm clearly both.

Judy: Can you hold one of those in one hand and one in the other and have them talk to each other a bit for me?

Jenny: The Philosopher would say to the Fool [laughing playfully], 'Oh, you know, dance! For God's sake, relax! You're always thinking.' And the

Fool would say back, 'You're right. I don't really need to weigh everything out, or to think everything out so deeply. I mean I really could be a lot more spontaneous.' [Jenny pauses a bit, as if pondering with a wry and thoughtful face, and then continues more to me than to the photos.] I think that this Philosopher is a little worried that sometimes spontaneity gets her into trouble. I think that must come from the past, being a little girl that got into trouble, through just doing what she wanted to. I don't think I did what I wanted as a child very much. I feel like I was a typical good girl. I really pleased my parents. And now I really don't want to [grimacing], but it's a struggle. It's a struggle. [makes a sound like a gasping intake of breath, and continues with voice cracking] Oooh, that's a tough one [sniffles, smiles trying to lighten up a bit, which turns into more of a hysterical smile/sob and pauses for a few minutes of contemplation]. You know, I feel like I'm looking after them right now [teary eyes overflow at this point]. Yeah, I am looking after them right now [grins/grimaces through tears as if trying to regain emotional control]. And I never wanted to [said forcefully through gritted teeth]. And it makes me sick [laughing, crying, and gasping simultaneously; seems on the verge of hysterics]. It's like what I always feared, was one day I'd have to look after my parents, and it's like I looked after them all my f__ing life [another gasp-laugh-sob], and I know that I am looking after them again, and I didn't want to, but I suppose I thought, if I do it with awareness I could do it. I just can't give them up, I suppose.

Judy: [approaching closer to Jenny and speaking much more softly] Which one of these [versions of you] do they know?

Jenny: I think they know both.

Judy: Would they know who belonged to those feet?

Jenny: Yeah. Yeah, they would. [begins to really cry]

Judy: Does your mother ever dance? [this was a bit of a wild hunch on my part, but Jenny had discussed her dynamics with her mother previously and it seemed like a good possible parallel to explore, especially because the Fool would dance]

Jenny: Yeah.

Judy: What was she like when she danced?

Jenny: [less tears, sniffling a bit] She was a little more "loose" [smiles briefly at memory]. Not too much, still pretty uptight, but, you know, she could loosen up a little. She still can, when she dances a little bit.

Judy: She knew she was a little too loose?

Jenny: Well, she only danced for me. She only dances for me.

Judy: Was she concerned that dancing for anybody else might get her into any difficulty? [I asked this because of the parallel established above]

Jenny: I would say so, yeah.

Judy: So what did she do for you to protect you from that?

Jenny: She told me not to do certain things. You know, not to do anything. My mother said basically don't swim, don't run, don't climb, don't skate, [just] don't. You might fall and break your neck. You might drown. For God's sake *don't do anything* [voice quite angry], and you might stay alive or something like that. So I finally broke free of her and my father when I was twenty and came to Canada. Twenty years later, I bring them here to look after them.

Judy: What do you think she'd do if you gave her that picture?

Jenny: I think she'd laugh. I think she'd like it.

Judy: Do you think you've convinced her that you've heard her, and that you don't fall down and break your knee or skin your nose, or whatever else she was worried about?

Jenny: [laughs out loud] Almost, but I feel like I didn't tell her everything, and that is what's hard. I want to tell her everything. I want to open my big mouth and say I smoke and drink, I do things that you never did, but I'm *not* dead. I'm still alive.

Judy: What do you think she'd say if you did that?

Jenny: I've already tried it. I've already said it. I've done *that* one.

Judy: What did she do?

Jenny: Freaked!

In discussing the session afterward Jenny summed up her feelings about the Philosopher and the Fool: "The Philosopher is the worrier who worries about what others think, the one who wishes to please, the one who analyzes how to please, the one who is very alert, very present, wakes up with the sunrise. The Fool, however, is without a brain, is spontaneous and was spontaneous as a child, [and] hasn't a care about what others think."

When I asked her to reflect back on what happened when I asked her to hold up the two photographs facing each other and have them speak to one another, she remembered their dialogue a bit differently. She remembered the Philosopher saying, "I am alert and tuned in to people. I understand them because I listen so attentively. I please many people. I am a good girl," and the Fool saying, "I don't want to be a good person. I want to have fun, dance, play, and laugh. I want space for myself. I love to be alone with the sunset."

These responses were not what she said, but rather what she remembered saying; this is an example of why videotaping sessions can be so useful. Her later remarks are in the same vein as her original comments, yet they revise the details and shift the possible meanings. She said she remembered me asking her if it is safer to say she is a "Fool" than a "Dancer" (as the Fool appeared to me in the photo to be more of a dancer than a jester), and says she responded by saying "I have to admit that I would love to be a dancer and do love to dance, but it would seem conceited to say I am a dancer, since in a traditional sense I am not. Yet when I change the words to 'I am a dancer' instead of 'I am a Fool,' I experience this smile throughout my whole being which finally is expressed on my face." About my question regarding her mother dancing, she thought she answered, "The times that stand out for me were my mother dancing in the living room and trying to kick up over the door knob. She would laugh and express joy as she danced, and she would appear worry-free for once. She only danced for her children though. She certainly *didn't* dance for my father."

One point that came up in discussing the process we'd done above was that Jenny explained to me that her mother had been schizophrenic, and she remembers several times standing alone as the ambulance men carried her mother out strapped to a stretcher to take her to the hospital for a "cooling down" time. It turned out that when her mother was the most loose was also when she was heading into a manic state, so for Jenny the spontaneous playfulness she wished to experience herself and see in her mother had embedded in it this edge of danger and unpredictable consequences.

This knowledge made her two cardboards even more "loaded" for further processing possibilities. She found that what she was trying to do for herself in her relationship with her mother was somewhat parallel to wanting to be more spontaneous and less analytical, less concerned about how she would react. She said she wanted to get to the point where she could feel anger and express it. "I do disagree with my mother sometimes, but it doesn't mean I don't love her. Maybe I blame her and say that she doesn't allow me to express what I need to express. I blame her for being crazy. The times when she's being schizophrenic or out of touch with reality still happen and I still feel uncomfortable. But I don't want to express that [because] I guess I have the belief that I could throw her over the edge. I wouldn't want to do that; I wouldn't want to take the risk." This is the direction I thought further therapy could help her go.

Final Considerations

One quick introductory self-portrait assignment, with no conditions or limitations except that it truly be created by self, produced instant-print photos stuck onto cardboard for Rita and Jenny. The initial assignment was the same, yet the contents and processing were very different owing to the nature of the women's distinct identities and issues. It becomes clear that the reality and truth of photographs exist only in the eye of the beholder, and that there can be great therapeutic benefits to using these stimuli to connect with emotional material that clients may not be aware of.

Synchronicity plays a large role in PhotoTherapy, such as Jenny "just happening" to leave off her feet in the first photo, or her memory being triggered by the image of the woman gazing out the window. These sorts of "accidental" happenings are ripe with possibilities if the therapist uses them as catalysts.

SAMPLE EXERCISES

There are two basic stages to working with self-portraits. The first involves creating the snapshot itself (or at least imagining such an image), whether or not further embellishment is added using writing or art materials. The second involves interaction with this self-portrait based on the therapist's suggestions and questions. The exercises presented in this section follow the same sequence, first giving readers suggestions on how to direct clients to make their self-portraits, including art enhancements if desired, and then a section of questions that can be asked about these images once their creation is finished. In fact, these questions can be effective with any photos clients feel are true depictions of themselves, including those that exist only in their minds, in fantasy or memory.

Preliminary Considerations:

The most nonthreatening kind of a self-portrait is one that involves no expectations, such as the kind I ask participants in a group or workshop to make to be used simply to introduce themselves visually, instead of using only words written on name tags. This can be easily adapted to individual psychotherapy settings; a client might be asked to just "play around" with the therapist's camera and take a photo that captures who they are or how they are feeling that particular day, with no rules given about what to do or not do.

If that still seems a bit too direct or threatening, clients can be asked to take a "generic" self-portrait that shows who they usually are, what they are like in general. If clients are clearly told there are no conditions or expectations apart from this photo needing to be their very own creation and not influenced by others, then they really are free to do whatever they want; any result will be acceptable and won't be judged.

As an easy means for getting started, therapists might suggest to clients that they examine a list of choices for self-portrait topics, such as those listed below, and choose the ideas that most interest them (or if none do, then to feel free to make up their own). This is not an exclusive "finished" list; readers may want to compile a selection appropriate to each particular client's needs. But this somewhat generic collection of suggestions often serves to show clients the range of possible choices. Often there will be therapeutically relevant information just in the reasons clients give for picking certain topics and rejecting others.

Initial Self-Portrait Assignments

The following is a good selection of beginner-level assignments. The instruction to the client is "go photograph any of the following that interest you."

1. The me of today (who I am right now, me as I am by myself)
2. The me I like (and, if desired, the me I don't like)
3. The past, present, and future me
4. Me acting out my goals, hopes, dreams for the future
5. The me my neighbors see; the me my boss, co-workers, friends, teachers, and/or strangers think I am (or will be)
6. The me nobody knows; the me my parents don't know
7. The less-obvious me; the secret me
8. Me as symbolized in other objects or places
9. Me showing some of my strongest feelings (both "good" ones and "bad" ones, like anger, sadness, happiness, love, hatred, jealousy, etc.)
10. My strengths and weaknesses (good points and bad points, what I do well and what I don't)
11. The young and old aspects of me; the masculine and feminine aspects of me
12. The me I would be if I weren't being the me I am now
13. Myself in twenty (ten) (five) (forty) (__) years (*choose any number of years to put in the blank);* or, me when I become my mother's (or father's) age
14. Me showing the changes I'd like to have happen in myself
15. Myself as I wish others could or would see me
16. The me I want my children or grandchildren to remember me as being
17. Myself if this was the last photograph ever possible to be made of me (or if it were going in a time capsule to the future hundreds of years from now)

Additional Initial Assignment Suggestions:

Even less threatening are assignments such as asking the client to make self-portraits showing themselves in different situations or settings, such as photographing themselves at each hour of the day and night, or at certain times each day of the week, or on the same day of the week every week for a month—just to get an idea of the variety of the client's activities and "who" he or she consistently is.

Similar self-study assignments might be requests for photographs of just their eyes or mouth; face only; head and shoulders only; full body;

back view; standing with eyes closed; lying in bed with eyes open and eyes closed, from above and from the side; in bed dressed; in bed with nightclothes; standing dressed (front or back); in their favorite chair; in their favorite place or room in the house or their favorite place outdoors; alone and with significant others, such as spouse, lover, family members, parents, grandparents, or friends; themselves expressing different emotions; themselves with a photograph of someone close who is now dead or living very far away; themselves with a pet, hobby, job, car, sport, favorite books, food, occupying their usual roles at work or home (or other roles), and so forth.

Clients could even be asked to photograph themselves in places where people are not usually photographed at all (routine places such as the grocery store, the dentist's office, the bus stop, the church, the laundromat, and so forth). All these suggestions are ways for people to begin to get fuller pictures of their own lives for themselves, and the actual assignments are limitless in possibility. Often clients themselves come up with good ideas for further assignments.

If these kinds of assignments are still a bit too abrupt or directly confrontational, one even less threatening way self-portrait work can be started is to ask clients to take self-portrait photographs in which they do not physically appear. In other words, the therapist can ask them to do the above assignments using stand-ins for themselves, such as objects with personal meaning or that represent them (clothing, books, coffee mugs, and so forth). They can produce metaphorical self-portaits that speak clearly of themselves to themselves, even though the client's face and body are not included in the snapshots.

In explaining to the therapist how each photo completes the assignment, clients can begin to reflect upon and present signals of their inner values, beliefs, cognitive mapping structures, and so forth, which the therapist will need to learn about anyway. This can be a rather safe way for clients to provide some of that information without feeling as much violation of personal boundaries as when directly questioned.

More Complex Levels of Self-Portrait Assignments

Once clients have photographed the comparatively simple projects from the "beginners list" above, the therapist can begin to further tailor additional assignments to better mesh with the client's own particular situation.

The suggestions that follow, which are much too open-ended in design to list as step-by-step assignments, are a sampling of the many branching directions the therapist can take once therapy is fully underway. Clients can be asked to answer the following kinds of questions by means of actual or imaginary self-portraits. These will constitute visual responses, which, of course, can then be further "worked" through additional questions such as those given in the final part of this section.

1. Photograph yourself showing the things that are most troubling you right now, how you are coping with them at present, and the things that are blocking you from solving them. Try to use the camera to make clear pictures of these problems for yourself (and the therapist), in order to see them better and gain some control over them. Photograph yourself as you are now and then as you would be if these troubles were not part of your life.

2. Do you feel any strong pulls within you that could be expressed as dualities having, for example, positive and negative components or that contrast realities such as past and present or real and ideal? These could be polarities, or "warring factions," within you, such as your needs and your wants; the good and bad, right and wrong, or angel and devil parts of you; the "light" and "dark" sides of you; your actual and fantasy parts, liked (wanted, desired) parts and disliked (unwanted, undesired) parts; young and old aspects of you, child and adult aspects, your mother in you and your father in you; or emotional extremes, such as happy and sad, future-fearing and future-anticipating. Try to get a single self-portrait that captures each polar extreme as a different quality or part of yourself and your life. You could also try to get a photograph of yourself that manages to encompass both aspects at once.

3. If you were to have your picture taken as a gift for someone you love (spouse, lover, friend, or even yourself), how would you like it to look? How would you dress? What sorts of background or special objects might you want to include? Would you include any props or other people? What sorts of postures or facial expressions would you want? Would you want to include only your face (head-and-shoulders) or more of your body? Take a moment to build this image, and then, keeping it in your mind, contemplate whether this image would also be acceptable as a gift to one or both of your parents (or grandparents), or whether you could easily give it to your boss or a stranger. What would have to change? Would you want those people to have your photo? If so, would you be willing to change to meet their conditions in order to do it?

4. Imagine that you are going to a family or school reunion and have been asked to make some photographs that would describe yourself and explain your life to people who haven't seen you in ten years. What sorts of images and information would you want to make sure got included?

5. What if you were taking photos of yourself to send to a relative who has never met you? How would you want to pose and what would you want to make sure to include? What if you wanted to send photos of yourself to someone who expressed interest in dating you? What would these sorts of snapshots have to look like to express your attractiveness? Would these be different from the earlier kinds, and if so, in what ways would they need to differ? What if you had reason to want to express how unattractive you could appear to someone? Could you picture what this would look like?

6. Is there any aspect of potential in yourself that you have never risked exploring and would now like to, such as being of the opposite sex, being an animal or an object, yourself in a highly erotic pose, in a bath, asleep, as a movie star, in a past or future life, before your birth or being born (or even after your death), yourself as royalty or the richest or most powerful person on earth, you if you were the therapist instead of me, you if you were your own parent or child—in short, yourself in a completely different identity? If so, why not try it out? No one is watching, and you don't have to show anyone, including the therapist, if you don't want to.

Debriefing the Self-Portraits Produced During Assignments

Once clients have in hand some version of a self-portrait, the second stage of the process can begin; this is reviewing and discussing the image and the client's experiences with it. The numerous illustrative examples and transcripts that have accompanied this chapter indicate the sorts of things I think are important to probe in the particular situations given, and the suggested questions provided in the section "Working with Clients' Self-Portraits" can also be helpful guidelines. But as mentioned before, these are all just stimuli to therapeutic process, and each therapist must tailor interventions to particular clients' needs.

This process can be as simple as asking the client to tell you about a new photo of him- or herself, using open-ended "request" questions, like "Tell me more about this, please." Or "Why was this the self-portrait you decided to make?" In addition to taking note of the persons shown in the picture, it is often useful to take careful note of background details and other potentially important information, by using such questions as: "Why did you pick that place to be photographed?" "What is it about these particular surroundings that made them your first choice for posing and placing yourself?" "What might you be wishing to additionally signal by choosing this location, these props (or objects, pets, or even other people), which you consciously included in your own picture? What part of you does this additional information give clues about?" "What things in the photo—except for your body—are included accidentally rather than intentionally? Now that you have discovered them, can you shed any light on what they might convey? Of the things that you did consciously pick to have with you in your portrait of yourself, why did you select these things in particular, and what other layers of meanings or messages (family, cultural, secret others) might they be carrying in addition to their individual personal ones?" "If the person in this photograph (yourself) died or moved away, and this photo was viewed by utter strangers (perhaps many years later or in a foreign country, or [my own favorite] by someone from outer space), what would they learn about the person in this photo? What would be forever lost to them, in their lack of understanding of the special coded details in the picture?"

The client's photo can stand alone as referent for the questions suggested below, or the client can be asked to include additional art expression and/or written elements in combination with the snapshot. The questions listed below should not be asked all together in the same session. Some might be sequenced within one day's encounter with the self-portrait; others might be better used in combination with other techniques, like album or projective work.

Begin by asking the client to study the photo (or photo-art production) and use *it,* not themselves, as the basis for responding to the following items.

1. Three things I like about this photo:
2. The most obvious thing(s) about this photo:
3. How I would describe the person in this photo to someone unable to see it:
4. Three things you wouldn't know about me from this photo:
5. My title for this photo (or a caption for it):
6. The message of this photo:
7. The secrets in this photo:

8. Three needs this photo has or might want to have:
9. Three feelings this photo has or might want to have:
10. Three feelings stimulated in me by seeing this photo:
11. What, if anything, is missing from this photo? (If the photo is incomplete, what is needed in order to complete it?)
12. Who or what this photo reminds me of, or stimulates in my memory:
13. Looking at this photo now, it seems that it was taken for ____ (specify person or persons) because:
14. Three ways this photo fits and doesn't fit my general way of being in my regular daily life:
15. If this photo (or person in the photo) could speak, what would it say or want to say? (Imagine words coming from it, as in the comic strips with speech bubbles.)
16. If this photo (or person in the photo) could come alive and be able to move what might it do or want to do?
17. What might I like to ask this photo, if I could? What might it want to ask me?
18. What would I like to tell this photo, if I could? What would I like it to know?
19. What would this photo like to tell me if it could? What would it like me to know?
20. Three things this photo would like to change about itself (or that I would like to change in it):
21. Things I expect will (or will not) change in it or I hope will (or will not) change in it:
22. If I could give this photo to someone, I would give it to ____ (or, I would *like* to give it to):
23. I would definitely *not* give it to ____ (a person who definitely could *not* have it):
24. If either of my parents (or: my close friends/lover/child/my significant other/strangers) saw this photo, they would likely react by: ____.

    They would likely say ____, think ____, feel ____, do ____, or worry about ____.
25. If I were the therapist for the person in this photo, I would probably have the following perceptions about my client: ____. I would also want to ask the person (or the photo) the following questions:

Assignments for self-portrait work frequently mirror and even often duplicate assignments given to clients to "go photograph x or y," for the simple reason that when the assignments are self-focused the client's body often ends up being included in these pictures. So in considering self-portrait work outside the immediate therapeutic session, therapists should probably take time to consider commentary and suggestions given elsewhere regarding photos taken by the client and photos of the client.

The self-portrait image used as the referent for the above list of questions can also be "worked" using most of the questions suggested in Chapter Three, on projective techniques. Therefore readers might also want to review that chapter when engaging in reviewing and discussing self-portrait snapshots. For example, clients could be asked to pretend they can expand the borders of their self-portrait, to discover what else might have been included if the "frame" had been larger. Similarly they can be asked to imagine how they might choose to crop the picture if they had to cut it down to half, a quarter, or even a tenth of its present size, without the important part of the image itself being reduced. Put another way, if the client could only have a portion of the image, where would the smaller rectangle have to be placed for the photo to not lose its identity, meaning, or essential communication of the subject? Such partializing questions (first presented in Chapter Three) can be helpful in assisting clients to focus their visually embedded perceptions of themselves.

If relationship or family issues are what is being therapeutically explored (or if the therapist prefers a systems/cybernetics therapy approach), other questions could be added or substituted to probe these extra dimensions, such as asking the client to answer questions in the above list again, this time as they think their mother (father, lover, other significant person) would.

Changing viewpoints can also be done as a family self-portrait exercise, so that the family poses for the photo and then answers the questions as a single unanimous unit. The process of coming to agreements about poses and answers can be a great exercise in family dynamics, alignments, interactions, power struggles, triangulation, fusion, and other nonverbally communicated facets.

5 Seeing Other Perspectives

Examining Photographs of Clients Taken by Others

Readers may find the following comments quite familiar. "Wait a minute. My hair's not right." "You like that photo of me? Uck! I think it's dreadful!" "I don't mind you having a snapshot of me, but only from the shoulders up until I lose more weight." "Oh, I can never relax in front of the camera. Just hurry up and take the picture anyway 'cause it won't look right no matter what I do." "No, it's not all right to take my picture." "Wow, you made me look absolutely wonderful! Thank you!" These kinds of comments are likely to sound familiar to anyone who has ever tried to take a picture of someone else. Most of us have opinions about how photographs of us will or should turn out, and most of us nevertheless cooperate with the photographer, unless we strongly dislike the person wanting to capture our image on their film. Sometimes we arrange to have photos taken of us, for example, in portrait studios. However, these are in a sense like self-portraits because we keep most of the control over production and possession of the image.

This chapter is about those other kinds of photos made of us by friends, family members, or even strangers: snapshots made for other people's reasons rather than our own. Although we are often permitted to view the results and sometimes welcome to give our honest feedback, the photograph is theirs, not ours, to keep. And while it is a photo of us, it shows us through someone else's eyes and perceptual filters.

The key word in speaking of photographs is *take,* and in a sense, photographers "take" us; we become partly theirs, at least metaphorically. Their "having" us is a demonstration that some sort of a relationship or interaction between us has occurred. If we know them well, or at least trust their intentions, we may be more comfortable letting them "catch" us unposed than if we are not certain about their purposes or expectations. Regardless, most of us will, perhaps unconsciously, want to compare the picture that was taken with the one we had imagined in our mind. It is human nature to scan dozens of photographs of parties, family gatherings, and the like, unconsciously looking most for our own image, to compare it with how we thought we would or should appear.

We don't usually view photos of ourselves and think "That's my friend's version of how I look." Rather we look at those snapshots and think "That's me! That's what I really look like," forgetting that we are seeing through another person's perceptual filters. Particularly if we are dissatisfied with the image, we will often turn our criticism inward and perceive ourselves as *being* unattractive, clumsy, unlovable, and so forth, instead of recognizing that we are only viewing one split-second of our life's possibilities pulled from the flow of time surrounding it, and in addition, it is someone else's constructed version of us that we are examining. Although some people prefer not to look at photos of themselves, or are quite adamant about not wanting to be photographed at all (both of which might imply deep psychological process about self-perception or self-esteem), most people are interested in seeing how they appear in photographs.

While reading this sentence, ask yourself the following question: if you knew you were having your photograph taken at this very moment by a friend, by a stranger, by someone you trust (or don't), would you still be in exactly the same physical position or frame of mind? It is likely that the idea of a camera pointed at you makes you suddenly self-aware. You are probably more conscious of yourself and your body. To the degree that you are aware of the camera, it is an invasion into the ordinary flow of your life and personal privacy. Taking someone's picture without their permission is always to some degree an act of violation, no matter how well-intended. The intrusion is always there in the form of objectification, no matter how innocent the photographer's desire to possess the image. Even when the subject is willing and the photographer's goal honorable, there is a shift of interpersonal power that puts a relationship out of its natural balance.

"Accidental" metaphoric extensions of us in the form of our personal surroundings, background environment, and other people are simultaneously appropriated as being part of us when someone photographs us in our own setting. In reexamining photos of us to look at everything except our own bodies, we may uncover patterns or themes about what or who we habitually surround ourselves with—things we may be so familiar with that we haven't noticed them before as being significant. Such patterns can help us in our search for better self-knowledge.

This potential dissonance can be therapeutically beneficial, especially when used constructively to contrast our view of ourselves with others' perceptions of us. Sometimes what other people treasure most about us is something we may not even be aware of (or worse, that we dislike about our appearance, like freckles or a pug nose). Sometimes what we think is an important nonverbal signal to others may not even be noticed by them.

How we think we are seen is usually very different from how others see us. We think we control their reactions to us by how we present ourselves, but that is just the first of many layers surrounding our ideas and feelings about our appearance. It can also be therapeutically useful to reverse this process; that is, to recognize that what we perceive about them may not be what they think they are showing us. Thus it is useful to compare others' visual documentations of us with our own inner pictures of ourselves to see what else we can learn from looking at ourselves from an outside viewpoint.

HOW THIS TECHNIQUE WORKS

This chapter will focus on photographs made of clients by other people. These are usually spontaneous situations or at least moments when the subjects had little or no control over component details shown along with their own bodies or faces. Photos taken by others of someone or something else, where clients were included only by accident are also in this category. These photos can be of potential therapeutic use, even though they may not have resulted from any direct action by the clients.

The Photograph of the Client

When people are consciously posing for photos, they sometimes are concerned not only with how their bodies and faces appear but also with having certain people, pets, objects, or other symbolic "markers" in the photo with them. Conversely, sometimes people want to remove certain objects or evidence of others' existence from the camera's gaze to prevent their relationships with these objects or other people being discovered by later viewers; for example, daughters may not include any sign of their live-in boyfriends when having friends take pictures that their parents might see. These are the kinds of things that happen when a person has some control over what appears with him or her in a photograph. Such managed pictures are somewhat like self-portraits in that there has been some degree of collaboration with the photographer. The things and people included in or excluded from self-directed portraits connect metaphorically to the self-image the subject hoped to communicate to others.

When a snapshot is not self-directed, however, but is rather taken unexpectedly, with no preparation, the environment around the subject will be captured along with the person by virtue of accidental association. If someone passes by with a camera and spontaneously takes a person's picture, much more than the person's corporeal figure will be encompassed by the lens.

The camera records everything that its viewfinder "sees," but people see selectively, especially when focusing on a person of interest. Thus in daily life we unconsciously tune out parts of the environment that are not relevant to what we are attending to, such as telephone poles behind people, which appear in photos to be growing out of their heads. The camera may seem to "mischievously" insert facts into the frame that we are not conscious of when seeing the "live" image; sometimes these can produce therapeutically useful surprises in the finished print. These surprises can be positive as well as negative in effect, such as presenting visual proof of desired physical changes.

One client told me that she had arranged to have some publicity photos made for her company brochure. She wanted the usual head-and-shoulders professional image. She rejected the resulting photographs, however, because in rearranging the books and knickknacks on the bookshelf in the background, the photographer had made visible an artistic postcard of a naked man a friend had sent her as a joke. This accidentally included background detail completely altered the professional image she had wanted to present.

Another woman had her desk at work covered with photos of grandchildren and pets, all sitting on little crocheted doilies. Work was her home away from home, and she had made it as "homey" as she could. She was photographed at her desk for the company's annual report, and that picture allowed her to see her environment as others did: cluttered, unprofessional, and too heavily decorated to leave space for her work folders.

When subjects ask photographers to explain why they organized a picture as they did, or why they picked one particular image from the whole roll of possibilities to have enlarged for the subject, people can learn how different parts of their identities are valued. For example, one man was told, "I chose to give you this one snapshot because it was the 'real' you, because you weren't smiling. I think you use your smile to cover what you are really feeling, and it's only when you're quiet and still and without a smile that I feel I am seeing the person you really are inside, the one I want to know." A client who is very overweight told me of her pleasure in happening to overhear her husband showing his recent snapshot of her to a friend and saying, "This is my wife. Isn't she beautiful?"

When a client shows a therapist photographs of him- or herself, it can often be helpful to ask that person about the background elements that appear in the picture, such as room decorations, furniture, or the landscape. Any such objects, pets, people, or details like plants or curtains may have significance, either by plan or synchronistic, "accidental" inclusion. All could be potential communicators of important information, feelings, memories, expectations, and so forth.

Sometimes ordinary photos of us can speak for us when we cannot ourselves find the words, as the following anecdote illustrates. During a three-hour plane flight, I sat next to a woman who spoke no English. After we exhausted smiles and nods, she reached into her purse and pulled out a paper-wrapped collection of photos. Laying them out on the food tray, she managed to convey to me not only where she was from (photos of her standing in front of a mosque, carrying a full basket in a field, and sitting beside a doorway of a farmhouse whose windows were filled with flowers), but also where she was going (herself hugging adult children and numerous giggling grandchildren in front of Disneyland and seated on an overstuffed couch surrounded by most of the same group). Hugging the photos to her chest, she conveyed to me with her smiles what her words could not: she loved them all and was loved back in return, especially by the grandchildren. She pointed again to the photos and then to me with a questioning look, so I fished out my wallet to show her my comparatively meager collection of pictures of my personal life and loves. With much pointing, nodding, and smiling, we had a great time "conversing."

It is, of course, important to observe and explore the client's choice of pose, clothing, adornments, such as jewelry, hats, makeup, class ties, and so forth. What reasons a client can give for deciding how to dress, pose, smile or not, make eye contact or not, and so forth, can be therapeutically relevant information. The way emotional affect is shown and expected to be perceived by others is a major consideration in exploring photos of clients. Can people read their expressions in the way they wish? Can they clearly communicate their feelings when they wish to, and not when they don't? These are also important aspects of photos of the client. Of course, it is also important to pay attention to the actual body and facial image presented by the subject.

People have different identities, images, scripts, gestures, and so forth, depending on the situations, social settings, and perceived expectations they encounter. They may use one rather "generic" neutral facial presentation when they do not have enough information about the people they are with to fine-tune their responses. This "public" identity may not let anyone else know who is "inside there." Because people often alter their physical and emotional presentations depending on who they are with and what they are doing, snapshots of them (particularly unposed ones) may well show strikingly different identities being revealed to different photographers, but not consciously. Photos of a client by different photographers may also vary according to the client's interpretation of why the photographer is there in the first place.

There is never just one single version of the truth of ourselves. Images of us may vary widely and none are particularly more privileged than any others. Photos of us by many various friends will show many different "truths" of our identity. Liking the resulting portrait does not necessarily make it any more truthful a depiction of us than those we strongly dislike. Even finding out *why* the photo of a person was taken in the first place can be useful information. For example, one client told me that as the only child of divorced parents, she was always being photographed by each of them. She sometimes felt that each wanted the pictures to show an ideal happy child who loved them rather than her true self, who was often unhappy and unable to express her feelings to either parent.

Many photos are taken of people merely to document their having been at a certain place; I call these "me-ats" (me-at-the-zoo, me-at-my-mom's, me-at-the-office-party, and so forth). Such photos may never draw much interest, or they might be retrieved from storage, perhaps to be re-examined or compared with later snapshots, because they provide a missing piece of a puzzle (as illustrated in Chapter Two in the story of my strong response to a photo of my husband-to-be and myself holding hands.) If a person knew she or he was going to be photographed and was given some choice in arranging the setting or pose, there could also be value in exploring the meanings embedded in those decisions.

Not only should the things in photographs of the client be considered, but attention should also be paid to any other people captured spontaneously in snapshots along with the client. How we relate with others when we don't know we are being observed can be very different from our behavior when we know that other people are watching. A photograph makes interactions between people permanent; the proof will last as long as the photo does, even if the actual interpersonal dynamics changed long ago.

Just as the significance of details may not be recognized until long after the fact, aspects of relationships may not become conscious until a good deal of time has passed. So many of our inner processes, conflicts, and feelings take place below the level of conscious awareness that we often do not become aware of them until we can see ourselves from an outsider's point of view. These are usually things which we have been censoring from our minds, even though our bodies have long been trying to get us to listen.

A woman told me that she had decided to break off with her boyfriend because "there was just too much manipulation from him in the past for me to be able to interpret anything from him as anything other than just more manipulation. He thought we should be married right away, no waiting, because he didn't want to be alone after his divorce. It didn't take me long to figure out that he was totally unable to accommodate another person's self. He used up all my patience and emotional energy, and you know what? One of the things that prompted me to make my final decision against any sort of permanent liaison with him was the sudden awareness that in every single picture of the two of us together, taken by other people or his camera's timer, he was grasping my neck, possessively, smotheringly, insecurely. Every damn picture—I felt I was under attack all the time, totally sapped, all my strength used to reassure him. My friends would comment about the photos, [saying] things like 'he certainly sticks close,' but I didn't really hear them."

Snapshots taken spontaneously of the client with others can demonstrate dynamics of relationships (what you are like when not aware you are being observed), and examining this "proof" can strengthen those bonds and enrich the connections of the relationship depicted. We tend to believe that what is photographed is made permanent: a client told me he didn't mind being with his new girlfriend in public but shied away from any snapshots friends wanted to take of the two of them together because they weren't yet a couple; their private relationship wasn't fixed; and he didn't want to risk documenting something that might not last.

Worried statements about photos that show relationships are likely to indicate a fairly conditional arrangement. A client's willingness to be "frozen" permanently on film with another person is likely to indicate mutual comfort and trust. Clients with low self-esteem can work on raising it a bit by being photographed with people who are significant in their lives and using the pictures to explore what such relationships are or aren't (really and/or potentially) like. Sometimes the excuse that "my therapist gave me this homework to be photographed with you" helps to break the ice and permit the bonding that clients themselves might not risk initiating on their own.

For therapists interested in family systems perspectives, photos of clients with others, especially family members, can provide a wealth of information about family power alignments, triangulation, emotional cutoffs, mirroring, and other behaviors. Certainly these sorts of photographs can serve as the stimuli for many questions about the feelings surrounding the viewing of photographs that other people have taken of the client.

Systems-oriented assignments can be given, such as asking the client to bring in (or make) new photos that show her or him with each member of the family or with photos of deceased ones. These can be used later to explore similarities and differences among people and to discuss intergenerational patterns. The client may be able to communicate difficult information by discussing photos of themselves taken by each family member, either old or new ones, possibly ones assigned by the therapist to illustrate a variety of themes (you at your best or worst, as they think you are or as they think you think you are, as you are alone or as part of the family, and so forth). Client and therapist then compare all the images to see what emerges. A good deal of the significance of such photographs rests in what they mean to each different family member and the conversations and feelings they precipitate.

Theories of objective self-awareness discussed earlier with regard to self-portrait work have relevance here as well, in that examining photos others have taken of us, even ones we requested or posed for, gives us a view of ourselves from an outside position. It is obvious in all PhotoTherapy work that participant-observers looking at something they are part of (including photos of themselves) will see and understand things differently than outside-observers will. When one person tries to play both roles simultaneously, the consequent cognitive or emotional dissonance can push him or her into the therapeutic process of confronting and changing his or her internal self-image.

It is difficult to argue with what a photograph shows you of yourself. When a photograph shows you the opposite of something you have long believed to be true, your mind can rarely hold both concepts without some synthesis or compromise taking place. Either one reality or the other will usually undergo quick and unconscious redefinition and reframing in memory. Blaming the photographer is one frequent explanation of this; however, clients quickly discover that this excuse brings on its own confrontational issues, as well as additional dissonance if one perceives oneself as having been visually distorted by more than one or two photographers. They cannot all be out to "get" the client.

I have found it particularly interesting to observe clients' cognitive duels when confronting photos that do not match what they think they look like. I have frequently heard comments like, "I know what this photo shows, but it really wasn't like that at all" or "I know there are lots of photos of my mom hugging me and playing with me, but I know she really didn't love me and didn't want to spend much time with me." When a photographic record of a person or event collides with the participant's radically different perception of the same moment of real life, therapeutically exciting consequences can result.

The Relationship with the Photographer

One significant difference between self-portraits made by clients and photos others create of them is the differential power relationships between the client and each person who photographs him or her. The reality of the moment will have been filtered and mapped by the photographer in a way that differs from the subject's perception. The purposes and timing of the photo lie within that photographer's control, and the subject may find him- or herself a relatively powerless object of the photographer's manipulation, rather than a person whose rights and needs are acknowledged and respected.

When we examine photographs, we may forget that we are seeing the photographer's construction of a reality. We cognitively perceive people in a photo being as they really were at that moment, rather than as they may have been asked to pose for a photographer. Children and teenagers in particular seem to blur this distinction, which makes them more vulnerable to advertising and also sometimes makes them confused about the power of the photographer to actually alter the subject's reality (and the subject's right to refuse to let this happen). Many people, particularly youth, often unconsciously blur the distinction between what is pictured and what simply is, and may reverse the causality; then they may be encouraged to buy a product because the people pictured using it seem so happy.

A rather poignant example of this was given by a client who was permitted to use the family camera when she was around nine or ten years old. Her parents noticed that she kept photographing her younger sister, with whom she had a very close relationship. This sister had Down syndrome, and had told my client that she was always sad because people made fun of her all the time. My client had taken all those photographs of her sister because, she told me, "All the photographs I had ever seen of people showed them smiling and looking happy. I truly believed that being photographed *made* people happy and thought that I was an utter failure because no matter how many snapshots I took of my sister, this never cheered her up like it was supposed to! Sometimes she even smiled in them like she was 'supposed' to, but this alone didn't produce the happiness that I believed was supposed to result. I was disappointed a lot, because although she looked happy, she wasn't, and this was too much confusion of reality to me. To this day, I don't trust photographs people take of me."

Sometimes spontaneously taken snapshots, where the photographer gives little forethought and the subject has little warning, take on altogether different meanings when viewed years later. One client brought me a photograph she had kept since childhood. It had been taken by a neighbor, who was a professional photographer, at her family's home swimming pool. She was just entering puberty, and the photograph was made to document her wearing her first two-piece bathing suit ("But you'd hardly call it a bikini!"). Her whole family was in the pool, splashing around.

Her father, "who liked me best when I seemed still a little girl," was treading water near the edge of the pool where she was standing. "I was clowning around with him, and I playfully pushed his head under water with my foot, so that the only thing you see in this photo is my coquettish pose, smiling triumphantly, with this hand coming up out of the water like a drowning man grasping for help. This image has always come to mind for me when thinking about the hard time my father had with my growing up and starting to date and wear makeup and all that stuff. He was horrified with this picture and forbade me to wear that bathing suit anywhere but at home. I think our neighbor probably saw it as a 'kiddie cheesecake' kind of shot. To me this photo, more than any other, shows the change in our relationship and the end of his control over my budding womanhood."

Allowing oneself to be photographed requires that one have some degree of trust in the photographer, no matter how tenuous. It requires (and results in) a relationship of some sort in order for the photographic interchange to occur at all. It is itself a form of communication, no matter how willing or unwilling either party may be to the photo-taking process. If you aren't comfortable being photographed (giving someone with a camera some power over you), then this will likely be communicated nonverbally somehow in the resulting image, regardless of how much you try to hide it or whether it is obvious to anyone looking at the snapshot later. The discomfort that existed at the time will always constitute a facet of the meaning of that photograph for you.

Sometimes a hint of discomfort has pointed the way to helping clients get back in touch with abuse issues from childhood. Reviewing old photos they appear in, we talk about the feelings they recall, such as how it felt to be photographed that day by that person, perhaps what the photo would say if it could speak its own truth, or perhaps how the client would have really posed for that photographer if given a choice about doing so. Many underlying power issues and imbalances are recalled through such discussions, and it is sometimes useful to have the client actually go back and reconstruct the images (revise their "truth" or even rephotograph it) to create a more honest representation of that moment. Issues of control are often crystallized through the dynamic of who is allowed to photograph whom, when, and under what conditions.

When clients have been abused, it is not uncommon to find numerous snapshots of them in poses that demonstrate distancing from others, avoiding eye contact with the lens, turning their face from the camera, attempting to hide or diminish their size or visibility, covering their face or key body parts with their hands or other objects, or being partially behind furniture. However, although such signals seem to me to appear frequently with clients having suffered abuse, I would caution readers not to draw any conclusion from this that any such image automatically means that abuse has actually happened. Things are not this directly correlational in PhotoTherapy or in life.

Persons posing for a snapshot that also includes other people, such as relatives or friends, would not be likely to voluntarily stand close to those with whom they had an uncomfortable or mistrustful relationship. An unposed candid photo would capture people naturally grouped with those they feel comfortable around. If, however, the photo were being composed by the photographer, people might be asked to stand close to, or even touch or make eye contact with, others with whom they would never do this naturally. Thus the "reality" the photographer creates through personal direction is always an artificially constructed one.

Posed photos like these can demonstrate several layers of reality coexisting simultaneously. When such a photograph is debriefed, the client may begin to interact with each of these layers verbally, nonverbally, or even through rephotographing or imagining. One client told me that she would like to redo most of the serious family portraits in her album so that she got to stand next to her brother and father more often, because the unspoken family rule for generations seemed to be to seat all the women and girls and let the men and boys stand behind and beside ("more free to move and breathe"), and that she didn't feel like being a girl in that family all the time.

Some people express horror at the idea of being photographed at all, but especially at being caught by the camera unprepared. Such strong reactions might be probed to see what lies underneath them. Perhaps there was abuse in the past by those who photographed them. Perhaps it is as current as not liking how they look. Or maybe it is relationship-based, as when people resist being possessed by others. Any of these possibilities might be true, or none.

If being photographed becomes a personal issue for the client, the therapist must come up with ways to help the client to desensitize this concern, if this is the desired goal. Various partializing, self-esteem, assertiveness, or relationship-enhancing techniques (discussed elsewhere in this book) can be adapted to this process. It is also true that if someone wants a picture of you (especially if she or he chooses to display it to others), this signals that you are important to this person. This aspect of photographs of yourself that others like can also be used to therapeutic advantage with clients who need more positive self-regard or more belief in their value to others.

Most of us (myself included) have some photographs of ourselves that we like a great deal, but for various reasons cannot or will not show to others. Sometimes the pictures show naked bodies, sexual arousal, or other taboo topics. Sometimes they show aspects of us we don't ever want anyone to know about. Some people trust the photographer enough to have such photos made of themselves, but don't want anyone else to see these pictures for a variety of reasons, some of which are quite acceptable and necessary, and others of which might indicate negative self-attitudes, which they hope therapy can help change.

For example, the new girlfriend of a client of mine feared his showing his family some photographs of herself because she was afraid they would not like her once they found out she was of a different race. Another woman, who had told her parents she had recently fallen in love and had been seriously dating a new person in her life (but *not* that this person was another woman), found herself having to censor the photographs from her recent birthday party to make certain that she wasn't accidentally exposed. Clients who believe they must take such precautions with photographs are expending emotional energy in maintaining such secrets and cautions. Sometimes it is useful to ask them "what would be the worst thing in the world that might happen if this photograph were to be seen by the person you most fear seeing it?" I have found that pursuing this process of imagining the worst possible scenario can sometimes be a good way to purge the secret of its unnecessary power.

As an example, with a photograph such as 5.1, of a tender moment between a couple who happen to both be men, I might ask questions like "What would it take, what would have to change in your life, for you to risk letting your parents see this picture?" or "If you did show it to them, what would they say or do, and how would you respond? Would they still love you anyway? What would happen if you just left it out on the table when they came to visit?"

To face their biggest fears of others' judgments, people must begin to find ways to educate those they love most without alienating them.

Photo 5.1

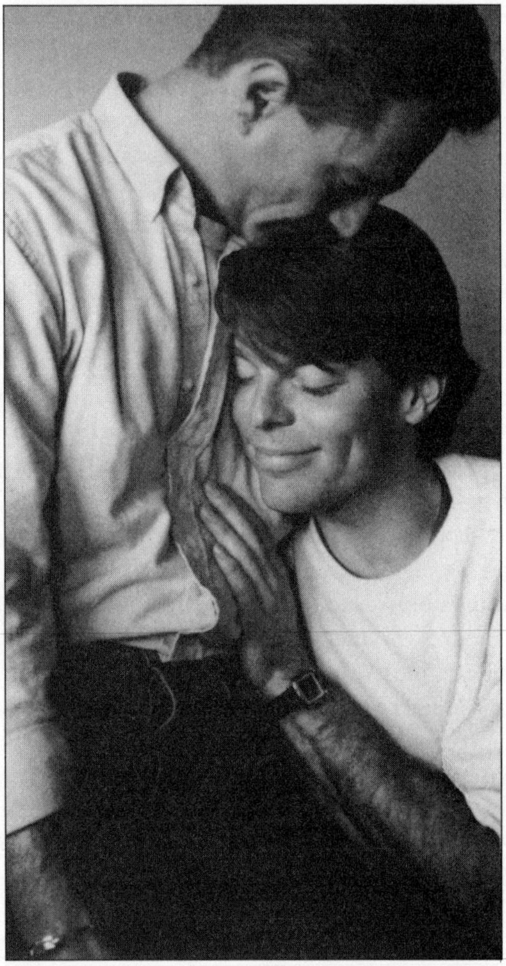

Sometimes the results are as awful as expected, but they can be survived, worked through, and repaired. Others times the feared reactions exist only in their expectations and don't emerge in the actual encounter.

I found myself in the position of having to ask a friend of mine, who was soon to be dying of an AIDS-related disease, if there were any particular things in his home (clothes, books, snapshots, and so forth) that I should not ship to his parents after his death. At first he giggled and told me not to send the how-to-improve-your-sex-life books, and then his voice became very quiet, yet angry: "Yes, the ones of me and my lover kissing and hugging. They never met him. They never approved of my homosexuality at all and thought I was a sinner. He and I are so close we feel that our insides touch, but I could never show my family these pictures or they would never speak to me again. Now that I'm dying I don't want them to have that happy obviously loved part of me. No way will they have the right to my relationship that they refused to see when I was alive. I'm tempted to send them these photos now, so that they can see how other people love me even though they set rules to their own love of their son, but I don't want to have the photos tainted by their judgments, so please give them to my friends to remember me by."

Other Applications Using Photos of the Client

The significance of a photograph taken of someone may lie in none of the above reasons. It could be that a snapshot becomes therapeutically relevant not for what is pictured within it as visual contents, nor for what that might mean, nor for what the photo expresses about the relationship with its photographer. Rather, its importance may lie in what the client may do with it or use it for later or in what it means to that person as a transitional or communicative object on the way to something else in therapy.

A good example of this was a session with a client who had brought in some photos recently taken of her by a friend. She commented how she appeared happy and relaxed in them, and how unusual this was for her these days because she was terribly upset by her sister experiencing the advanced stages of cancer. "She won't talk with me about anything serious, and when I try to bring up my feelings for her, she doesn't want to hear it and changes the subject. It's hard to remember those carefree days when we were younger and stuck together like twins. I love her very much but she won't let me tell her how much I'll miss her, and she won't let me help her at all. Maybe I'll give her this photo of me and tell her to look at it, and it could tell her how I feel. I love her very much, but I don't think she knows it, and I just can't tell her directly out loud. I'd be too embarrassed and so would she—we wouldn't know what to say next. Maybe she would tell it that she loves me, too. Also, I'd like to have a photo of myself together with her before it's too late, but she doesn't like to have her picture taken, so it would be quite the battle and I wouldn't want to force her."

Photos that have been taken of people living their ordinary daily lives can also be useful. This is another, and less active, form of PhotoTherapy, but it is therapeutic, nevertheless. Photos taken of a client over a period of time can give visual proof of actual physical changes in their bodies or surroundings, good and bad alike. Clients can see for themselves deterioration or improvement in their physical health or appearance. Clients can look at issues regarding aging, consequences of alcoholism, or body-image disorders, for example, and can study these directly without feeling blamed by others. Positive aspects of this can be the discovery of desired or expected changes in physical conditions, such as a child growing taller (standing next to the same table three years in a row) or the results of weight-training classes.

Photos of people, especially photos that show place, time, and familial or relational contexts, can provide proof of family roots and history, and as such can be particularly useful for those undergoing enforced and undesired dislocations in their life. Several agencies include programs to provide adopted or foster children with photographic records of their past journeys, and the visual proof that they were truly loved along the way, so that their life can have a more permanent memory-trace than their young minds might be able to retrospectively recall later in life. Life-books, foster-placement albums, and similar collections are established by caring adults who maintain these pictures of their wards in each home, each family, and each location where they must live before being more permanently placed in something that will become "home." Many people with erratic childhoods, owing to factors like parental alcoholism, homelessness, or repeated marital breakups, have no consistent life story from which to form their identity. They have lived in the chaotic upheaval of the immediate present for so long that the past consists of only fleeting moments in memory. Photographs of places where they have been could partially help; however, photographs of themselves being there and taking part in whatever was happening at the time would provide much stronger connections for those fleeting memories.

In my work with people experiencing the last stages of AIDS-related diseases, who know they will soon be entering the hospital with some degree of certainty that they won't come out again, I often assign photos to first be made of them with their loved ones, their pets and gardens, their treasured objects—so that they can take them to the hospital to look at and escape into as they lie in bed. It is one thing to have photos of special people, places, or things. It is altogether different, and much better, I think, to have photos of oneself with these things.

Similarly, for grieving friends and families mourning the person's death, it's been my experience that it's not as helpful to have a photo of the deceased person alone as it is to have photos of the friends and family members with that person, touching, interacting with them, being together and being seen being together. Being together in a photograph helps people remain together in memory.

AIDS in particular has produced its own body of imagery in the field of critical art discourse and sociological representations (for example, Atkins, 1989; Crimp, 1990; Grover, 1989a, 1989b; Howard, 1989; Ray, 1990; Watney, 1987). Most photographs of people who have AIDS-related conditions picture them as passive sad victims rather than life-pursuing survivors. Yet, many people have begun to live a long time with their HIV-positive diagnoses, and photos of them can be life affirming for themselves and for others who hope to match their survival rate (Probus, 1988; Yankovich, 1990). Many art therapists have already begun using inner imagery, and in many cases actual personal photographs, as part of their interventions with clients who have AIDS (Fenster, 1989; Howie, 1989; Probus, 1989; Rosner-David and Sageman, 1987). Successful therapy with people who have been traumatized or who are suffering the results of stigma (Goffman, 1963) has often begun with having clients attempt to visually create an external representation of what being "tainted" means inside their minds, and then designing interventions that can begin to implant ideas of empowerment rather than resignation. Taking charge of what is being done to one's body is often the first step in seizing the will to live. Initiating photographs of one's physical and emotional changes is a step toward self-recognition and the ability to react to what is happening.

What is done PhotoTherapeutically with images of any client taken by other people will, of course, depend on the therapeutic focus. These photographs are tools and must be employed with the therapeutic goals always in mind. Their particular benefits arise in helping clients to understand how others perceive them and what they can do to alter these reactions by changing how they present themselves to other people.

WHAT TO DO

The debriefing of photos of the client taken by others can be approached from a multilevel-framework perspective. First there is the level of the actual visual contents of the picture: the images of the client and everything else in the photo. Next there is the probing of the meaning of those details for the client, both as he or she may originally have reacted to the photo and also as these meanings may have later shifted. There is also the level of the photographer's role. Finally, there is the level of what might be done with these images later. The following list of intervention suggestions is structured in parallel with this framework.

Understanding the Visual Contents of the Picture

One of the best ways to therapeutically debrief a photograph of a client is to ask the client to tell you about all the details in the picture. Discussion can encompass the making of the photograph, reactions to it by the client or others, what it is of and what it is about. Questions such as the following are useful:

Where were you when this was taken? What were you doing there? Why were you there? What was happening? What is the story of this picture? Who else or what else is in the photo? Please tell me more about them. What occurred after and before the moment shown in this photo? What are the most noticeable things about this picture? Did you like being photographed there, at that moment, or with those people? What might have you preferred as a result instead of this picture? If you had brought a camera to that moment, would you have been taking pictures yourself at that place or time? Why or why not? If you were someone else with a camera at that moment, do you think you would have photographed yourself as the photographer did? If so, would you have changed any part of it? Which parts, and why? Do you think viewers can tell what you're thinking or feeling by looking at this photo? If so, what would a viewer learn about you from it? What can't a person know about you by looking at this photo?

Sometimes it can be helpful to ask the client, What would you have wanted to have appear in this photo that isn't there? How would the photo be different if that "missing" part were added? What do you wish hadn't been in it? What would be different about the photo if that part was removed? How would these various changes affect your feelings in reaction to this photo?

How the Original Meaning of Details Changes over Time

It would be helpful for most clients to learn about which visual details are consistently important enough to them to make a difference and find out whether these are the same ones others notice when trying to understand them and their nonverbal messages. Questions such as the following may at first seem to be about the contents of the image, but they quickly bridge to the client's feelings about those contents and nonverbal expectations about what those details should communicate to others.

How does the picture compare to how you thought it would turn out? Does anything about you look different from what you expected, and how do these unexpected differences change the meaning of the photo for you? Do you like the mood and tone the photographer captured (playful, formal, serious, flirtatious, sensual, suggestive, and so on)? Is this a true representation of yourself, or does it seem that this photographer may have defined you in a way you think isn't right and needs to be corrected? How was this spontaneously captured moment different from or the same as most other times in your life? Can you imagine how changing different aspects of your physical presentation would alter the effect of the photo? Is this your natural spontaneous self, or is this your "posing behavior" (how you act when you know someone might be taking your picture)? What parts of yourself did you have to adjust when you knew you were being photographed? How did you know how to pose for this photograph? Did you succeed in conveying the image you wanted to? Why or why not?

What is this photo's message? What does it say about you? How do you feel about this? What could be revised in your behavior to make it more honest or realistic, so that candid photos of you would capture a different image or communicate different information or emotions? What things appear in the photo that you didn't expect or that altered the photo's meaning? Are these things new to you, or are they things that are always part of your life (like a messy room, always-present cigarette, squinting eyes, over-stuffed bookshelves, and the like)?

Would someone have to know you well to understand you from other people's pictures of you? Do you see yourself as being fairly consistent from one social encounter to the next, or do photos of you differ markedly depending on the situation or the photographer? How do you feel about photos of yourself? Are there parts that you wish wouldn't look as they do? Do photos give an honest representation of you, or are there parts you always hide? Will candid snapshots of you be different once your life has changed in some way? If so, what differences might be visible in those photos? Looking at this picture now, are there any parts of it that you are unhappy with, or feel taken advantage by, misrepresented by, or want changed? Is this a photo you could give to someone you love (or who loves you)? If so, who, and what would they say about this photo? How would you feel about this? Is there anyone who you would never show it to? What might they say about it if they did see it?

Basic facts and information about the client and his or her surroundings that are made visible in the picture can be examined for their significance. Visual contents that appear repeatedly in numerous photos can be especially useful. When we share snapshots that others have taken of us, we nonverbally signal to others that we do actually have relationships of trust and friendship, or even deeper intimacy. These photos constitute proof that we have mattered to others. The caring that these images can signal is sometimes overlooked in the detailed investigation into the visual contents of an image, yet its meaning for the subject of the photo must also be considered at all times.

The Photographer's Role

Most people immediately examine pictures of themselves to judge them by their expectations of how they think they should look. What they sometimes forget is the photographer's influence on the final image. How the picture turned out depended a lot on the subject, of course, but the photographer also intervened and translated. Because any such intervention is also a filtering process, it can be included in the PhotoTherapeutic exploration.

People who do not like pictures of themselves often find it logical to blame the photographer for creating bad pictures. They say, "I would never have looked that way naturally. It's the photographer's fault I look awful." It can be a delicate problem for a therapist to explain that the photograph shows the client's own face and body, and that no matter how unhappy the person is with the result, the truth is that for a split second, she or he really looked this way or the photographer could never have put it on film.

Some trust, no matter how hesitant, is always involved in the appropriation of a person's image into someone else's camera. To take someone's picture (even with permission) is to take something from her or him. If the subject's permission is not secured before their picture is taken, he or she can truly feel assaulted, intruded upon, or even robbed. Thus photos of the client can be probed for what they might signal about the subject-photographer relationship. To further explore this aspect, questions such as the following might be asked:

Does this photo capture the "real" you? Did the photographer get it "right"? How much of what we can learn about you from this photograph is put there by you and how much do you think was the photographer's part? Do you think the photographer's input was intentional or accidental? How can you tell? Did you find any surprises in the contents of this photo, and if so, do you think any of this might be because it was taken by this particular photographer? How might the photo have turned out differently if some other person had created it? What would be different about you in this photo if some other person had taken it? Imagine photos of you, taken at that time and place, by a good friend, a parent, and a stranger. How might they be different? How might the whole process have felt different?

What does this photo communicate about your relationship with the photographer? Does it show your true feelings about him or her or about being photographed? If not, how do you feel about that? How do you feel about that photographer? If the same person were to be photographing you again some time, what might you want to do differently to prepare for this recapturing? How would your alterations in dress, pose, posture, facial expressions, gestures, or prop inclusions change the personal meaning being signaled to viewers? Regarding those parts that you don't like about your own image—those the photographer "got wrong" or "messed up"—what might have been the reason this happened? What could you do so that this wouldn't happen again?

If we know we are being photographed, we have some degree of input or control as to the amount of manipulation of the photo (if we exercise that right). In that sense, what ends up in a photo of us is at least partially under our own control, though ultimately at the whim of the photographer. The photographer's power has been at least partially accepted by us. To explore compliance and its significance, it might be useful to ask clients the following questions:

Why was the photographer there? Why did that person take your picture? Did you know it was being taken? If so, how did you feel about this? Did the photographer ask you first? Did that make any difference, and did you feel pressured to agree because the person asked your permission? Looking at it now, are you glad that you agreed? Would you prefer they had not done it, and if so, what did you do to try to stop them? Did you want to see the results? Did you mind if the photographer showed your photo to other people? Why did you want to see the finished prints? How did they make you feel? Did you try to affect the results by altering how you were photographed? Did this work? What did you do to change your visual (nonverbal) presentation? Would you let this photographer take pictures of you again? If so, under what conditions? Would you like to be able to photograph the photographer, or be photographed with him or her by someone else? How do you think the photographer would feel about this? If you could photograph that person, what would you do and what would you want the process to be like?

Later Uses of Photographs of the Client

The invitation to my twentieth-year high school reunion asked those attending to bring twenty slides or snapshots that described "my life as it is now" and "what I've done or experienced since high school." Frequently when attending wedding receptions, I watch while the families show home movies or slides from the bride and groom's childhood years. These are good examples of the kinds of creative uses that can be made of photos that people have stored away. Photos of ourselves, no matter how or why they were first made, can stand as statements about our life, even if we did not initiate them originally. Any time we view a photo of ourselves, we almost automatically give thought to what others will think of it, what they will do with this print, who they might show it to (or want to show it to, even if they don't actually do it), what it would mean to others to see it kept out for display, and so forth. How we feel about these pictures at the time we first see them is worth exploring; how we feel about them later—even years later—can also be valuable to probe. These later encounters, long after the original photo-taking, are the focus of this section.

Clients might be asked to go look through all the photographs of themselves they have gathered over time to find their favorite or least favorite ones—those that present them well or poorly, those that hold a secret, those they would like to do over, and so forth. The goal is not merely to confront the images, but to use them as stimuli for processes related to therapeutic goals. For example, if a client is working with a photo he or she has selected as a favorite, the therapist could ask, "If this photo could speak, what might it say to you?" "What might it say to others or the world?" "How would it describe you if it could?" "Who else might think it was good enough of you to be a favorite of theirs, too?" "Who would definitely not agree, and why not?" And so forth. If it is a photo—

even if only a remembered one—that the client strongly disliked, the therapist could ask, "What is this one like, and why don't you like it?" "Is there someone who does (or would) like it, and why would they like it even if you didn't?" "Would that person's response change if he or she knew you didn't like it?" and so forth. Therapists will want to craft other questions like these to guide the process in the desired direction.

Many of the exercises suggested for self-portrait work can be easily tailored for work with photos of the client taken by others. For example, images of clients in snapshots can be enlarged and used as masks, speaking for the client when direct expression might be painful or risky. The client can also address "that person" as a separate identity, or pursue observation, dialogue, and other interactive or objective self-awareness goals by working with it.

In looking at photos of themselves, clients of course are also projecting, and thus projective PhotoTherapy techniques can be usefully applied. Similarly, snapshots of clients taken by friends and family and included in collections on walls and desks, in albums and wallets, and so forth, can also be worked with through the techniques described in the next two chapters, on photos gathered by clients and photos in albums.

A colleague (Stechman, personal communication, September 26, 1990) shared with me (with permission) the experiences of one of his clients, a successful therapist who had felt all his life that he had not really belonged in his family, that he didn't fit in. He had at first thought he might have been adopted, but he resembled his parents too much for this to be likely. A deathbed secret told by his mother to his sister (and then relayed to him) informed him that his mother had tried and failed to abort her pregnancy with him and wished he had not survived. With this revelation, things began to make sense, but his unconscious pain kept emerging and overwhelming him.

In reviewing photos of himself at different stages of his life, he noted a lack of bonding or closeness with his parents. He looked through several family albums and kept coming back to one picture of him at age eight, alone with his bicycle, far from home. Looking at it, he expressed feeling validated as a "sole" survivor, as an individual who really had not been part of the family in the way his siblings had, and who had truly been alone in his childhood.

He looked a long time at that little boy beside the bicycle and commented that he had finally found himself, the little boy within him who always knew he was alone, even though others had always assured him differently, and he realized he had never fully attended to or comforted this child within himself. He said his work had always been focused on helping other people, and he now understands that it was at the expense of ignoring this inner child. In retrospect, he said, he thinks he became a "care-oholic" through avoiding the anguish of exploring his "own" child's pain and anger. Now this man carries this photograph with him and looks at it when he feels himself becoming too involved with his clients. It serves as his talisman for emotional health and validation.

ILLUSTRATIVE EXAMPLES

The first anecdote related here ties together childhood photographs of the client and images she chose as metaphoric self-portraits in a projective exercise. The second involves a twenty-year old snapshot from a holiday fishing trip. A client's later reexamination of it revealed meanings which could not have been perceived in it earlier. The third example involves photographs of a client that held secret messages that no one else could see, but that were useful in her therapy. (This woman was another colleague's client, but my own personal friend. In this case, I was the photographer, but not the therapist.) The fourth and final presentation is a monologue by a man regarding a photograph of himself and a second photograph of a woman, both perceived as unflattering images. His responses provides clues to the aspects of gender that photographs of people can suggest, without either photographer or subject being aware of them.

Case Example: Penny

Photos of the client that document ordinary real-life activities can later be explored by people in those pictures and their meanings probed. Penny found that early photos of her showed that her life changed significantly when her baby sister was born just as she herself began puberty. Many photos of her at age eleven showed her as a tomboy, playing in trees, shooting arrows with her bow, fishing with her dad. At age twelve, Penny and her brother are pictured holding their new sister, beaming down at the baby parentally and happily ("she felt like a special treasure"), and there are fewer photos of her freely playing. She moved into early womanhood and added responsibilities. "I didn't really want to grow up, but I enjoyed helping my sister grow up. I enjoyed being a 'little mother,' but I missed being part of the boys' gang."

Penny had previously chosen for her projective exercise two photographs that seemed most like herself metaphorically: a gathering of small ducklings and a naked child "riding" a broom in play. About the first she commented, "Soft young cuddly creatures, all snuggled together for protection, waiting for their mom to feed them," and about the second, "Exploring, the whole world is waiting for you to find it, trust, innocence, total unbounded curiosity." When I had asked Penny to speak about this image, she expressed, "It's about something I've lost, there's that early sense of innocence and trust that I no longer feel, that time of unconditional love, when life was only an adventure and there were no commitments, and the world was safe and open. This all changed when I became a teenager and encountered all those expectations about my behavior and school and church." These two techniques (projective versions of herself and actual photos of her) brought forth the same underlying themes in her thoughts and reflections; this demonstrates how significant information will present itself, regardless of the technique selected to activate it.

Case Example: Eva

Eva, in her sixties when we first met, showed me an old photograph taken twenty years earlier that showed her leaning over the railing of a pier, gazing at the sunset across a calm ocean, arms spread apart. That is what *I* saw, but it turned out to be a picture of sunrise, not sunset. This simple misperception of mine led to a rather important discussion of how each sunrise is also a sunset, somewhere on the other side of the world, and that the actual physical moment was simultaneously sunrise and sunset, depending on where you were viewing it from. This turned out to be very significant for Eva because she was feeling herself entering what she termed her "twilight years" and was becoming depressed about life drawing to a close. She had earlier used such metaphors about life and time, saying she was entering her "sunset years" and that she was fearful of the unknown "eternal night, looming a few years down the road."

This photograph had been in her personal collection for years as a memory of an enjoyable fishing trip with her husband (who was now deceased). She had brought it in originally in response to my request to see images of her during happier times in her life. What particularly caught her eye in this photo was that the rising sun bisected the horizon and was also centered on a strong vertical between its reflection on the water's surface and the clouds above it. Eva said this seemed to her to resemble a cross, adding that this imagery gave her comfort. I noticed a parallel "cross" image in her stance along the railing, but wasn't sure if she had noticed this (nor whether she would feel that it had any significance for her if she did perceive it).

I decided to work toward this possibility "sideways" by asking about any other forms visible in the snapshot. She noted all the parallel lines of the pier's walkway and the railing lines, all converging toward a point on the horizon. I asked about any other verticals, and she immediately responded, "Myself standing there—why?" I replied that to me, her outstretched arms along the top rail seemed to form a cross with the vertical of her body mirroring the horizon, but added that she might not agree. However, she immediately exclaimed, "Wow! You're right! Look at that! I am the same! I am that sun. I am part of that flow of time," and she rushed into the other room to get the photograph she had selected from the projective pile in an earlier session.

This second image was of a twig in a snowbank, with a shadow making a contrast line, but Eva had seen this as a surface of darker and lighter sand at a beach (photo 5.2). She said this "sand picture" had originally attracted her "because of the division line that seemed to go through it, like a yin/yang symbol. When you asked me where I might like to go inside that photo, I wanted to be sitting cross-legged right on that dividing line, with one knee in each side."

This seemed to me a possible expression of Eva's ambivalence about aging and her present discomfort in accepting that natural process, but I didn't want to inflict my assumptions on her, so I tried asking why she thought the two seemed to fit together so well. She replied that the sand picture had provided some therapeutic processing, but it wasn't until viewing the fishing trip image that some of what she had said earlier came into better focus. When we looked again at the fishing trip photo, which she had originally shown as an image of happiness, she realized that the imagery she was now finding so powerful had been there all along but she had not construed those meanings before this session. Eva said she took great comfort in finding out that these things were not new but had

Photo 5.2

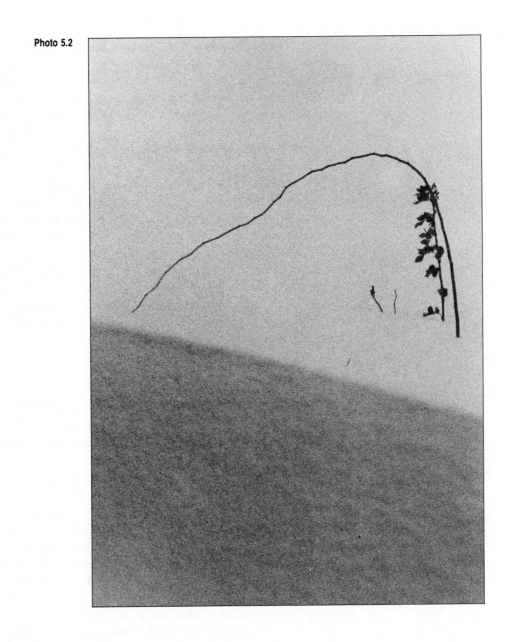

always been there, even though she had not been of a mindset earlier to notice them.

The thing that made the final connection for Eva between her fears and the fact that the flow of time wasn't external to herself was seeing that in her snapshot she appeared to be straddling lines, just as in her fantasy pose for the projective-choice (twig) image. Although she was standing on the pier, her head was centered on the same horizontal line as the sun, the horizon line passing directly through her eyes and ears ("the sun is like my third eye"). Additionally, not only did the horizon line bisect her head but the railing her arms were resting on (forming the horizontal of "her" cross) "goes right through my heart. My heart is right here on earth, but my head is becoming part of what else might be out there. Maybe it's not so separate after all! What's funny is that it's all been there all along in this photo, but I just now noticed all these other layers of meaning. Maybe that's why I liked this snapshot so much all these years. And look, I have my back to the camera. I'm already looking in that direction and it's OK that I'm not looking at the person taking the picture. I'm not usually that vulnerable."

Case Example: Maureen

People frequently notice things in photos of themselves that others cannot see. A photo can give visible form to internal processes known only to the person in the picture. Sometimes this knowledge is conscious, but other times it becomes conscious only when recognized in photographs. One of the best examples of this is the case of Maureen, a friend of mine who was receiving counseling from another therapist. At the time, my role with Maureen included photographing her for promotional purposes. She was a singer-musician and needed some publicity posters. After making the photographs for her, I found I had another half-roll of film remaining in the camera and suggested that she and her boyfriend let me use up the film in some portraits of them together. Both liked the idea and agreed. They posed spontaneously for these portraits, with no instruction from me as to what to do or how to look.

The results pleased me artistically. There were several frames that I liked, so when I gave Maureen the business photos, I also brought along some finished prints of the more personal ones as a gift. Maureen and her boyfriend were happy to receive these extras, and slowly looked through the two dozen prints of themselves. However, in viewing photo 5.3 Maureen's face changed markedly, and she suddenly jumped up to go make tea.

Maureen's sudden change of mood puzzled me, and I quickly followed her to ask what had upset her. She answered, "You are my friend, but I don't tell you everything. One thing I have been discussing with my therapist, but haven't told you yet, is that I am leaving him, ending this relationship, but I haven't got up the courage yet to tell him. He doesn't know

Photo 5.3

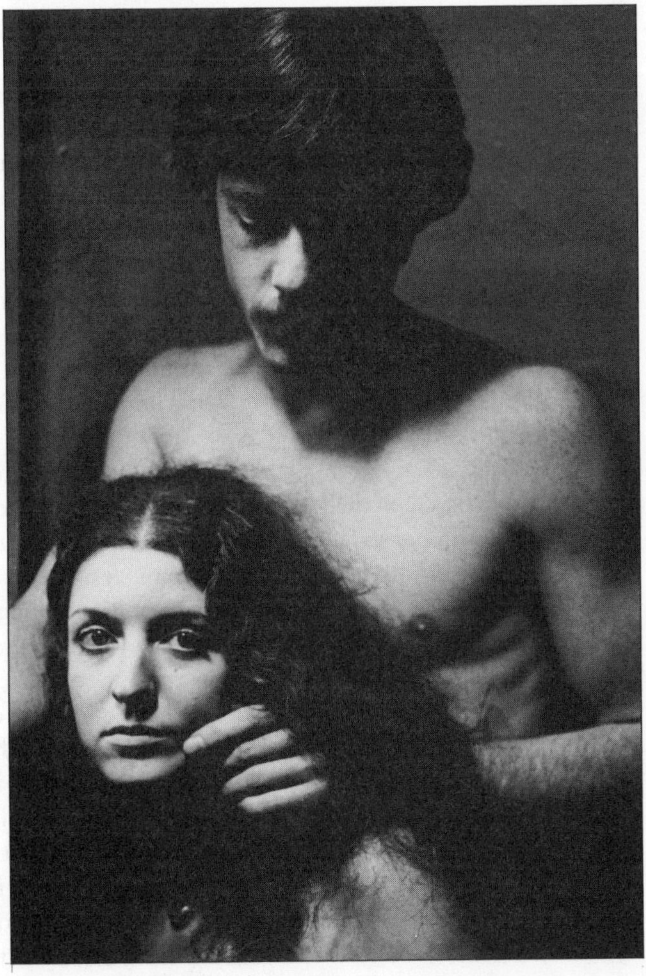

at all. I have to make my plans first for what I'll do and where I'll go, so I haven't said anything yet because I couldn't bear to stay on here after I tell him I want to end this. So I thought your photos would be some nice memories to take along. But my god, look at that picture [the one she had left the room in response to]. It's there in my eyes. He'll see it for sure. I'm leaving him, and my eyes say it all, and now he'll know." She burst into tears and turned away, asking me to leave her alone for a while. I returned to the porch to continue looking through the photos with her boyfriend, whose first comment was, "Look at this photo of us together and how much love her eyes are showing to me."

What was so definitively there for her was completely invisible to him, and to me, as well, at the time. The "reality" of that image was different for each of us. Had I not been there when Maureen first viewed it, I might never have known of its additional signals or that she might take it to her therapist for use as a potent symbolic communication. Looking at this photo again years later, I now think I can see what she meant, though I didn't understand at the time what she had found in her eyes. The photograph hasn't changed at all; I have.

Maureen and her boyfriend benefitted from using that photo as a therapeutic focus point in their counseling process; they then released it to me for PhotoTherapy demonstration purposes. As such, this image has become almost an icon in workshops: people frequently have strong yet different reactions to it.

One couple argued about the photographed couple's power relationship based on their hairstyles! The wife, who had long hair and was wearing a hippie-style loose dress said, "They don't fit as a couple. She's bored, and he's sort of wimpy, in a domineering sort of way. I'm getting that from their appearance because her hair is long and mother-earth style and his is short and kind of fashionable and dressy." Her husband, who had a stylish haircut and conventional clothes, retorted, "I don't really see him as a wimp. I could see, though, that he could be seen as a wimp, but that's not the impression I get. I get that he's more deceptive, and I think she looks more depressed than bored. I can see that she might look apprehensive. I get the picture that he would be leading her on, that she would realize it and be in a sort of depressed state. I think it's because of the hairstyles and so on that I'm just reading into it. He looks like he's been to the hairdresser, and she hasn't, and he looks as though he's more stylish, so—I feel that he would be the more deceptive one." I thought it would have been interesting for that couple to look into a mirror and hold the photo under their own chins.

One client commented that the man looked as if he was forcing the woman to smile by pulling her lip with his finger. Some people see the two as a very loving couple; others see her as being in an abusive relationship. One woman stated, "I can identify with her, but I can't identify with him. I wouldn't mind being her, but I wouldn't want him as my mate. Why? Because he seems too soft, somehow." When I asked what he would have to change for her to like him, she replied, "I think I'd like him better if he looked up and out, rather than down that way. It seems submissive." When asked to "voice" each of these optional poses for him, she answered, "When he's down, he would say, 'You mean everything to me, my world revolves around you,' and if he were looking up, he'd be saying, 'You and I are partners!'"

One man responded intensely and angrily to this photo by saying that the fellow, being slight of height, small-shouldered, and so on, was "obviously under the woman's power; she's probably a real bitch, and he frequently has to say 'I'm sorry' a lot. It looks like he is holding a facemask of a woman, and about to raise it up to cover his own face. This is probably how he protects himself in the world, by hiding behind women. They have all the power anyway." Later he added that "perhaps he had cut her head off and was delivering it on a platter." This client seemed to me to be communicating some strong assumptions about women, demonstrating how he has experienced their effect on his life and defined their roles, and signaling some unresolved anger toward them. Our discussion about his strong reactions led to a journey back through his family photos to explore what his mother's relationship was like with his father and with himself as a child.

Case Example: Joseph

Joseph commented on some publicity photos of a woman. He perceived the pictures as "very unflattering." He discussed them in comparison to photos friends had recently taken of him. He said, "Photos that are chosen to depict a person should flatter that person. When I see those [pictures] of this woman, they don't seem flattering to me, as a male. Some photos could be, but those aren't, and therefore I find myself wondering why she picked those. Any picture of an individual should be flattering, but especially of a woman. A male could be macho or show a business side or other qualities, but females should have more emphasis on how they appear. Some part of her photo should be more flattering."

When I asked him to clarify what he meant by "flattering," he said that it means "some physical quality or inner quality that shines through as opposed to those of a male representing his empire or business, portraying his role. The female would be more conscious of how she appears. It is conceivable to me I could look ugly in my picture and still maintain or project some kind of quality that compensates for the ugliness. I'm not expected to look attractive, but I would expect that she would be more conscious or sensitive about how she is portrayed in a photo to be seen by the public. Therefore I expect she would have chosen a more flattering picture. I think that traditionally women are more conscious of how they look and their impact of presenting themselves. Why? Because an attractive looking woman holds a man's attention longer, or is likely to, and therefore she is more likely to gain attention. The typical male tends to overlook a woman who is unattractive or doesn't command attention."

He continued, "Now, I know I'm a male viewer. I'm even aware that most photos of women are assumed to be taken to please the male viewer, and that worthwhile viewers are assumed to be male—I'm aware of these politics in my head, but my heart likes to enjoy looking at women! I think a woman sees different qualities when viewing another woman. I assume the goal of this photo was to attract viewers' attention and hold that attention, and I think a male viewer will pay more attention to a photo of an attractive woman, or the most attractive photo of any woman. If I see a 'bad' or 'different' one, if I see a bad photo of an ugly woman, I'm not going to spend a lot of time looking at it, though I might wonder for a moment why she picked that one to show people, because women are judged so much on their appearance, not their abilities."

He added, "As this is not a good photo of [her], I think embedded in this photo is a coded meaning that it was chosen by a woman to be viewed by women and therefore the attractive image is not only not the goal, but would be a handicap. Our socialization has mandated this perception, but it is not genetically programmed, nor necessary—but that's the way life really is out there, no matter how politically unpopular the perception may be. I think gay men often do the same sort of staring and judging of photos of other men, just like I realize straight men like me probably objectify women by their looking at them. I think photos of women for other women would avoid 'pretty pictures' and that flattering ones would not interest them as much as those showing the opposite aspects like strength or skills. I think that women may more consciously process images of women initially more intellectually than emotionally, and I have no idea whether lesbians objectify in their gazing or not, but I'll bet that some of this happens, regardless. It's how life is. That's how I was raised. I can cringe and be horrified at the realization and try to outgrow it, but in the end, it's true for me, even as liberated as I try to be, and however much photos of me don't have to look nice, I'll still be drawn to photos of pretty women!"

This man's comments express with great clarity widely held biases about how photographs of women relate to their status in society and point to the kind of work that can be done using photographs to expose and examine stereotypical thinking in general.

SAMPLE EXERCISES

These exercises follow the same framework as the sections in the chapter, and so I have attempted to keep the accompanying instructions to a minimum. However, there are times when the way the therapist initiates the exercise may be as important as the actual questions asked later once the client is holding a finished photograph. Therefore some of the sections of questions below will begin with "stage-setting" introductory comments. Also, readers may notice that some of the questions within those lists may have already appeared within the chapter as occasional illustrations of the kinds of questions that therapists might ask. As I anticipate that most therapists reading this book will probably return primarily to the "Sample Exercises" portions of chapters for independent referencing of quick practical suggestions, I made sure to reinclude those key question-examples mentioned earlier so that the list given here is comprehensive and complete, and so that readers would not have to go back to find those listed separately on other pages of the chapter text itself.

Preliminary Considerations

Clients can be asked to go back through their personal collections and bring in those photographs that best answer what the therapist assigned them to look for. These can then be explored in discussion with the therapist for both the visual details contained within them and the meanings that these details build in the client's mind. If clients do not have photographs in their personal collections that will fit the assigned topic, then clients are often requested to go have them taken (but given clear explanation about how these are different from self-portraits).

Sometimes in having new pictures taken of them by other people, clients also serendipitously encounter a different quality of interaction with the photographer than occurs in just face-to-face interactions. Since this itself may turn out to be therapeutically useful, therapists may actually want to tailor the client's being photographed more for the purpose of what will take place during the process than for the resulting pictures.

Questions may be asked along any step of the process, from clients selecting photos that were taken earlier of themselves or having new ones made according to the therapist's assignment to the active investigation of these individually or in combination with other photos, art enhancements, written accompaniment, and so forth, as the focus for therapeutic discussion and mutual review of the image and all steps of the process involved in having it in hand. It is preferable if the client can examine each image from two different viewpoints: knowing he or she is the subject and also viewing it as if looking at a stranger. In either case the client is asked to respond to the image in the snapshot rather than to speak about him- or herself directly, and also to try to interact with the "self" in the photo as if dialoguing with another real person. As techniques of projection and self-portrait PhotoTherapy underlie a lot of this, I will not repeat these components in the following lists of questions, as readers can back-reference the sample exercises from the two previous chapters for that information.

The role of the photographer is also important therapeutically, as that person is the reason this picture of the client exists at all. When the client and therapist discuss any photo taken of them, both are also discussing their projections about what was going on in the photographer's mind, that person's intentions and goals, as well as consequent feelings when seeing the finished photographic result. Also, they are discussing the relationship between the client and that particular photographer (as contrasted with others who may have taken the client's picture), and so there is also a section of questions below for these components.

At the end of the sections of recommended questions, there is a simple exercise so that readers may begin to learn how to use client photographs in more active and interactive ways. This is one of my favorites, and so I offer it as a "sample"; dozens of other possible combinations of these applications are equally possible.

Existing Photos of Clients

Clients can be asked to look through their personal collections to examine and bring in photos taken by others in response to questions such as those below:

1. Bring a couple dozen images of yourself that you think could best explain to a stranger who you are, that could catch a far-away friend up on the past ten years of your life, or that tell your life story.
2. Bring in photos of yourself that you like and dislike. They can be photos others have given to you as being very flattering or funny, that you think show you at your best and worst, or that demonstrate the range of feelings others have captured you showing, perhaps some you wish had never been taken.
3. Bring in photos from your family's or your own past that you think would help show or explain why you are now having trouble.

Having New Photos Made of Clients

Clients can be asked to have photos taken of themselves by family members, friends, or even strangers in response to assignments such as those below:

Simple Assignments. Have yourself photographed:

1. in your favorite place; with your favorite person
2. with a good friend, a pet, a stranger
3. at home, at work, at play; involved in a hobby or a favorite activity
4. with your family (parents, siblings, or "family" as you define it)
5. dressed up, costumed, nude
6. walking, talking, sleeping, thinking, daydreaming
7. as you think your parents perceive you
8. as you have always wanted to be seen
9. thinking of a special person or place

Complex Assignments

1. Have someone play at being a detective by following you around for a few days photographing you, as if trying to figure out who you are and what you are like from the snapshots they take of you.
2. Have yourself photographed by each member of your immediate family as they choose to picture you. You should not be posing.
3. Ask a family member or significant other (spouse, lover, or best friend) to photograph you while you are being what they think is your best and your worst over the course of a week. Try not to pose. The following week, have the person photograph you as *you* wish; pose all you want, and feel free to discuss the posing with them.

Debriefing Photos Taken of Clients

Once the client has brought in snapshots others have taken of them, the second stage can begin: reviewing the photographs, discussing the meanings embedded in their visual contents and in the interactive process of having them taken, as the following suggests:

The Visual Contents of the Photograph. It is usually a good idea to remind clients to use the photos, not themselves, as the basis for answering the following questions.

1. Describe this photograph to me as if you were explaining it to someone who cannot see it. Start with what is most obviously noticeable and then add any other details you find. Who else and what else emerges there as you look at it? What do these communicate?
2. Where were you when this was taken? What were you doing there? What was happening? What happened just before and just afterward?
3. Were you surprised at anything that appears (or doesn't appear) in this photo? Is there anyone or anything in it that you wish weren't there after all? How would it be different if those parts weren't there?
4. If something seems to be missing or appears to need changing now that you look at it closely, what might these be? What would be different about the photo if it were now different in this way?

The Meaning of Those Visual Contents. The questions here are designed to begin with the contents of the photograph and quickly bridge into the client's feelings about the contents and expectations about what they should communicate to others.

1. What is the story of this photograph? What is its message?
2. What does it tell about you, and are these things you like? Do you think other viewers can understand this just from looking at it, and if not, what would you have to add to help them understand? Can other viewers tell what you are thinking or feeling by looking at it? What might others be able to learn about you from looking at it? What couldn't they know about you from viewing it?
3. What secrets lie beneath the surface appearance of this photo? Who in your family would know this, or agree with you? Who could you safely tell this to who would understand? Would you want to?
4. Why was this picture taken? Do you think the photographer got what he or she wanted? Why or why not, and how do you feel about that? Do you like your apparent mood (playful, formal, serious, flirtatious, sensual, suggestive, and so forth)? Would someone have to know you well to understand you from this picture? Is this a true representation of you, or does it seem that this photographer may have a different definition of you that isn't right and needs to be corrected?
5. What emotional expression is being signaled by you in this photo? Do you think a viewer can truly know what you were feeling? What were you feeling there? Which aspects of your physical presentation could you change to alter the emotional message in the photo? Looking at this picture now, are there any parts of it that you are unhappy with? That take advantage of you? Misrepresent you? Need to be changed? To make this a better or truer photograph, how should its visual contents or the way you are presented be changed?
6. What do the faces and body language of others in the photo convey to you?
7. What seem to be the differences between pictures of you that you like and those that you don't? Why do you think this has happened?
8. How are these photos of you different from self-portraits or portrayals of you in family albums? How do you feel about these differences? What would have to change in your family for your favorites of these photos to be included in your family's albums?

9. Is this a photo you could give to someone you love (or who loves you)? If so, what would that person say about this photo? Is there anyone you would never show it to? What might they say about it if they did happen to see it?
10. Focus on the background objects and details in these photos. If you were to look at them as an anthropologist might, what could be learned about this person from all those surroundings? What special knowledge would a stranger have to have to understand why some of the things in the photo were there with you? What else would a stranger need to know to understand what is in that photo with you?

The Photographer's Role. The following questions are designed to help clients think about how the photographer's perceptions of them filtered what they are seeing.

1. What was the story of the making of this photograph? Who took it, and why did she or he want to photograph you?
2. What do you think of how the photographer pictured you? Is this the "you" that you know and recognize? If not, what are the differences and why do you think they appeared when this photographer made this photo? How do you think this photographer sees your real self? If he or she didn't picture you satisfactorily, what could you do next time so that, even though this is the photographer's picture, you nevertheless could be depicted more to your own liking?
3. What do you remember about how it felt to be photographed that day by that person, in that way? Were you comfortable? Was the picture-taking all right with you? Did the photographer ask your permission first or not? What difference did this make on how you looked in the photo and how you felt about it later? Did you feel pressured into agreeing because the photographer asked first? Would you have stopped him or her if you could have? Looking at the photo now, are you glad you let the person take the picture?
4. Does this photo capture the "real" you? How much of what you see of yourself do you think was put there by you, as compared with how much was the photographer's part? Do you think the photographer's input was intentional or accidental? How can you tell?
5. How might the photo have turned out differently if some other per-

son had taken it? What would be different about you if some other person had taken it? Imagine that a good friend, a parent, or a stranger had taken this photo at that time and place; how might the results be different in each case? How might that process have felt different?

6. How would you describe your relationship with this photographer? How do you think this might have affected the photo? Do you think this photo conveys your true feelings about the photographer? About being photographed by him or her?
7. Since this photo was made by someone else, it belongs to that person, not you. How do you feel about this? Do you mind if that person shows it to other viewers without your knowing?

The Client's Role. The client's role can be explored in two parts.

In Terms of Photographs Specifically Discussed

1. In which of the photos we have just been examining were you aware of being photographed? How can you tell, from looking back at them, which were posed and which were not? Can you show me what you mean? How does your posing behavior differ from your usual way of being? What parts of yourself did you have to carefully change when you knew you were being photographed?
2. In those candid unposed shots, is who is with you and what you are doing different from the photos you knew were being taken? If so, who or what, and why?
3. How did you know how to pose for this photographer? Did you try to alter the results by doing something on purpose? If so, what did you do to try to change your visual presentation? Did you succeed in conveying the image you wanted to? If you don't like how it turned out, how could you change your interactions or behavior to make photos of you more honest or realistic in the future?
4. Would you like to be able to photograph the photographer in return, or be photographed with that person by someone else? How do you think the photographer would feel about this? If you could photograph that person, what would you do? How would you want the process to be?
5. If you learned that the same person were to be photographing you

again sometime soon, how would you want things to be different? Would you let this person photograph you again? Under what conditions or circumstances? Would you want to be alerted in advance or just let the person catch you unaware?

In Terms of Photographs Taken in General

1. Who do you permit to photograph you? When? Under what conditions? If you were to be photographed soon in the way *you* wished, how would that portrait have to look to satisfy you? What pose, clothing, jewelry, and other adornments would you choose, and why? Would you dress up or be informal? How would you pose your body, express your face, and handle eye contact with the photographer?
2. Of all the people you know, are there any who you wouldn't let take your picture? Why not? What would have to change for you to let them? If these people did somehow take your picture without your knowing about it, how would you feel? What do you think those photos would look like?
3. Are there any people who you would refuse to be photographed with? Why not? If you found that you had to be photographed with them despite your unwillingness, what might happen and how might these photos be different from other ones?
4. If you had been at a reunion of your entire family, and you knew you were going to see all the snapshots everyone had taken there, including many of you, what sorts of things would you expect to see in these nonposed candid documentations of all those interactions? Would you be worried about how you would look with certain people? If so, which ones, and why? How would you be feeling in anticipation of seeing those photos?
5. Are there photos of you that you cannot show to others? If so, which ones, to whom, and why? Is this because of something the photographer did when arranging or taking the photo (would the photo be acceptable for showing if someone else had taken it), or some other reason?
6. How do you feel in front of the camera? What would be your ideal picture-taking situation? What is it about you that photographers would have to know in order to get a good photo of you?

What Else Can be Done with Photos of the Client

By now readers should be familiar with how to combine photos created using one technique with those resulting from others. Both making and talking about snapshots can be therapeutically valuable; however, with many kinds of clients' photographic products, additional exercises can be designed to use them as artifacts to create even larger "pictures" of clients' lives (and the processes surrounding their interactions with themselves and others), as the following two-part exercise explains.

Part One. Select a photograph that someone has taken of you that seems typical, make two photocopies of it, and then attach one to the center of a large sheet of paper. Look at all the visual details in the image besides your own body, circle each one, and draw a line from it onto the paper. Write a description there of your own connection to each one, whether object, person, or animal. Can you create a narrative relating all the external parts of the photo to yourself in a story?

Part Two. Use the second photocopy of the picture to remove yourself from those familiar surroundings by cutting yourself out. Place your disassociated figure on a neutral blank background, such as a sheet of newsprint. As you now have no other visible context, and the "new" photograph of you has no other visual content, you are free to create one using art materials, other snapshots, images from magazines, and even words, if you like. You may also change your clothing or other adornments, and so on. Compare your new image with the original one. Note the differences and what they mean to you. If you wish, you can use versions of this exercise to create alternative identities or other contexts free from the constraints of photographic reality.

6 Metaphors of Self Construction

Reflecting on Photographs Taken or Collected by Clients

Years ago, my cousin and I traveled together, visiting the same places, seeing our relatives, and having a nice adventure. We took lots of snapshots, sometimes standing right beside each other so that we wouldn't have to depend upon each other's mutually-questionable talent. Upon returning home, we noted how so many of our photos of the same subject were so dissimilar that we often seemed to have been visiting different places. Each of us had forgotten places that to the other were treasured memories.

Our snapshots taken at various family social events demonstrated the different relationships each of us individually maintained with our various relatives and the differential perceptions we each had of them, neither of which were we previously aware of, nor ever thought to discuss between ourselves. When our two collections were mixed together, our close friends were often able to correctly identify which photos were taken by which of us, though they found it difficult to explain exactly how they knew this. Our own photos seemed to describe us as well as what they were taken of.

This experience demonstrates how when people take photos their unique personalities can invisibly "appear" within the borders of the finished prints. For therapeutic purposes, this is equally true for photos in magazines, calendars, books, greeting cards, and posters that people have found and kept—because each was found by the "taker" to be important and worth noticing.

A remembered image can also be suggestive of the things that are important to a person. These are among the reasons that this chapter defines "photos by the client" to include not only snapshots taken by the client but also any other photographic images the client has "taken" metaphorically by acquisition, whether done spontaneously or in response to the therapist's instructions.

The photos people take and keep serve as tangible extensions of the self and as, quite literally, personal constructs of reality in the fullest definition of the term. They signify the photographer's relationships with objects, people, places, and things. They reflect our self-concept, give access to our projections, and document our perceptions. Taking pictures can be conceived of as an active decision by the photographer to record a scene, or as a more passive receptivity by the photographer of a scene that calls to him or her, demanding to be recorded. Not unlike Jung's (1971) dichotomy of the origins of art (springing from the artist's intention or forcing itself upon the artist), photographs are taken in response to one or both of these influences. The unconscious, though influencing both modes, seems to push strongest when given most opportunity in those situations where the photographer had not consciously planned to take a snapshot but found him- or herself doing so simply because the moment *felt* right.

When we take photos, or even think about taking them, we assume a different stance in regard to life itself. We transform from being involved participants unaware of our own position to being observers. We no longer are part of what is going on. Thus a scene that we examine and try to document is irrevocably changed as a result of our observation of it and our removal of ourselves from its process. To really be involved is to be unaware of participation. To be aware of our part in it is to become self-aware and construct a boundary, no matter how permeable it may be, between us and whatever we are looking at.

Most photographers do observe the scene in front of them as objectified, to be manipulated, captured, frozen, and otherwise used for certain purposes. Eyes experiencing the world do see differently when there is an additional agenda of potentially turning what is being naturally viewed into becoming a fixed photographic representation of the real thing. In fact, if the photographer had not thought this moment worth rendering permanent, we would never be seeing it at all. People often forget the strong influence that the intrusion of the camera or the photographer places on the subject matter, even if only scenery.

Sometimes our photographs later show us things we didn't realize at the time we pressed the shutter. People taking pictures sometimes encounter their own personal patterns of symbolic expression (as well as more universal archetypes) appearing "accidentally" in spontaneously taken snapshots. The images they gather in their personal collections sometimes reveal themes or patterns not apparent in individual acquisitions made months or years apart. Yet, seen as a whole, they come together to make more sense than when just viewed one-by-one. Personal photos speak very powerfully about their owners in ways never intended or planned. As a colleague's client nicely expressed it, "The photographs I take become the 'me' that can then be examined by the 'I' [that I am]" (Combs and Ziller, 1977).

Regarding the critical photographic moment, I usually take photographs more because of what I feel than what I see, or rather, how what I see "makes" me feel, but this is certainly not a process that is cognitively pondered at greath length while holding the camera. I have found this out only after pausing to retrospectively examine my own particular style and rationale of photo taking. Some of my most insightful photographs have occurred at moments when I was not even conscious that I had pressed the shutter, and for me, though not necessarily the same for anyone else, this is not an infrequent happening. Much the same as Cartier-Bresson's "decisive moment" (or, in Minor White's phrasing, "the moment waiting for the photographer it has chosen"), my camera has pointed out to me what it is that I have been observing and attending to about what is already there (or, at least, is seen to be there) in front of my eyes.

All media mediate; it's just that often we don't notice these filters because they do not noticeably intrude. In being a "reflective" medium, photographs can also suggest information to viewers about the self who took the pictures in much the same way that self-portraits do. It's just that the "self" being represented in the photos being taken may not have an actual duplicate bodily correspondence appearing on the film as subject. Nevertheless, the "self" of the photographer appears in every photograph he or she has ever taken.

The idea that the visual scene is always "just there" waiting for anyone's camera to objectively capture it, with the photographer making no qualitative difference on the moment being captured, is simultaneously both true and untrue—and this paradox comprises a major theoretical underpinning for this chapter.

I am occasionally asked if it means anything if a person doesn't take or keep any photos. No, this fact doesn't signal anything on its own. However, in therapeutic situations, I would want to know if not having photos matters to the client. It is fine if a person has none and doesn't miss them, need them, or want them. But, does the person want to take photos but feel that she or he can't or isn't good enough? Would the person take some if she or he knew that the prints would turn out all right or that certain results were guaranteed? Has a past experience in photographing or being photographed precipitated a decision to not make any photos now? Other considerations might be that the person's photos have been lost and the task of replacement seems overwhelming, or the person may feel rejected or abandoned by his or her family and feel they don't have a family to belong to. There are many different reasons why people may not have photos, and those reasons and the feelings associated with them might have therapeutic significance.

HOW THIS TECHNIQUE WORKS

When things aren't going quite right or when life isn't flowing as ordinarily expected, people instinctively construct stories to explain to themselves (or others) why things aren't proceeding as they were supposed to. In trying to make sense of it all, people tend to try to "normalize" what has interrupted their natural process of living in order to reduce its degree of strangeness and enhance their position with regard to the threat. People's attempts to make life more comprehensible place them in the role of outside observer of their own life. This perspective can help give them a better sense of control over life's unpredictabilities.

This is one reason that therapy works: the client takes the time in a safe setting to tell his or her story to a stranger and, in doing so, often gets a better understanding of it. In naming, labeling, and otherwise trying to explain what is going on, people gain insight and acquire understanding and control over what may have previously escaped their conscious grasp. Taking a photo of "it," or creating a story about "it" from already-existing photos (their own or those taken by others) can be another way to give something form, cohesion, and sense that it originally appeared to lack. The therapeutic advantage to asking clients to take pictures or share the ones they have is that constructing and presenting a visual story of what is going on in their lives can help them to understand it more fully.

Taking photos is a form of self-expression and creativity; when this is done on assignment, and there is no way the photo can turn out wrong, because it is the personal communication that is sought, the results are extensions of the self that assist in explaining that self. Taking snapshots can enhance self-esteem or assist people to clarify goals. Picture-taking can be useful in visualizing future realities such as desired outcomes, jobs, accomplishments that seem vague when mentally considered, without any tangible vision to assist in practical considerations. Photos can be taken as a means of trying out changes or relationships; fantasies can be explored by photographing them; consequences can be rehearsed and communications practiced, all inside a camera.

In more specific terms, photo-taking assignments can help clients to bridge generational, cultural, class, racial, sexual, and even political differences. To increase tolerances of differences, those differences need to be reframed as being nonthreatening characteristics. Shooting pictures instead of guns or word-darts has proven successful in a variety of situations; it becomes nearly impossible to do random violence to those with whom you have established a distinctly personal (and hopefully positive) relationship. When people stop seeing each other as strangers or interchangeable ciphers they take on emotional dimensions for each other and can communicate more easily, especially if they have shared experiences in common.

For example, when working with a group of teenagers who were robbing local corner stores, I established a program whereby part of their court sentence was to make photographic documentaries on the lives of other stores' owners and staff. I also asked them to be photographed with these people, both in the stores and in other locations. As the emotional distance between the two groups diminished, they began to form a few personal bonds; finding themselves required to communicate in order to make the assigned pictures, they often discovered interests in common. Discovering that some of the store owners were once themselves teenagers who had trouble with the police helped my clients to believe there might be a positive future for them. It also made the store owners more real and individually human. Vandalism in the neighborhood soon dropped markedly. Similar projects have been assigned with youthful fire-setters, graffiti artists, shoplifters, and so forth, whereby they had to return to the scene of their crime and photograph its consequences as victims had reported them to be. In personalizing the crime and interacting with its consequences, my clients reexperienced their actions from a different viewpoint. In looking at photographs someone else has taken, a client becomes able to view the world literally through another person's eyes.

When we take photographs, we have some degree of control and power over what we frame in the viewfinder. This can be helpful when considering therapeutic interventions with clients who find it difficult to make choices or commitments, or who resist being responsible for the consequences of their own actions. Clients who have experienced loss of personal power in the past, through abuse, enforced hospitalization, or a handicapping injury, can benefit from the metaphoric power they wield when they take snapshots just as they wish and when they wish. The personal statements that result are inarguably theirs, and they know that no one else has had any part in creating them. This often frees up expression and increases feelings of empowerment and self-confidence.

A collection of photos given to the person by others, and those taken, made, or gathered by themselves, borrowed from walls or tabletops at home and selected out of albums, when viewed collectively can serve as a retrospective summation of life and can be very useful for positive reframing of a person's life when it seems to most strongly consist of only gloom and doom. It can animate depressed clients to rediscover and reflect on the good parts of their lives, and find reassurance that there are people to whom they are special, who will miss them or who are willing to accept their changing life conditions. It can be empowering for them to take charge of a part of their identity when so much of it seems to be ruled by others or "fate." For people whose lives seem to be tumbling out of control, it can provide useful structure to create a life line, a cogent summary of who they were before this medical crisis and use this to nonverbally signal "if there was a way in, there may be a way out." Even if the prognosis is definitely terminal, such life-affirming positive reminders of good times can sometimes assist clients to reconnect with good memories and to prove that their life has mattered.

Taking Photographs

We make a conscious decision to take a picture when we want to put onto film an image we see (even if only in our minds). We may actively intervene in a scene to set it up or arrange it for the camera. Taking a picture can also be a less conscious act, wherein something we notice calls to us, seeming to "want" to be put in photographic form. Either of these situations can occur spontaneously or in response to assignments given by the therapist or others; for example, news photographers either search for specific images to fill a particular assignment or just go photograph whatever catches their eye and later form a story from those images. Sometimes the story later formed by several photos is far different from what the photographer originally thought she or he was working toward.

The pictures we take often carry deeper meaning than was apparent when we quickly snapped them. For example, a client once showed me several of his art photos, and I noticed that a lot of them seemed to feature pairs of things or people, such as a picture of two people walking near two trees along a path where only two lampposts were standing, and there even were only two clouds in the sky. In another, two houses had two sets of steps climbing to two matching doorways between identically paved entry paths with matched shrubbery and mirror-imaged handrails and porch details. There were so many examples of two-ness that I commented on this pattern and asked him if he also saw it. He looked at what I was pointing out and commented that yes, he did see what I meant, but he didn't think there was any particular significance in it. So I dropped the topic.

Weeks later, he did a self-portrait assignment to photograph reflections of himself, either literally in mirrors or windows or symbolically in objects or nature. One set of photos from this assignment showed him reflected in a mirror so that he appeared to be standing beside himself; he titled this group "Double Exposure." In viewing these, he seemed to be thinking about something quite deep. Then he looked at the next group of photos, for which he had posed with his back to a large picture window facing a beautiful sunset. He had wanted the photo to look as if he were outside, but he had mistakenly used a flash, so the resulting print showed no outdoor scene at all. Instead, the background appeared completely black, and a ghostly image of himself was reflected, as if from outside the window.

He grew very pale staring at this photo. "I thought I was going to see myself alone with the sunset, and instead I find my dead twin staring back at me. I was born with a twin brother, but he didn't survive very long. I've always felt that I wasn't complete, that there should have been two of me. He should have lived, too, or else we both should have died.

Why did I live and he didn't? It's always bothered me, but I'm only beginning to realize how much he is a part of me even now, even if only inside my mind." We explored some of the issues around this subject, such as survivor guilt and unachievable expectations, and then we returned to re-examine the photos he had shown me earlier that had included so much two-ness and to explore what might have been going on deep inside his unconscious mind when he had been taking them.

This case illustrates how in taking a picture we literally symbolize ourselves. Each photographic decision is based on inner criteria; we create the meanings in what we see because of how that visual information signals meaning to us. Every photograph we take also communicates about ourselves because the camera actually encodes meaning ("focuses") in both directions simultaneously. Thus the image can provide therapeutically relevant insight to the person who decided to photograph it because it communicates about what the person is drawn to or what matters in his or her life. In reviewing several years of snapshots in her personal album, one client communicated her sudden comprehension about her just-ended marriage quite succinctly: "Look at that! I'm in the final stages of a lousy marriage, and lo and behold, no matter what the subject matter of my photographs [from those years], they all have common elements: barriers and confinements! I should have listened to my photos instead of my mother, who kept urging me to try to make it work!"

Layers of potential meaning are always embedded in each snapshot someone takes, and each layer is of potential therapeutic import. Each person's reasons for choosing to take a certain snapshot, to freeze a particular moment in a particular way, can be as personally significant as what the photo is actually of. In photos taken by clients, we see not only what they have seen (or at least a representation thereof), but also who *they* were when the photos were taken. Explicit content is just one of several important aspects to focus on in discussion; it serves as only the starting point for exploring images' meanings and purposes from clients' perspectives.

In some cases, we may never completely understand why we are almost magnetically drawn to certain pictures until years later. Sometimes we never do find out.

Collecting Photographs

A client once told me she felt struck "by a lightning bolt" with the realization that her marriage might be on the rocks when she visited her husband's office and noted several photographs displayed on his desk. They were pictures of his boat, a favorite fishing trip, his new sports car, and even a few of himself with the children, but none of her. She noted that her own desktop office snapshots were all of family and friends, including several of her with her husband. Looking at them more closely, she noticed for the first time that in all these "couple" photos, she was looking at him, touching him, hugging him—while he was gazing at the photographer and expressing, in her words, "a 'closed' body posture" toward her. She told me that it was that essential difference between the kinds of snapshots she and her husband displayed at their workplaces that first signaled to her that trouble had arrived.

Traditionally, people have placed photos of relatives and family events in albums or displayed them in their homes or worksites. But people may not always want treasured photos in permanently unalterable formats, glued to pages or framed. One man has maintained a long tradition of quickly snapping instant photos of his friends and family, and he likes to keep those pictures visible. He has created a collage of more than a thousand instant photos on a wall in his living room (see photo 6.1). Finding out what photographs or collected imagery clients keep around them in their ordinary daily living or working spaces can be a good beginning point for determining what is important to them.

When he moves, he removes all the photos and replaces them on a living room wall in his new home. He says that when the wall is full, he will start a second one. Some are arranged in chronological order; others are placed by relationship or past connections. The therapist of a client with a display like this might want to make a home visit. For the purposes of PhotoTherapy work, such a wall could be a rich source of information about the life and values of the person who put it together, as it is clearly more than simply an "album."

The symbolic significance of some photos in clients' personal collections may lie not in the images themselves but rather in the way the photos serve as bridges connecting them to whoever took, or gave, them the photos. I have a Christmas card showing a glass bauble tree decoration in a gift shop window reflecting a city street-scene in Paris. The card is visually attractive on its own, but its significance to me is in its connection to the person who gave it to me—a close friend who died recently. Though the card itself could have had any photo on it at all and still have been equally special, I now can no longer see Christmas cards with that kind of decoration without remembering her. The trace has been perma-

Photo 6.1

nently etched in my associative memory. In this way, photos take on layers of meaning for the people who collect or encounter them.

It can also be interesting to explore parallels between the photos a person takes and those they collect or respond to. A friend, discussing my photographs with me, pointed out some definite connections between what I had photographed myself and what she noticed in my collection of other people's images (artworks on my wall, favorite greeting cards on my desk, and so forth). She noted what she termed a quality of "stillness," and on closer examination, I agreed. The people in the pictures appeared to me to be pausing in suspended time; they seemed to be inside themselves, not involved with the myriad distractions around them. I described this as "being" rather than "becoming." Suddenly, while saying this, I made a connection that I had not understood previously: I was reaching a point in my life where my years of training were ending and I could go out and *be* the person I had been preparing to be. The phrase that popped into mind was "getting ready" has turned into "start." This was accompanied by an image of myself having been treading water for fifteen years and finally reaching shore. Perhaps I should have then gone out and photographed myself in that scene to use it as a reminder!

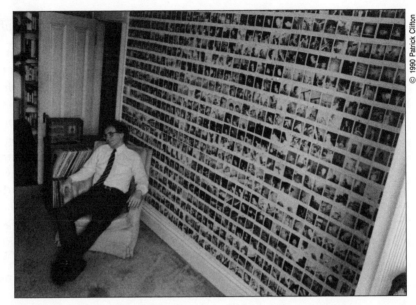

Assigning Clients to Take or Collect Photographs

When I have a hunch about something that might be going on in a client's life, I may design an assignment for her or him to do right in my office or later, as a homework assignment, because I think it will help uncover more emotionally relevant information. Such assignments may even include the somewhat paradoxical-sounding instruction to "go photograph what you can't remember" or "go photograph the secret you've never told anyone," which, if not consciously censored, can often result in clients starting on a path of discovery. Often I take my ideas from the photos they have already brought from home or from their responses in doing self-portraiture or projective work. Thus sometimes photo-taking assignments may include reusing or even reworking other photos or incorporating their processing into the design of the new photographing tasks.

These assignments can be open-ended ones, where I cast a wide net to see what comes up in clients' minds and cameras, or they may be more specifically focused on particular topics that I believe the client needs to explore further. The exercises at the end of this chapter provide examples of both photo-taking and photo-gathering assignments. These assignments may appear simple at first, but they can provide powerful personal insight, emotional resolution, and unconscious synthesis when we review and discuss both the process and results of that assignment.

Assignments can thus be tailored to client needs; for example, they can give clients a measure of control over impending closure, death, separation, fostering out, and other such issues by using photos to make transitional stages. Photographic documentation of such events helps make them real, and assists clients in accepting them. It is hard to move on to new situations if the old ones have not been cleanly "finished."

I have used such techniques in various situations. For example, I asked a mother whose adult son was very close to dying to photograph him in his hospital bed and to go to his home and photograph it as well. The stated purpose of the assignment was for her to have photos of these places for her own memories and also to take him photos from home for comfort at his bedside. My unstated, and more therapeutic, purposes included her coming to terms with the fact that her son was not going to leave the hospital and that his home she walked through did not contain him in it (and never would again). The process of taking the pictures was as therapeutically important as working later with the finished prints.

I have assigned children in divorcing families to photograph each parent and themselves with each parent. If there was to be a joint-custody arrangement, they were to photograph all the rooms in each home, in order to precipitate a bit more conscious contemplation of the changes that were about to happen and to help them to better emotionally occupy various newly revised identities. Each family member can be asked to take a number of photos of anything they want (including themselves) to give as a gift to a departing parent or sibling and, in explaining why these were the ones selected for taking, help to individualize and personalize the relationship being explored. In such ways, clients of all ages can gain a bit of understanding and control over life events beyond their usual expectations.

As a simple example of this, one young client found herself very hesitant to take a Saturday job and was unable to verbalize her reasons; she just knew she was worried and the vague anxiety was interfering with her job interviews. I asked her to go photograph a wide variety of jobs, to go make photos for a week of everywhere she found people working. I designed the task so that it would not interfere with anyone's work, and in case anyone got nervous about a teenager with a camera in their store, I gave her a "cover letter" on my letterhead stationery that explained (without defining her as a client) that I had requested her to complete a photo assignment for my office on students working at weekend jobs, and included my phone number for verification.

Thus freed to stare without staring (by looking through a lens and the later prints), she could test out the world she was so hesitant to enter. Several things emerged from her snapshots; for example there was a surprising preponderance of clocks over the heads of various employees. Noting this, I asked her about any possible significance, and she replied that as someone who had always been chronically late, she was very afraid of not making it to school and appointments on time and had begun to always locate the clocks anywhere she went, as a matter of habit so that she wasn't always seen glancing at her watch as if bored with the person in front of her. This small photo-based detail that revealed a bit about her worries illustrates how information can be catalyzed for therapy even from unplanned contents of snapshots.

Taking photos of a situation or person deemed difficult can help get a clearer focus of the problem or the relationship that appears insurmountable. For example, clients may be instructed to photograph the person with whom they have a difficult relationship or members of their family who they really secretly dislike, or to go photograph a representation of their childhood abuse (the room, the visual reminders, the perpetrator if possible), and so forth. These are assignments they may not want to complete because they expect them to be emotionally difficult. If they will risk it, even if it is necessary to tell themselves it's only for the therapist's reasons and doesn't count as self-initiated or desired contact, they often find that the worst thing they encounter is their own fear of trying. They may learn that it has been their own fear and resistance that has prevented resolution. The results of such assignments can be intensely powerful, not only in the resulting prints, but also in the actual process of beginning to symbolically take back the power over something or someone who the client previously felt crushed by.

Assignments can sometimes result in clients touching on that strange synchronicity that often appears in therapeutic processing. Although I don't understand the phenomenon, I have encountered it sufficient times to trust it. For example, in the morning on the first day of a two-day workshop, I asked participants to spend an hour photographing any topic on a list I provided (such as those in the exercises accompanying this chapter). The rest of the day was spent with other training activities, and the students didn't get to see the photos they'd taken until the following morning. They had other exercises to do in the meantime, including working with photos from their personal collections or albums they had brought to the workshop with them.

For one woman, the combination of exercises "accidentally" contacted some unconscious connections between her past and current life. These are her words:

> My grandmother was a very special person in my life. She raised me for my first five years, as both my parents worked and did not have time or energy to be with me. One day when I was five, Grandma went to the doctor and died in his office. I later learned that she had a heart condition, but at the time it was a huge void and unexplained mystery. Throughout my growing-up period, and now in adulthood, I retain so many memories, phrases, and personality characteristics of my grandma. When you asked us to bring important photos with us to the workshop, I brought an old picture of Grandma taken when she was in her early twenties. I value it because there is such a strong resemblance to me

at the same age (at least I've been told this). I often feel that she is with me somehow, even now.

Anyway, when we were asked to take photos around one of the themes presented, I chose "what I would like to be in forty years." I had misgivings about finding anyone in their seventies in this industrial part of the city, and even less hope of finding anyone I would want to be like. Nevertheless, I went out into the parking lot, and this sprightly, elderly woman came toward me on her way to the bus stop at the corner. I took seven shots of her from quite a distance, as she seemed apprehensive about the camera, and I don't blame her! She got on the bus and disappeared from sight. [See photo 6.2.]

When I returned home that evening, the image of this woman at the bus stop was really bothering me, as it seemed to jog so many memories of my grandmother. I searched and found this [photo] of my grandma in her winter garb in front of her farmhouse. Her coat and hat, as well as her general demeanor, are

Photo 6.2

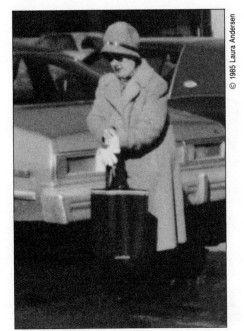

amazingly similar to those of the woman I photographed. I had not even been conscious that I possessed this particular old photograph. It had been years since I'd seen it, but obviously somewhere in my memory the image was stored. [See photo 6.3.]

So thirty-one years after the death of my grandma, the images were merged and dealt with. The next day when we got the photos back from the overnight lab, all these "coincidences" were confirmed. The sequence of photos appears almost to be a "hello to good-bye" statement; I even titled my collage of the bus stop photos "Good-bye Grandma." I still cannot quite believe the power behind and in this event. This is the strongest illustration of synchronicity that I have ever had, and I find it affirming and exciting.

This example illustrates how much more there can be to photo-taking PhotoTherapy techniques than the examination of preexisting photos that clients have brought with them to the therapy session. I have found that carefully tailored assignments to take photos or rework old ones can be exciting and valuable.

Photo 6.3

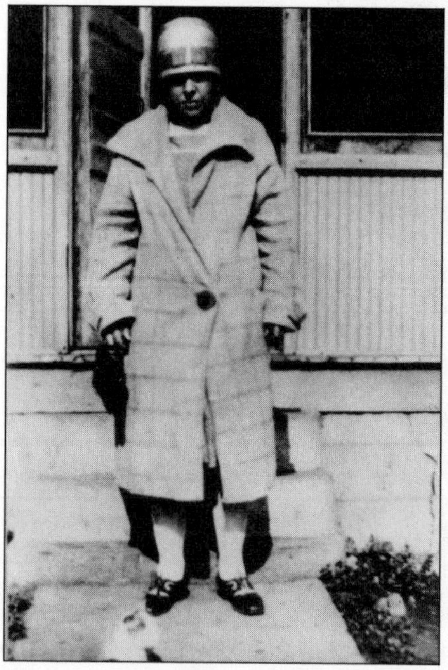

Other Aspects of Client-Created Photographs

I am not only interested in photos clients take or collect, spontaneously or on assignment, but also usually even more curious to find out how these can be used even further as representational artifacts in more complex processing. As these are discussed more thoroughly in both the following section about what to do with these images once the client has provided them, as well as covered within the various exercises recommended at this chapter's end, I will just briefly mention here that these additional combinations and permutations exist and can be very effective adjunctive tools themselves.

Clients can be asked to describe invisible photos, such as those lost though still remembered, or even those not ever really made, for instance, "If I had taken photos during the past year, they would show ____"; "If I were to take photos of my life to introduce it to my future in-laws before we actually met, these would be of ____"; and so forth. Asking clients to describe in words the pictures inside their minds will usually produce a lot more emotionally contexted information than just having them verbally answer questions about something. I have even asked clients to go photograph their dreams or what they are unable to tell in words.

Taking photos can itself be healing, just by virtue of the very nature of the creative art-making process. Similarly, darkroom printing of previously taken film can be itself selectively communicative and creatively expressive, in that what is printed will have been personally chosen, arranged, and kept, as is illustrated with the example told me by a client who didn't realize until a week after he had printed a photo of his family, that he had cropped his father totally out from the group and that the father's "not being in the picture" had remained completely unnoticed by him and his siblings until their mother pointed it out!

As our culture changes its attitudes towards those growing older or encountering terminal illnesses, they begin to be seen as individuals rather than a diagnostic group having no individual variances. Efforts to maintain quality of life are an increasing focus for geriatric and other traditionally disempowered populations, and life-review work has often been used to strengthen self-esteem in a variety of therapeutic applications with people of all ages. Life reviewing is a natural process most often taken up by those anticipating that life for them could end or change drastically, and thus "the elderly" become a natural group for using PhotoTherapy techniques to recapture the value of past years and relationships.

The PhotoTherapy literature, though documenting numerous applications of this chapter's techniques with all age groups, has paid particular attention to the usefulness of such techniques with geriatric groups and those dealing with loss-of-life issues (for example, Walker and Cohen, 1984). It is the life-affirming and memory-evoking purpose that photographs serve for such people that makes PhotoTherapy a particularly useful intervention with these populations.

Most of the various PhotoTherapy techniques that can be applied individually to counseling people can also be useful for larger groups or residential settings with only minor adaptations, and this is useful to remember when one is working with geriatric or terminally ill populations and with other people in sheltered living situations. A lot of the PhotoTherapy literature documents applications with people in either hospital settings, group living situations (retirement or nursing homes), geriatric day programs, community center activity programs, and even joint situations involving elderly and preschoolers together.

In such situations PhotoTherapy interventions have often been designed to help return a sense of individualism, personal meaning, and awareness, to provide a vehicle for making social contacts and validation for accomplishments, to engage previously untapped creative ability, to help people regain a sense of their own life's continuity and importance, and, in reviewing their life, to both stimulate communication and better accept the perspective that it is likely drawing to a close. Thus PhotoTherapy work with some of the just-mentioned populations would be done for different purposes than the traditional psychotherapeutic goals of individuation from family identity or improvement of interpersonal communication skills with others, because the needs and expectations of these people at different developmental stages or ability levels are usually quite different.

WHAT TO DO

This chapter treats photos by clients in terms of taking photos, collecting photographic images, and carrying out photographic-based assignments. However, in practical applications, these distinctions often blur and overlap. For example, in life-review work, I ask clients to bring in all sorts of photographic imagery that has mattered to them. This usually involves a variety of photographic artifacts, often including photos they themselves have taken. Assigning them to then do something with these images, such as collage work or active-reflective contemplation, further blends these facets.

I often start "working" this technique by just simply inquiring of the client what sorts of pictures do they seem to usually take, what are these usually of and about, and why do they think this might be the case? Do they like the photos they take? What do they like to take pictures of, and when? How can they tell when the moment is right or when it is something they will want to keep? When they do take photos, do they usually get the results that they expect? If not, what seems to usually go wrong? When they look back at their photos, what stories do these memories seem to construct of their lives, and how does looking at all those photos make them feel? This can itself be a very good, and yet relatively painless, way to start self-examination.

There is always one more person in a photograph than you usually find when counting. This is the photographer, who is always part of the moment, though often invisible or sometimes only noticed as a shadow. As a consequence, clients should be asked to probe each photo in their collections that they did not take themselves with questions such as "Who do you think made this picture?" "Did that person get what they hoped for or wanted as a result?" "Why or why not?" "Did they make it for a particular purpose, and what might that have been?" "What were this person's reasons for wanting to stop time at just that moment or permanently fix this place or person onto film?" "What might they have said or thought about it when they saw the result at first?" "What might they say about that picture now?" and other such questions directed toward finding out what different answers might occur should the client imagine herself or himself as the originator of that snapshot. This is how working with photos taken or collected by clients can be combined with the use of photo-projective techniques: sometimes pretending they took a photograph can release feelings or information in clients that may not have been available through working solely with their own pictures. All photographs we take are simultaneously personally projective and self-portraits as well; the techniques suggested for "working" each kind can well be adapted for application with any other.

Photos taken by the client can, and should, be debriefed to explore the possibilities offered both by pictures the client planned to take and by pictures the client took spontaneously, in response to an appealing subject. The client's reasons for wanting the planned photos, the circumstances involved, and how the results correlated with preconceived expectations all need to be considered. With regard to the second type, questions should focus on what in the visual and emotional contents of that moment attracted the client's attention so strongly that he or she felt compelled to photograph it spontaneously, without prior thought. In any case, when a client describes a photo and what it means to him or her, the therapist may have different perceptions or reactions. If these are shared nonjudgmentally as alternative possible interpretations of that photo, they can be helpful in exploring how and why people might have different perceptions of the same visual stimulus.

Working with Existing Photos: Reflective Techniques

If the therapist can get clients to share what it is about the contents of a photo that makes taking or having it special, the therapist may learn a great deal about what the client values in life. To get started, ask to see clients' wallet photos, desk or tabletop or refrigerator photos, and request them to bring in scrapbooks of photos or collections of pictures that have appealed to them, even those taken by others. Looking at these, it is quite natural and nonthreatening to ask questions about them and ask clients to tell you more about them: Why was each taken? What is it of as compared with what it is about (and how might this be different now than on the day they took or first saw it)? What memories are associated with each? What feelings arise when looking at them? How is the particular photograph you are looking at similar to all your others? In what ways is it different from them? How does it compare with photos in your family albums?

What is sought is information about what the client has photographed and why she or he has taken each picture at the chosen place and time. Also, what might have altered these decisions? Clients may also be guided to think about their influence in the role of photographer; that is, what do they attribute to the snapshot that might communicate about or reflect themselves? A very useful question is, if the client had to pick only one of these photos as most representative of him or her, which would it be and why?

Whenever I am shown a large selection of photos that a client has taken (or even just a contact sheet of proofs from one roll), I try to notice whether there are repetitions of images, symbols, or themes. When I begin to sense a rhythm or regularity to the client's visual interests, I often will state my perceptions to see if the client agrees. If we are noting similar things, then I might work to assess patterns as possible personal symbols or probe deeper for archetypal meanings. I might use direct interactional techniques, such as requesting the client to ask such photos, "How are you a portrait of myself in equivalency?" "What parts of myself do you represent?" "What parts of me are you trying to communicate with?" "What do you say about my own life?" "What do you want me to notice, speak about, tell, ask?" "What are you trying to tell me (about myself or my life)?" The client can answer for the photo (and even dialogue with it), either out loud or silently.

As the client begins to explain why he or she took or kept a particular photo, many things the person has never thought about before begin to become conscious. Questions at this stage need to deal with information and feelings about why the client took that photo at that time in that way with that content: "Why did you choose that moment? Why was that the 'right' moment and how did you know that? How did you decide what, who, and how much to include? Did you get what you hoped for or expected (which are not always the same thing)? Did you photograph instinctively or by plan? If photographing instinctively, did your hunch succeed in giving you the photo you wanted or thought you would see? If by plan, did it meet your prior expectations? How do you know this? What in the photos affirms this or disappoints you?

"Would you do it differently next time, and if so, why and how (or why not)? What were you hoping the photo would capture conceptually and/or emotionally? What did you hope it would bring forth in yourself when later viewed? What did you hope it would call forth mentally or emotionally in others when they saw it? What reactions do others express when they see it? Is this similar to what you thought other viewers would see or feel? If so (or not), why do you suppose this is the case? (Perhaps the client could ask those people why this is different.) Are reactions by other people to one certain photo consistently different from your own but consistent among all those other people? Why do you think that might be, and what might be the reason for such dissonance? What do other people tell you they think your photo(s) say(s) about you? What do you think about this and how does it make you feel?"

Certainly, what people take photos of is important, but so is what they don't photograph or don't notice in those they have taken. Probing in this direction can also be very useful; questions that ask about clients' usual photographic rules can shed light on their value systems. What they unconsciously or consciously exclude (or include but don't notice as making any visible difference) can be at least as significant as what they consciously include or pay attention to. Therefore I sometimes question whether there are any images that they avoid taking, or whether they have suddenly been surprised to find things in their own photos that they weren't previously aware were there. Sometimes they can bring in "found" photos to represent certain themes or feelings when they themselves would never have gone out and actually taken them; if it is too threatening to confront things directly (including one's own self-images) collecting or collaging previously published imagery can serve as a good transitional object for beginning to explore such things.

Much as an earlier section addressed using remembered or imagined images, clients can be asked to think about photos they might have taken or found and to talk about these. *They* will be able to see the images quite clearly, even if the therapist cannot. This can be a safe way to start questioning in this mode, as it can be less threatening than dealing with photos that the client is responsible for having made or brought in. An informal tone is most comfortable: "Are there any moments in your life you wish you'd had a camera to record? If so, what would these have looked like?" "Now that you are living in this new foster home, what pictures might you take if you could to show your parents what your new life is like and how it is different, better, or worse than living with them?" "Think of all the snapshots you took on your last holiday trip—which do you most treasure now in your memory?" "If you could make five changes at work, and take photos to show me those changes, what might I see differently?" "Are there any photos you've seen in my office that you'd like to have copies of (or wish you had made yourself)? What are these like? Why would you want them?" "If I gave you a roll of film (with free processing) with the instruction to go use it up by the next appointment, what kinds of photographs would you take?" And so forth.

Having Clients Take Photos: Active Techniques

Before asking a client to go out and take pictures, we need to be sure he or she is willing to do it. Some are comfortable photographing scenery or objects, but not other people. A person may feel intrusive, awkward, or afraid of being rejected if he or she asks permission to photograph other people (which, of course, clients should do). Clients who don't like to be photographed or feel that being photographed invades one's privacy may assume that others feel the same way. However, if social contact with a human subject is part of the therapy goal, then such dilemmas can be resolved through a variety of anxiety-reducing methods, such as rehearsal, photographing in large public gatherings or from a distance, photographing only in the mind's eye (no camera involved, just visualizing images), and so forth.

If the client is shy or unassertive, the photo-taking tasks can be designed with this in mind: first assign wide-angle shots of places or people from far away. Then begin to move closer to the subject, first by using a telephoto lens to visually (but not physically) get closer, and then later, when it's more comfortable, a normal lens, while the client gets physically closer to the subject. Or, begin with photographing crowds of people in public and then slowly have the client reduce the physical and personal distance (over many weeks) to a close-up of one person in a more private setting.

Socialization skills are worked with simultaneously as clients interact with subjects, observers, and later viewers of their pictures. Shared experiences occur on which friendships are often later based, as most subjects will want to see their pictures. Clients do not need to tell strangers that their therapist has requested such activities; they can simply say it is a "class assignment in photography" without bending the truth very much!

Completing assignments is sometimes the first indication clients have that they can create something that pleases them or others, or that they can take pride in. And they cannot argue with it if they, too, like the photo. This boosts self-esteem and self-confidence as they recognize that other people are impressed by what they have created, and especially as they know they themselves completed the process without being told what to do or how to do it. It is a tangible representation of their abilities to nonverbally create something that other people admire. Clients not usually expected to communicate, such as autistic or intellectually limited people, can find themselves enjoying picture-taking, even when they bring in snapshots of subjects that don't mean much to others, such as the blurry tops of trees, dead-end streets, or garbage cans (Hopper, 1990).

When beginning work with clients who may initially be hesitant to take pictures, I often start with extremely open-ended assignments, such as, "Go use up this roll of film on anything that catches your attention." "Go take pictures at the park or at the Little League ball game." Or "Just take some snapshots at that party or your family reunion." I emphasize that I would just like to get a better picture of their life by "seeing about it" instead of only hearing about it. I stress that there is no hidden agenda, that I have no secret ulterior motives, and that I'm not going to be searching for anything in particular when I look through the prints they bring in. It's just that I want to have a better idea of what they are interested in and who the people are in their life.

Photos clients are assigned to take can be oriented toward capturing specific events, places, objects, and so forth, that form their daily lives, or can focus on capturing more abstract concepts, such as feelings or memories. In asking clients to go photograph their feelings, either as an open-ended assignment or with a request that they capture particular emotions other people are expressing (such as fear, anger, sadness, frustration), several things happen that can be of therapeutic benefit. Clients not only get a chance to find out what these feelings look like on others, but also discover that others can manage to express them appropriately. They literally get a good picture of what these emotions look like and can also examine them at arm's length and see if they fit for themselves. Feelings that are feared must be confronted before they can be risked; things people hate must be confronted before any change can happen. Generalizations must be individualized if they are to be neutralized. Phobias can be desensitized by photographing and rehearsing encounters with the visual evidence first before facing the real thing.

Assignments can be innovatively created by therapists who wish to have clients explore their feelings. I may ask clients to take pictures of whatever makes them feel sad, happy, angry, worried, safe, frightened, or depressed, or just go shoot things that make them have strong feelings of any kind. These assignments validate clients' right to have these feelings and signal them that I am certain other people have them, too (without being crazy). In seeking, finding, and documenting these feelings, clients must cognitively map and define them in order to examine them consciously.

I may similarly ask them to photograph their problems so that I can better understand them, or photograph their hopes, dreams, message for the world, what no one really knows about the real person they are, and so forth.

I may use general wide-focus assignments such as "take at least one photo a day with the instant camera and then write about it or talk into the tape recorder about it, bringing me the week's worth when you come next week," or more narrowly concentrated topics, such as, "Photograph people who seem to be feeling the same as you." I particularly like asking clients to photograph "my life in twenty pictures or less," "what's wrong in my life," "things about our relationship that make me mad and frustrated," "what I would like to change about my significant other," "what I really want out of life," "things that bother me," or such self-reflective topics as "the me nobody really knows." These are self-portrait in nature, of course, but they are also photos that clients consciously construct, and usually are not of themselves directly. Regardless, these photos will indicate what is important to them and what matters in their life, their underlying values, attitudes, belief systems, and so forth.

My procedures can range from lending clients my cheap and practically indestructible cameras to use until the next appointment, to requesting that they use their own camera, to asking them to make photocopies of pictures in their personal collections that will furnish answers to the assigned questions. I may even ask them to draw representations of photos that would exist if only they could have taken them. I may request a specific number of photos to finish the assignment, or simply tell them to use up a roll of film on one or all of their choice(s) from a list of possible topics. Sometimes I give no specific topic, but rather just ask them to go shoot themes of their own. (Many clients have come up with very good ones by themselves, such as, "I love you and you don't seem to know it," "What this family means to me," "When school is over, I will ____," and others.

In addition to these possibilities, clients can benefit by using their cameras or, more often, their photo collecting, to take or find photos that can help them summarize their daily life or reflect on their personal history. This can be in a right-now sense, such as "please create a scrapbook about yourself that you might use to send to another country to tell your pen pal (or distant relative) more about you and your life," or it can be in a life-review summary sense, as when I ask clients to consider that they have been given one (three, six, whatever) months to live, and must try to put together a photo collection which would represent their life's journey or value, create a visual will or construct their visual legacy. Sample assignments in this case might include: "things that are still unfinished in my life," "things I want to do before I die," "if this were the last roll of film on Earth or the last photos I know I can ever take," "photos to show people of the future who I was and what my life was like (to those born a hundred years from now)"; "the visual legacy I'd like to leave to my grandchildren," "a document showing what I've done with my life so that it can be seen to have had a purpose," "a document that shows me as the pivotal bridge between past and future generations," "how my life got to where it is today (markers in my own life's story)," "my accomplishments (even though perhaps not significant to others)," "things I've done to make the world a better place (or help people)," and so forth.

The snapshots resulting from these assignments can be therapeutically worked as images on their own, or, as the following section discusses, they can serve as the basic artifacts for further PhotoTherapy or art therapy combinations in processes such as the creation of a personal time line or other collage work.

Instant-print cameras can be used in the office in the midst of dialogue with the therapist to provide an immediate visual expression of something the client has just said or tried to express. This immediacy can be used to great therapeutic advantage when, for example, a specific client needs the extra factor of immediate visual feedback. Using "invisible" cameras can also be helpful, as when clients "take" (or remember) photos in their mind and sketch or describe the images. One colleague (McDougall-Treacy, 1979) has developed a useful exercise based on these principles, her "person-as-camera" experience; it is revealing and enjoyable to participate in.

Later Uses of Images for Complex Applications

Using photos they have taken or collected, clients can make collages, time lines, visual stories, and other creations. These can then be worked using much the same procedures as have been described in previous chapters. In this milieu, however, an entire collage can "speak" with the client, exchanging questions and expressing feelings. With younger clients it is sometimes helpful to ask them to create a comic book with the images and write scripts or dialogues below, or onto, the finished photographs or photocopies of them to create stories.

Instructions from me that might produce such useful material might be ones such as, "take all the photos you've brought in as a response to the assignment and lay them out on the tabletop (or large sheet of newsprint) in such a way that they make sense to you; now that they are there, perhaps share with me what sorts of feelings or thoughts come to mind when you view these all at once (which might be different than when seeing them individually)" or "Now that they are taped down in the arrangement that makes best sense, try connecting them with lines, shapes, colors, words, or even other pictures in such a way as these connections help to support or explain the first layout." Using art materials and snippets of magazine images or words, or constructing visual/verbal narratives to help fill in the blanks or further detail their overall reaction to the entire collage, clients can provide very useful information and emotional details that may not have been available in discussions of individual snapshots.

For example, one client laid out a collage whereby the central five images were brightly lit and full of color and those bordering those five, placed closely to the four corners, were somber, dark tones in contrast. She drew dark lines between these corners to form a border encompassing the bright ones. She herself appeared only in the corners, and the central ones were all of various lovers she had known. Either PhotoTherapy or art therapy could help here, but in combination they could suggest so much more to any therapist trained in both processes.

Numerous images (not fixed to paper), spread out in front of the client, may be used in exercises that require the pictures to be moved or sorted. The client can even be asked to find other photos from magazines, family albums, or even my own always-ready collection of photos for projective uses. Photo-interactive exercises (for example, the Space Station exercise described in detail at the end of this chapter and the Rings exercise discussed in the next chapter) are usually done step-by-step, so that the client encounters the photos and their meanings and makes decisions about their personal importance or value in a structured context. The only requirements are that the images have personal significance for the client and that the clients think about their selection criteria when choosing images to use in the activity.

Once the photos are laid out so that all can be seen at once, I might pause to talk about the collection as a whole or the selection process (for example, whether the client encountered any emotional reactions or surprises in the selections or the process). But I much more frequently move directly into the active part of the assignment, as talking can be a strongly intrusive interruption.

In the Space Station exercise, for example, I ask clients to select six images from the larger collection (see the Sample Exercises for details) and to put the rest away. Eventually the client must select the one photo most meaningful to the terms of the exercise. These actually end up being prioritized in order of their value to the client (numbered from one to six, with number one being the single most important photo of the entire group). The number of photos at the start of the exercise is arbitrary; if there is less time, you may begin with four or five; if several hours are available, you might prefer to begin with ten or twelve. However long the prioritization process lasts, the client should remain silent; it is a nonverbal process, and if done well, the client will likely be in a trance-like state of intense focus on the photographs. (See photos 6.4 and 6.5.)

When this portion of the exercise has been completed (see the Sample Exercises following in this chapter for the exact instructions), the client is asked to talk about the process itself, as well as about each image. Using interactive questions suggested throughout the previous four chapters, the therapist should be well versed by now in the kinds of possibilities for therapeutically working with each of these client-taken (or found) images on its own, along with ways to have them dialogue or interact with one another while the client 'observes.'

The Space Station exercise can precipitate some of the strongest ther-

Photo 6.4 ***(left)***
Photo 6.5 ***(right)***

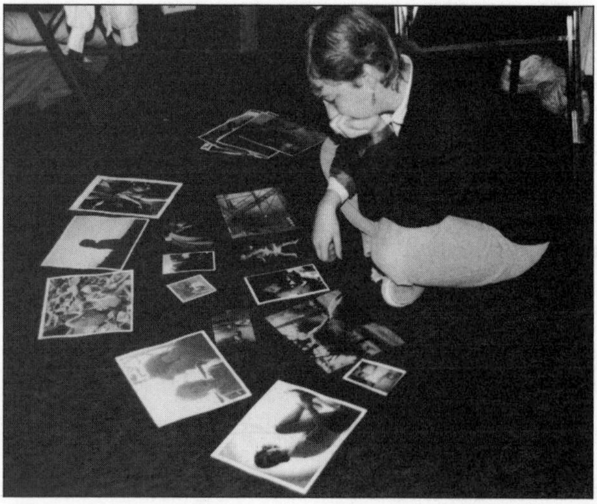

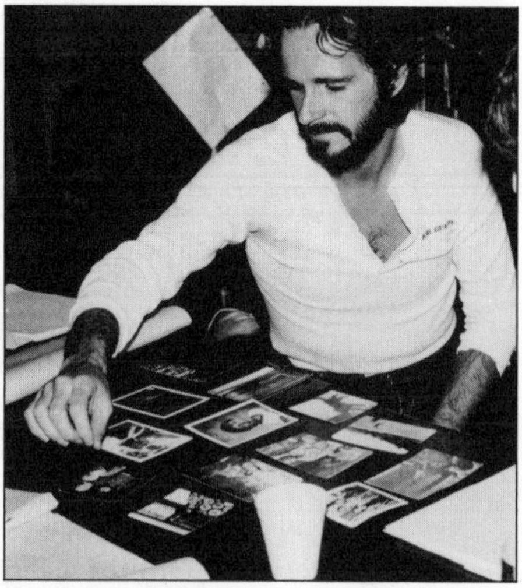

apeutic consequences I have ever encountered. It asks clients to consider that they have been granted their ultimate wish to travel in space and happily occupy a space station, alone and with no further human contact for the rest of their lives. They have to pack quickly and can only take along a few personal items—and no more than six photos—and particularly, that they are never coming back or seeing Earth or any of its inhabitants again. This preparation elicits serious contemplation of what is important in one's life; the exercise is also a clear, though often unconscious, metaphor for the death process and grieving.

Suddenly these thin pieces of paper become very dear stand-ins for those people and things important in the client's life, and knowing that they will never see these again can stir up major emotions and inner turmoil in clients not expecting to encounter them in such a raw fashion. As one client expressed it, "I felt like the final selection process was like my first aid training in doing triage work. This process of elimination began to feel like I had the power to decide who I was going to keep alive and who I must therefore let die. It felt like war, and it felt awful!" Another told me that it was all too painful to contemplate leaving voluntarily and that he would simply commit suicide rather than leaving all those he loved behind to never be seen again.

Doing this exercise individually with the therapist can be very useful on its own; however, sharing the results with significant others or family members can augment communication and introspection. Sometimes I ask the client to show those others the entire original collection—as many as fifty images before narrowing choices—and have the others tell the client which six each thinks the client would have picked during the actual exercise. Checking their expectations against the final order can also be very productive and emotional. Similarly, the client can be asked to guess which original fifty (or final six) their significant others might pick if they were doing this exercise, and then have the other(s) actually do it (alone or with the client witnessing, depending upon the situation). This, too, can be cathartic and informational. Regardless, this type of exercise allows participants to explore issues of significance, separation, loss, grieving, and death.

Often I hear such qualifier questions as, "Will I ever be visited up there?" "Will I actually never see other people again?" "Will I have a mirror to remember what I look like, or should I take along photos of myself too?" And "Will those left behind find out whether or not I've brought along their photo?" (from those for whom this will make a significant difference in terms of guilt). I usually leave these choices up to participants; how they decide can provide therapeutic material.

The strongest portion is usually the final partializing, where people find that they have to choose between photos of, for example, their mother or their wife, or one child over another. Encountering such forced choices has sometimes resulted in clients later making one photo that has everyone they love inside the single image. In finding out what photos are most significant to them, clients may also realize how terrible it would be to lose these to fire or theft, and consequently decide to have duplicate copies made of the most important snapshots.

Many go home to tell someone how important that person is to their life, and that they had not previously thought so or said so. Some people select photos of places because they know they'll remember the faces of loved ones; some find that they want only people photos because scenery isn't important to them. One person found that for the final choice (between photo number two and photo number one), he had to choose finally between a deceased lover from a past years-long relationship and the person with whom he was very much in love but just beginning to establish a formal bond. He said he kept running into his "shoulds."

Another found she had ranked her six not according to her needs, but instead by who needed her the most: her grandchildren ended up in first place instead of her husband or children. One woman said that, in trying to decide between a photo of her father and one of her husband (for the final first place position), that "I learned a lot about my dad and all my unfinished business around him. I found what I could and could not give up. I discovered finally that I could give up my past, which was a large surprise when I found myself doing it!"

Another discovered that, although his family made it into the final six, that ultimately when he narrowed it down to the one final photo that it was a picture of a stained glass artwork he had made, as it expressed something so deeply inside himself that he could not explain it in words, but knew that if he could only take one photo that this had to be the one.

One woman's final six were all of her dog and cat rather than her family or friends, and in explaining these selections, she reported, "They are the real loyal family to me. The dog always sits by my side in my studio (except when another dog goes by and she gets interested). The cat is so loving (except when he has a bird in his mouth and then I hate him)."

This woman had previously done a self-portrait exercise where, in discussing her results, she had commented on being the mother to her animals and mentioned that she would not give her photograph to either her husband or her daughter (with whom she lived). I wondered about this life where the animals were great except when they were acting like animals (their true nature), and began to probe her relationships with people, wondering if there were similar unrealistic expectations putting conditions on their lives.

Each person will do this exercise differently, but I have rarely encountered a client or workshop participant who did not find it intensely powerful and emotionally complicated. Many of them express feelings of deep sadness, of experiencing endings and leavings, of letting go and moving on while leaving parts of themselves behind, about giving up one's hold on some things in order to learn more. "It was like I was killing them off, one by one, like a concentration camp full of death; it was full of good-bye's," described one woman.

At its most extreme, the Space Station exercise precipitates feelings about death and bereavement, loss and grief, and a host of other relationship termination issues. If these intense feelings are too extreme for your clients' current situations, the exercise can be lightened by using different instructions: "You have just walked into your home and found it on fire; you have two minutes to select the six photos you can escape with safely," or "You discover that you must move to a much smaller apartment; in fact, it's so small that you can only take six photos with you when you move there."

ILLUSTRATIVE EXAMPLES

By now, readers should be quite familiar with the process of debriefing selected individual images by asking particularly-focused questions, and so I will not spend a lot of time now in this section repeating illustrations of such therapy involving single snapshots. This section will provide a bit more comprehensive demonstration of the wide variety of results that can arise (and be worked with) using this particular technique, as well as some feedback from those experiencing them as to what it was like to go through them.

Photos the Client Takes Independently

Many examples in this chapter illustrate spontaneous photos by clients; therefore this section concentrates on photos people take with conscious forethought, after arranging the scene, props, and so forth. The photographer's image may or may not appear in this type of picture, but when it does it is used more as a prop, consciously placed to help form the story of the photograph, rather than as a self-portrait. Of course, these boundaries are blurred, as many such photos can be both types simultaneously.

Photo 6.6 was created by a woman who sought to make psychological statements about gender oppression. She explained to me that she used mannequins because they were maneuverable and because they signaled the objectification and disempowerment of women's bodies and voices in traditional photographic practice (and life) (Newberry, 1990).

The next photo was taken for different, yet related, purposes: to visually present oppression and feelings of angry powerlessness. Yet both photographers reported to me that the planning and taking of their photos itself provided a degree of self-empowerment and helped give voice to inner messages and feelings. This second example deals with class oppression, yet its visual presentation is (to me) also clearly connected to gender. Again, the results helped reclaim the self of the person making the photos.

Photo 6.7 was made by a woman who put herself into the picture not for self-portraiture purposes but to express her feelings about being evicted from her apartment in a charming old building so that developers could tear it down to make room for condominiums. Her feelings about having to move concentrated into obsessive anger and unresolved conflict. She fought the eviction notice and won a four-month extension, but eventually she had to leave what had been her home for two years. Recognizing how much the experience was affecting her life, she addressed the issues photographically to explore them and to document what was soon to be only a memory.

I pondered the psychological territory for clues as to why this event had become such a critical one for her. As it happens, "her" house still sits there, empty and damaged. Tenants of other such places have refused to move out and still "squat" on, but she and other tenants did leave this place. Perhaps she felt guilt over abandoning her building, not protecting it, as she subconsciously thought she ought to (thus possibly tapping into leftover childhood issues or those relating to nurturing or mothering needs. She describes her childhood as one where the idea of a stable consistent

Photo 6.6

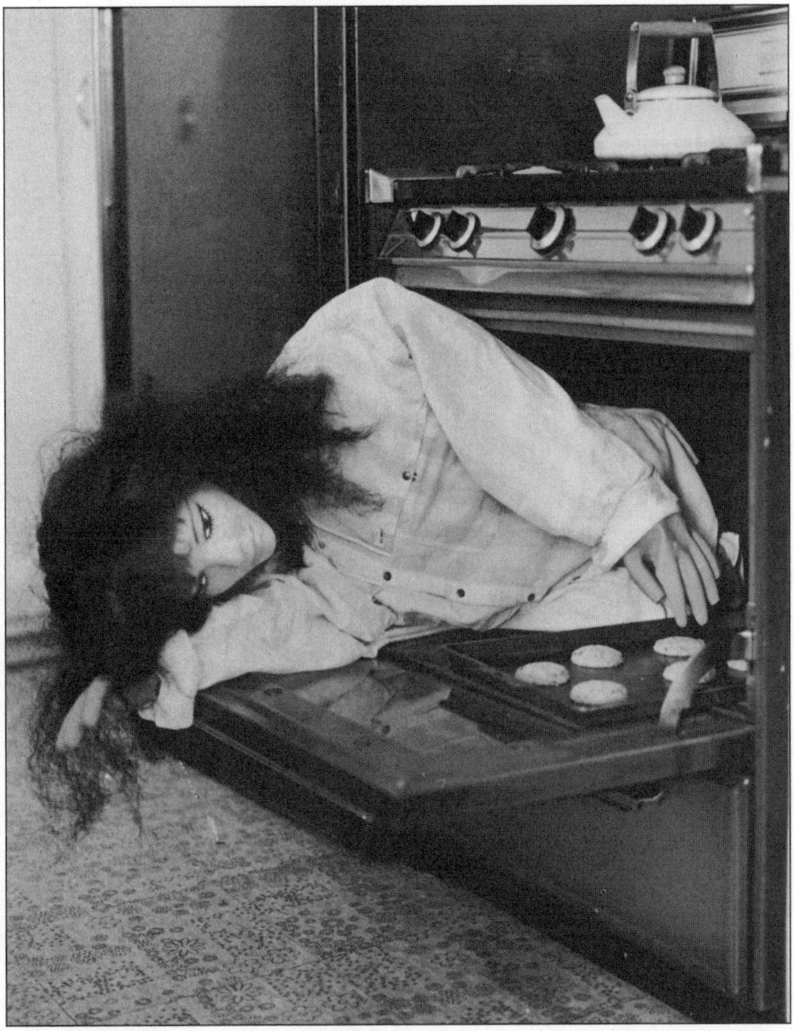

© 1990 Barbara Newberry

home environment was "a joke." Her parents separated and her family moved six times before she was eight years old. "Home" was carried from residence to residence. As an adult woman she has staunchly maintained her freedom and has continued to move frequently. As she puts it, "Other places I've lived in before, I left by choice. This is the first time my home rejected *me*."

Photo 6.7

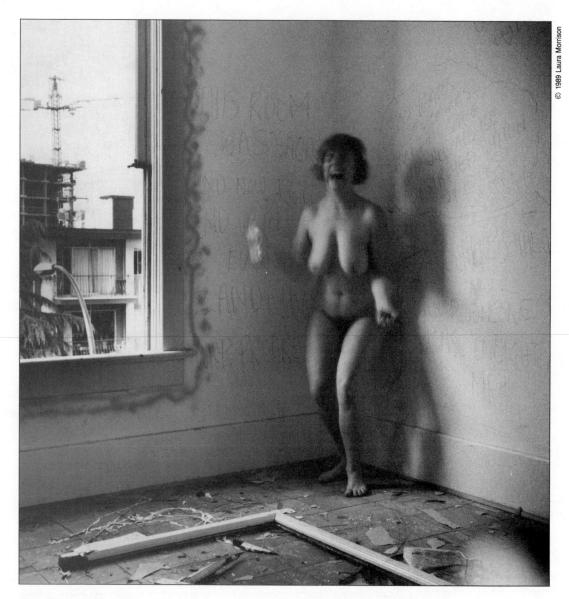

I asked her if the situation and her feelings would have been different if the house had been torn down immediately rather than still sitting there blaming her. She was ambiguous in response: "I've just been really obsessive about the whole thing and I feel caught because I want the place to be torn down so that it doesn't exist anymore, but I don't want anything new to be built there either." When I asked why, she replied, "The people who would buy those condos wouldn't have any idea of what they had replaced, and that construction would have permanently erased history. I feel regret that I didn't stay, really angry when I hear about squatters who've managed to successfully stay in theirs."

She expressed personal feelings of powerlessness: "What do I do with my rage? So far, I've taken pictures and talked to lots of people, but it's not been enough. Now I'm trying to organize a show on housing. I keep wanting some kind of damn good reason that this is happening, but there doesn't seem to be any except maybe I'm supposed to be learning to face something." In many ways the apartment had been this client's ideal home, and she felt outrage at having found it only to have it taken away by "enemy" forces who left her powerless. All of these were issues that she needed and wanted to explore, and she hoped that her photos would help her do this in therapy.

She added, "This experience taught me that when faced with power, I knuckled under. There was also fear. I was too committed to material things like my stuff being thrown into the street. I wasn't getting much support from other people for my fight to stay there. My friends got tired of hearing my complaints, [but] it all began to feel like an end-of-world frenzy to me."

In the photos she took initially to express her frustration, she found stimuli to communication about deeper underlying issues and more wide-reaching concerns. We agreed that she should do some therapy work around these issues to prevent them from becoming a permanent pattern in her life and protected her from associating love and involvement with the fear of loss.

Photos Taken in Response to the Therapist's Assignment

I assign photo taking for several reasons. Beyond the gleaning of additional factual information about who or what is significant in the client's life, and the benefits for them of the actual picture-taking process, there is also the reason that client photo taking can help me clarify things they believe they have already explained to me quite clearly, but which I am still left vaguely confused about. In the example that follows, I simply wasn't "getting the entire picture" of what Rosa meant when referring to proper mothering; viewing her photos, I began to understand what she was really telling me.

My client was a nine-year-old girl named Rosa. She had been physically and sexually abused and emotionally neglected by her birth father. For these and other reasons she had been in a foster home for the past five years. I found her to be cooperative and conversational, but her emotional relationships and expression of feelings appeared to me to be very limited and blocked. Her foster mother was concerned; she had just returned to work a few months earlier, when her youngest child was old enough to be placed in day care, and she said she wanted to have Rosa talk with me because Rosa had grown distant from her over the past few months. No matter what I asked Rosa, I couldn't get any helpful information verbally. She answered my questions nicely—and neutrally—and I couldn't uncover the cause of her emotional withdrawal. It was also possible that Rosa might not know consciously herself.

As it happened, Rosa liked taking snapshots, so I gave her a few assignments: knowing we were dealing with feelings and emotional relationships, especially between her and her foster mother, one of the many topics I assigned was to go to the park and zoo and photograph people of all ages. Another was to take pictures of mothers whenever she had her camera with her and saw them; I wanted to find out how she saw "good" and "bad" mothers, which kinds of relationships she was drawn to or fearful of, as well as any other information that might emerge. The subjects of the photos Rosa brought to the next session were mainly female. Most were photos of children playing with mothers nearby or mothers pushing strollers or holding toddlers or chatting with school-age children. No individual child or groups of children appeared alone without a female adult nearby.

I scanned through all her pictures and pointed out a few other women who also appeared in the photos, but who were either alone or with men or other women, and asked Rosa about their "motherness." Rosa's replies clearly revealed some clues as to what had been going on inside her mind, very likely outside even her own awareness: "Those aren't mothers at all, or else they're the 'bad' mothers, because their children aren't with them!"

In retrospect I could understand how this girl of an abusive childhood would naturally have felt vulnerable and unsafe when her mother hadn't been around to protect her, and how she might have internalized this in terms of the foster mother's having recently "abandoned" her own baby to day care rather than keeping the child with her at all times. The mother's act of returning to work sent a strong signal to Rosa. Also, working more, and with younger children to capture her attention when she did return home, the mother didn't have as much time for Rosa, who had lots of leftover issues with mothers who "weren't there." Rosa's photos pointed the way toward hidden information and helped open up dialogue and understanding between her and her foster mother.

Collage Work with Assigned Photos

If I take a picture of something or someone, then part of that thing or person in some ways actually becomes mine. I have made it mine by possessing its visual form, based on my personal motives for "taking it." If I see something in a photograph (whether or not other viewers see it), it is there for me; I can see it, so I know it is there. And if I have its visual representation in front of me, then I have some degree of control over it, even if metaphorically. This seeing-knowing-having concept contributes to the proof of the existence of the thing being examined. If I can see it, I know it's there. If others can see it too, even if only through viewing my photograph of it, the proof grows even stronger.

This aspect of photo making is particularly useful with clients whose memories or secrets have not been revealed to others or not validated by them. Having clients make photographs that illustrate such abstract concepts as "my abuse," "my fear of commitment," "my alcoholism," or other aspects of themselves, can help them gain sufficiently externalized pictures of those abstractions to begin confrontation, catharsis, and closure. Put concisely, to photograph something helps a great deal to make it more real, not only to others, but also to one's self.

The following collage was made by Sheila in response to a two-part assignment. First, she chose "the less obvious me" as her topic (from a list provided; similar lists appear at the end of this chapter). Next she took a dozen photos to visually illustrate that topic. When the prints were ready, she arranged them all on a large sheet of paper in a way that made sense to her, using art materials to further enhance the collage. (See photo 6.8.)

Photo 6.8

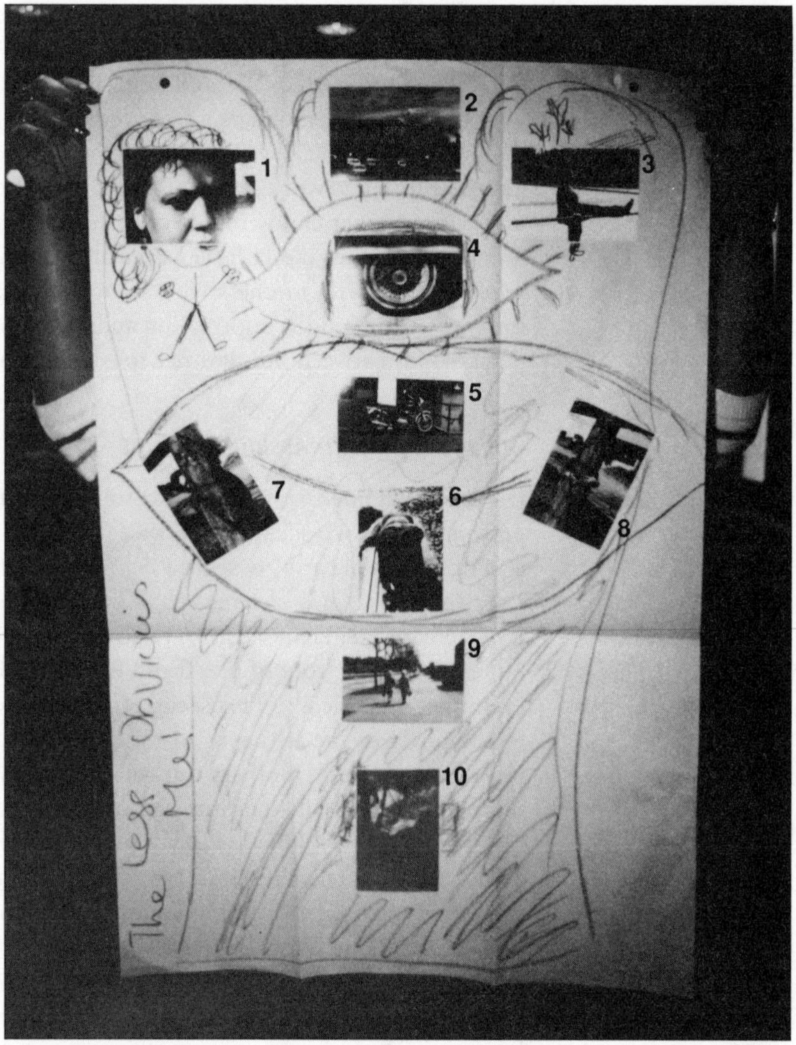

Sheila told me that when she viewed the list of topics, she had thought immediately of the terrifying sexual abuse she suffered from age nine to age seventeen by her step-father and another man. She realized that she was ready to see that trauma from a perspective outside herself, so she specifically went out to photograph her abuse.

Sheila used ten photos in her collage. (They are numbered in the reproduction here to aid this discussion.) She taped them onto newsprint and then drew a boundary form that visually enclosed them. She later described this form as a fist shape (the three bordering curves at the top that look like knuckles) and a face (a solitary eye and a closed but smiling mouth).

The overall shape, being such a strong, forceful, vertical form, seemed to me quite phallic, but I did not say so as I did not want to plant the idea in Sheila's mind. (In fact, when I first viewed her collage I did not know of her past abuse; she presented that fact later, while discussing the snapshot of the motorcycle.) The mouth is outlined in red and filled in with yellow slash marks. The "trunk," also outlined in red, is filled in with red slash marks. Above the mouth an outline is drawn in blue, including around the eye. The pupil of the eye is green. The title, placed vertically at the bottom left, is in black, as is the stick figure drawn around the top left photo. It is a person whose arms and legs descend directly from the neck (there is no trunk to the body) and whose hands are knobby fists.

Each of the top three photos is within one of the "knuckles." The photo at the top left (1) is of Sheila's face, but with no mouth (though she filled in her missing lip and chin in her drawing around it). The middle top picture (2) is of a stop sign. The top right (3) is herself sitting on a horizontal barrier or railing, in profile except for her head, the leg nearest the camera placed up on the horizontal support. In the center, immediately below photo 2 is photo 4 of the wheel of a car, with wire spokes on the rim; this forms the pupil of the floating eye.

Below the wheel is a photo (5) of a parked motorcycle (the image is obscure owing to the flash I used in taking this picture of Sheila holding her collage). Below, also in the center, is photo 6, a feet-first view of Sheila lying prone on a bench, with her head dangling off the opposite end; the two closest bulges are her knees, the next two are her breasts, and the farthest two are her shoulders (her neck and head are "not there"). These two photos straddle the lip line, and two other almost-matching photos of Sheila are placed at either end of the smile. These are both of her standing behind a tree so that its trunk completely covers *her* trunk. Part of her face appears from "underneath" in photo 7, and two arms are coming up and over it in photo 8. Otherwise, her body is blocked from view, as if being seen from above with a massive person on top of her.

The next photo down (9) shows two people walking away, and the bottom one (10) is a photo taken just after photo 6; but from the front of the bench and showing only Sheila's head and neck. An elbow is visible at the back left of someone off in the distance watching, but not involved at all. In this picture, Sheila has drawn, again in black, an end to the bench that cuts her body off with a vertical line right above her breastline.

When this collage was discussed step by step, Sheila responded spontaneously to each photo, telling how it related to the others and to the collage as a whole. She explained, "I wanted to go out and take these pictures and arrange them because arranging them was part of it, explaining them, and I wanted to put them on there and see what that did to me. When I took the pictures, I knew what I was taking. It wasn't one of those things where I just went out and took pictures. I wanted to challenge myself—because I had not done this kind of thing before. I hadn't done anything I could actually look at, myself. [My] abuse, to me, was always very far removed. I wanted to bring this a little closer. You know, you can go to all the therapy you want, but unless I deal with it, forget it! Right? So that's how I make it tangible to me. And it did wonders that way because I was able to look at it and say, 'yes, yes, yes, yes!' It was a way for me to bring it forward to me so I could look at it. The less obvious me is the victim me."

She went on to describe each of the photos individually. She at first described photos 7 and 8 as "me hiding behind trees," and then changed it to, "No, trees are strength but they are also phallic symbols, which to an abuse victim is also not strength to her, but strength of the offender. So in these, they come along and overpower me, because I know I'm looking around and trying to get around it." Looking more closely at the drawing around photo no. 1, she exclaimed, "Look at my hands—they're like this [making claw shapes]! I'm crippled; it's like I'm crippled! I have no hands so I can't push him away." The motorcycle picture (5), she explained at first rather passively as, "My step-father rode a motorcycle. That's where the motorcycle's from," but then went on to much stronger emotional discussion a bit later: "The motorcycle was quite by accident. I saw this bike, and I thought 'I remember this very well.' It was like the imperative to this whole collage because that was him symbolically. That was my symbol for him. I remember very much putting it in the center of that collage. Look, it's inside my mouth!"

I asked her, "Now, if you knew that you were going out to photograph all this, and knew you were abused, and you knew you were going to go photograph the victim you, the less obvious you, and you knew that you were looking for trees and things that would symbolize all this, if you knew all of this stuff ahead of time, why did you bother to go photograph it?" She immediately replied, "Because then I can visualize it all at once—and I'd have it to take home with me. I'd have it to keep. Why? Because I think—one can't always gauge their successes by just the here and now. It's got to be from where they come from, too. And I guess that would be why, that I am no longer overpowered by this person at all. And I can look at that and say that, yep, that's what was going on. But now, this is a different Sheila, this is a much different Sheila."

Looking again at photo 9, Sheila suddenly realized, "These two little old ladies walking away, they remind me now of my aunt and my grandmother, who were twins and completely shut their eyes to the abuse. Neither one told me he had been arrested seven years before we came to live with him. They never told me that, and they knew very well!" Looking again at photo 10, she described it as being up on a table underneath a body: "I would die like that. I felt many times that I was just going to die. I really did. Like I was going to die from it. There's my grandmother [photo 9] and I'd just died of the abuse," and then she pointed out how the abrupt end to that "table" reminded her of being boxed in, as if in a coffin. The stop sign, "was a definite [message]. I know what that means. It's just like, 'Stop it!' That's all it was. I needed it."

During the discussion, we gathered her fragments of information and reactions as we went from one photo to another. Then we built our next hour's dialogue on weaving them together. It was only in later stages, reviewing the collage, after the original exploration of it, that she began to find even more than she had noticed in her first descriptive encounter with it.

Pointing to the tightly closed red lips, and referring to the placement of the motorcycle and surrounding three pictures, which directly symbolized the abusive acts, she became aware that she was actually having trouble breathing while talking to me and said, "I have to catch my breath. Oh, this is very weird, because all that is on here is an eye, and mouth, and god knows what all the red parts are down here. All the abuse stuff is in my mouth, and there was a lot of oral sex involved. You know what? I didn't realize that when I did this. I know that I didn't draw that conclusion when I [drew] this. He used to stuff a sock or underwear in my mouth to keep me quiet while he fondled me or did whatever, and once he [put] a knife blade on my tongue. He just laid it there. He was a horrible man. Maybe that is why the mouth is closed and smiling. Right now is the first time I thought of it. I had not paid much attention [before] to the art work around it until right now looking at it thinking Holy Christ! But I'll tell you, Judy, I don't remember putting these all in the mouth. I really don't, and I didn't notice that until I was sitting here today."

A bit later, the closed mouth took on even further meaning. "This mouth, I just keep looking at it. 'No more! [it would say] No more!' It's probably why I have those tiny little fists [drawn on photo 1]. I had just died. No more. I think, when I was doing this, a lot of it was the finale of the whole thing. The finalization of it all. It was *all* over, it was *all* done, it was *all* out in the open. He'd gone to jail; he was out of jail. It was *all* done. It was *all* behind me. There weren't any secrets left. Everybody knows. We can all get on with it. And I know that's probably why the mouth is closed."

I asked again, "If it was all done, it was all over, he had gone to jail and was out, if it was done, why did you do this [make the collage]?" She answered, "I don't know. I needed to." I asked, "If you did know, what do you think you would have done it for?" She replied, "Because I wanted to see it there. I wanted to *see* it there. I think the victim comes to deal with it in your own way. I think because we're all different and it affects us differently, we take our own ways out of there. [Now] it's on paper. That difference is validation—putting them all there, and seeing it, and validating it through photos of myself. Before, it was like this happened and that happened and this happened. It was all rambling for me. This tied it together. Somehow all those little pictures all went [claps hands together several times] 'Done! Stop! Finished! Over! You know, done!' Before, I couldn't say to someone, 'Well, this is how I'm feeling,' but the pictures help explain that. It helped explain it to me. It did. I put it all there, and I tied it up."

Reflecting more about the original decision to photograph this subject and make the collage, she reflected, "I wanted to see what that would be like to look at." I asked, "Well, what was that like?" She replied, "It was damn shocking. I mean, especially because I had set out to do that, and I thought I was being really cool, going click click and all that kind of stuff, and yet in control of it all. And when I put it all down on paper, I remember going, 'Oh my god!' because then I saw other things in the pictures that I wasn't looking for, and had not seen before, and my facial expressions in the pictures at the time weren't what I thought they would be like. [Was] that the child Sheila or is that the adult you? I had a wonderful time taking the pictures. I was in control of what was going on, and when I'm in control I'm usually having a good time. Coming back and then looking at it all, the emotion changed. It changed to one of "Oh! Oh, you did do that, [and] you did that well. It's good. It's what you wanted to present. Yes!' But then I started looking at the facial expressions. Somehow they weren't what I had anticipated I don't think." She summarized her feelings by saying that looking at each individual picture was no problem but that the power of this process hit suddenly when she had viewed the collage as a whole.

When I asked her about the overall shapes she had given to the entire collage when drawing its outlines or borders, she was unable to see it as any kind of image at all at first: "Maybe I was just trying to find a frame for it somehow." Then, after looking a while longer, she said, "It's sort of like a tree, like, like this [showing me a fist], you know—like a fisty sort of thing—phallicky! phallicky-ish! Yes!"

When later reviewing this process, she said, "I have got a lot of strength from my past when things happened to me that weren't positive. Somehow or other I have found strength in those experiences. It was awful, but there's strength in it. If I could deal with that, I could deal with anything. I wouldn't want to have to handle anything else like that ever again, but if it should come, I'm ready this time. I know I could handle it." She had gone to photograph her abuse so that she could finally see it outside herself. She kept the collage for a while to remind herself that it was over and could not hurt her any more, and then she threw it away—"because it was finished now."

Much later, Sheila made a self-portrait in a place she liked, near a parked car beside a wall of graffiti. I found it very interesting that in this picture she 'happened' to pose under a sign that read, "Authorized parking only. Violators will be towed"!

A Client's Response to Using Personal Photos

This last example deals with William's experiences with the Space Station exercise discussed earlier and also in the Sample Exercises. His experience was fairly typical: he has not had a camera since childhood and had a collection of snapshots of people and places that he has casually gathered over the years in storage boxes and drawers. He asked me to work with him, as there seemed to be many unanswered questions about his childhood, and he wanted to explore some of his difficulties with intimate relationships.

When asked to bring twenty to forty photos to use in a version of the Space Station exercise, William did manage to narrow his large collection to a selected smaller group—sixty-three images stuffed into a carrying case. The exercise proceeded according to the specifications in the Sample Exercises. My memory of the experience is that it became very intense for William, even in the selection of the first ten. By the time I was asking for only one, his eyes were brimming and his voice was nearly inaudible. He spent a good deal of time at each step of the narrowing-down process, sitting with the images, occasionally widening his trance to include me (and "coming to" a bit each time this happened). Other times it was clear to me that nothing existed for him except the photos (in fact, he later expressed surprise when I told him the telephone in that room had rung; he had not noticed it at all). Unfortunately, we did not videotape the process (and both now sincerely regret this, as much detail has slipped away), but he offered to write down his feelings about doing this work with me for the purpose of this book, because he said, "People just cannot know how powerful this is internally for someone unless they hear about it from someone who went through it."

Also, later I had asked him to think about what the groupings would have been if I had said start with fifteen instead of ten. He had definite answers as to who would now be included and how they would feel about it. I also asked him if he thought he would change any of the originally selected group if we did the exercise again, and he said he really believed not. However, there is a new person he has recently begun to date; if they become close, at some point he might be willing to consider including that person's image and thus would know that he was symbolically letting them into his heart. It would be a big nonverbal signal about letting someone get that close to him again.

One particular detail of my doing this exercise with William demonstrates the flexibility PhotoTherapy processes can provide both client and therapist. In this occasion, he found that he did not have a photograph of one of the most significant people to appear in the final six, so I took a tissue from the nearby box, folded it into a snapshot size, handed it to him, and said, "There, now you have a photograph of him. I can't see it, but let's say that its 'back' is to me, but you can still see what's there, so now you can use it just like the other images that I can see." This tissue became a key focus for William's attention at several moments in the process, and at one time he even held it up about a foot in front of his eyes, glared at it, yelled at it, and screamed out some anguished cries; it had become that person for him and was given the reality that it needed at that time.

William describes what happened to him as "much more interesting than I had thought it might be. It was quite a task gathering twenty- to forty-odd photographs that meant something to me! The 'process' of the session had begun with this search. Why did the six-year-old 'me' with the neighbor's dog bring that warm feeling? Why did that Halloween photo make me grin with a flow of memories? Why did I find pictures that I thought I'd thrown away in anger? I arrived for the session feeling like I was carrying something very special in my leather carrying case, this collection of 'me.' It's funny too, because photos never really seemed to hold that kind of power for me. Laying them out on the floor was interesting in that the 'therapist' in me began wondering what this collection of photos was saying about me. I remember being quick to say that I wasn't the photographer for most of the collection, trying to lessen the responsibility or impact. Ha!

"Choosing ten to 'take with me to outer space' was fairly straightforward. Narrowing those ten down to five was much more difficult. Who (not *what*) could I do without? Narrowing from five down became a very anxious event. My parents are divorced, and in my collection of forty photos there wasn't one of the two of them together (interesting . . .). So as important as they both are in my life, I took a picture of each of them to space. I wanted to include a picture of an old boyfriend—my first. The photo has always been a reminder of the passion I have for life (among other things!). I had wanted to include a picture of another boyfriend (the end of that relationship had been recent and difficult), but I didn't own a photo of him. So you folded up a tissue into the size of a snapshot. With some imagination, I could picture him clearly in the whiteness of the tissue. I seem to have totally blocked out what the fifth photo was.

"Narrowing the number of photos was hell. No one could have convinced me that a picture could be such a 'key' to information, feelings, and memories. But they were a 'roadway' leading to well-defined (but well-buried) memories. In verbal therapy sessions I've spent a good deal of time *talking* about my parents. My shrink would be the first to complain that when I talk, I distance a certain amount of emotion. And yet here, with this picture of my mother four inches from my face, I'm feeling angry, unloved, alone, and four years old. Your probing questions kept me on track for much of the time, but also allowed me to feel in control.

"Back to the folded tissue. Angry, disappointed, unloved, and alone. This is what the last relationship had left me feeling. I had been the stable understanding one throughout most of the relationship. Here I was feeling alone again. And recognizing it in context with other relationships in my life. At times I couldn't see the tissue for the warm tears that flooded my eyes. The sadness and anger took the form of huge sobs, a crying from within my body that I'm not used to. I've been able to connect with this type of feeling in a traditional verbal therapy session, but not this readily!

"At a particular point, I wasn't willing to get near an emotion connected to this last lover. You asked me to hold the folded-up tissue and say how I was feeling *to* it, as if it were him instead. I wasn't able to admit those feelings to *myself,* let alone him! But you urged a little harder, physically pushing the tissue closer to my face (confronting it). I didn't want it (him) any closer than I had it. You pushed a little harder against my hand; I pushed back—there was no way I was going to have this man *in my face.* Pushing, resisting, encouraging, confronting, and eventually crying, I was in tears because of a stupid tissue! I was feeling all those things that I had felt when I had decided to end the relationship, and I was so sad, so disappointed, and *angry* because I had wanted this one to work. Damn him, he let me down."

SAMPLE EXERCISES

Readers are advised to consider all levels of photos that clients have taken or gathered together in order to integrate the probes given below with other interventions based on self-portraits and/or photos taken of clients, including those that appear in their family albums.

Preliminary Considerations

Photos by the client can be reviewed and explored therapeutically from a number of levels. The client and therapist can together look at photos that the client has taken or else collected over the years from other sources like magazines, greeting cards, calendars, and so forth (as well as those given by other people as gifts). These methods of working with existing snapshots I call "reflective techniques," in contrast with what I term "active techniques," which involve having clients take new photos. In addition, these images can be helpful later as artifacts used in more complex applications or interactive combinations with those techniques discussed in the other chapters.

The therapeutic "working" of client photos individually or collectively was presented earlier in this chapter. The list of suggested questions and exercises below parallels the framework used in the chapter's text and gives a more complete and comprehensive set of directions for several of the exercises mentioned earlier (for example, the complete instructions for the Space Station exercise). As these previous chapters were so detailed in their descriptions of the many different steps of exploring photographic images with clients, I am not including a separate section about this in this chapter. Rather, the discussion process is now built into each section that follows, and these now also will combine the assignment tasks with those questions I recommend be asked about them.

Photos the Client Has Previously Taken or Collected

Clients can be asked to look through their personal collections of photographs to bring in photos they have taken or found and respond to questions such as the following: What sorts of things do you usually take pictures of (and about), and why? What is the usual mood or tone in them? When do you usually take them (under what circumstances)? How can you usually tell when a certain moment is the right one to capture and keep? How do you decide what, who, and how much to include? Do you photograph primarily instinctively or by plan? If instinctively, do your hunches usually get you the photos you want? Do you usually get the results you expect? If not, what seems to be wrong with them? What sorts of visual or emotional contents of situations attract you so strongly that you find yourself taking pictures spontaneously? Do you usually like the photos you take (and if so, why)? What is your usual reaction to looking at pictures you've taken? To whom do you usually show them, and what have been their reactions? What sorts of photos do you find you consciously avoid taking? What sorts of surprises have you discovered later in photos you've taken?

When you examine all these in front of you now, what themes or patterns seem to appear in them? What topics, subjects, or symbols seem to keep recurring in them? What particular moods or feelings do they seem to express? What sorts of messages or secrets do they seem to have? What stories do these memories seem to construct of your life? How do these describe you yourself? What reactions are you having right now looking at all these? What, if anything, would you like to ask or say to these photos right now if you could? What thoughts or memories arise in you while you are looking at these? What might they be symbolizing apart from their specific contents? Do these remind you of anyone else's pictures? If so, whose and why? How do these differ from ones found in your family album? What can these snapshots tell the therapist (or a stranger) about you? How do they do this?

Looking at one photograph (or just a few) in particular, go over all the questions above, just rephrasing them to apply to given snapshots. Ask: Why this picture? Why at that time? What was it taken for? Who was it intended for? What result was expected? How does this photo compare with the ones you usually take? How is it similar and different from the rest? From other people's? Does it hold any secrets or surprise you in any way? If you could, would you create it differently now? How? What had you hoped it would evoke in later viewers?

Address any given photograph(s) directly (and have them address you) in dialogue: How are you a portrait of myself in equivalency? What parts of myself do you represent? What parts of me are you trying to communicate with? What can you tell about my life? What do you want me to notice? What might you want to speak about, tell, or ask me?

Look at photos in your collection that were taken by other people, but that you collected on purpose to keep. Select some and ask the above questions, revising them slightly to fit each photo.

Now think about the added role of the photographer in the creation of the photographs? Who was the person who originally began the capturing of those moments that attract you so strongly that you wanted to keep that photo (or copy thereof)? What do you imagine were the photographer's reasons, feelings, and expectations in making that picture? What common themes or patterns in the photos you have gathered into your personal collection reflect you metaphorically?

Photos the Client Is Assigned to Take or Collect

Photographs clients take or collect on assignment can be reviewed and discussed using questions in the preceding section. Therefore, this section concentrates only on those kinds of photo-taking or photo-finding assignments, from basic simple tasks to complex or multistage activities, that clients can be given. The suggestions below are in the form of general recommendations; therapists will wish to tailor these to each client's unique needs and goals.

Simple Assignments. Clients can be asked to take photos in response to the directions, "Go photograph:"

1. your favorite place(s), the place(s) that are most special to you
2. your favorite activity (activities), what you most like doing
3. your favorite person(s), the person(s) and/or object(s) which are most special to you
4. your home and domestic environment; your work and/or hobbies
5. your family members (however you define "family")
6. inanimate objects or artifacts that could serve as stand-in's (or equivalents) for you (or some aspect of yourself or personality)
7. things, events, or people that you have strong feelings or thoughts about

Complex Assignments. Clients can be asked to take photos in response to the directions, "Go photograph, according to the topics of your choice below:"

Focusing on Daily Life

1. Take photos every day for a week (or every hour for a few days) of things, people, events, moments, to create a visual diary of your regular life patterns (or of a typical day or week in your life).
2. Take photos of things, people, events, and so forth, that aren't part of your ordinary daily life.
3. Take photos showing who you are (pictures that describe your various roles; for example, mother, lawyer, gardener, and so forth).
4. Take photos that show what is important, nice, or interesting about you and your life.
5. Take photos that communicate what is missing in your life or what it needs to be even better.
6. Take some photos of your problems so that the therapist can understand them better; pretend you are photographing what is wrong with your life.

7. Take some photos that can communicate about your goals and dreams for your life.
8. Take a few dozen photos that can serve to nonverbally describe you and explain your life to an important stranger, such as a distant relative, blind date, pen pal in another country, and so forth.

Focusing on Fantasy and Imagination

1. Take photos as if these were the last photos you could ever take, or as if this was the last roll of film in the world and you have just one or two weeks (or days) to use it up.
2. Take photos of what you don't usually take photos of.
3. Take a couple of dozen photos that would be your contribution to a time capsule that will be opened in the year 2100.
4. Take photos of what you cannot say in words or what your mind doesn't want to remember.
5. Take photos of the way you would like your life to be and/or the changes you would like to see happen in your life.
6. Take photos of things you want to do or accomplish before your death.
7. Take photos of what it means to be a grown-up or a child these days, what "woman" and "man" mean to you, what maturity means, and what success is like.
8. Take photos of what you think your life will really be like in two, ten, twenty, forty, or however many years you pick, and then also take some of what you hope it would ideally turn out like if you could control the future yourself.
9. Take photos of those parts of your life that no one knows about or that you feel others don't value enough in you or don't understand about you, the less obvious or secret you.
10. Take photos of your memories.
11. Take photos of photos that seem to have been skipped or overlooked in the making of your family album, photos you wish had actually been taken or included, or which you think were taken but consciously left out.
12. Take photos of abstract concepts like the difference between "safe" and "not safe" or the difference between people you can trust and those you can't.

Focusing on Emotions and Feelings

1. Take photos that will show how you feel about the world, your life, your work, your family, your friends.
2. Take photos of people who seem to be feeling the same way you do.
3. Take photos of things that make you have strong feelings, including your problems.
4. Take photos that present the parts of you and your life that you don't show to anyone else.
5. Take photos of the secret(s) you could never tell anyone before now.
6. Take photos of the more abstract inner parts of you or your various issues or concerns, such as "my abuse," "my fear of commitment," "my alcoholism," or other aspects of your inner self.

Focusing on Interpersonal Relationships

1. Take photos that express your roots and family background.
2. Take photos of each member of your immediate family as you wish to see them, think they really are, or wish they would be. (Each portrait should reflect *your* ideas and not be influenced by the subjects.)
3. Take photos of family events: occasions that are regular moments of your family being together (for example, a day in the life of your family, both collectively as a family unit and also each individual in it).
4. Take photos of people with whom you have close relationships, such as friends or work colleagues, and particularly your significant other(s), such as spouse, lover, and so forth. Show them in typical settings, doing typical things.
5. Take photos of what seems to be going wrong in family or other relationships, or of what makes you mad or frustrated about those relationships.
6. Take photos of people who threaten your stability or happiness and those who help enhance it, those who would help you in an emergency and those who would make excuses not to.

Focusing on Life's Story

1. Take or find photos that can create an autobiographical time line or narrative of your life; for example, photos that can represent

the years before your birth, your infancy, childhood, adolescence, coming of age, adulthood and senior-age years (even if only as expectations), and perhaps even your life after or beyond the moment of physical death.

2. Take or find photos to illustrate your important accomplishments, even if unknown or insignificant to others, such as those things you've done to make the world a better place or to help other people by making a difference in their lives.
3. Take or find photos that can help summarize or reflect on your life retrospectively by showing how your life was meaningful to yourself and others, how it had purpose and relevancy.
4. Take or find photos that can be used to form your visual will or visual legacy to your grandchildren and others of future generations, that will explain you, your life, and what is significant about it so that others born after your death will be able to know about you and your life's meaning.
5. Consider that this is the last day (week, month, year) of your life. Go photograph what you wish, and also try to put together a photo collection that will represent your life's journey or value. Along with this, take some photos to illustrate what it is that you haven't accomplished that you thought you would, the matters of unfinished business left over (and with whom), as well as the people you wish you could take with you (or leave yourself behind with).

Exercises That Use Client Photos as Artifacts

The above sections concentrated on photos the client took or collected. This section provides suggestions regarding additional work that can be done using these pictures as bridges to more complex activities. Most of the exercises presented below can be done from both an individual and a family-as-unit perspective. It is also interesting to have the client's significant other(s) do the same tasks and compare both results, even if this is only an imagined process inside the client's mind. Clients should be asked to follow the instructions given under any of the following headings:

Exercise One: Interactions. Arrange the many photos taken or found in previous assignments in front of you as a collage that, taken as a whole, makes sense. Or lay them out one by one like a comic book that can tell a story; perhaps add scripts and dialogue. Have each of these snapshots talk out loud about itself. Have them talk with you or ask you questions, and then you do the same to them. Have them tell you about yourself, their photographer. Ask each one what parts of you it represents or is trying to communicate about, what each is trying to say or tell you (or ask you) about your life, and respond in turn. Ask each photo why it was taken, what it means to you, if it had not succeeded what would have been lost, whether it was what you wanted, and if not why not, what its role or purpose is in your collection, and other such questions.

Exercise Two: Elaborations. Start with the autobiographical time line or personal narrative created in the previous assignment section. Take or find other pictures that will help illustrate your feelings about this story of your life or that can provide more information, fuller detail. Feel free to use any art materials you wish to enhance the story with drawings, pictures, additional collage materials, and/or words, if you'd like. The goal is to elaborate the emotional context of that story.

Exercise Three: Mirrors. From your collection of taken or found photos, select those that you consider to be the most interesting and desirable, or strange and undesirable, and place each one at the top of a piece of paper. Caption each photo and then write a paragraph about each in the space below it. Next, look at the stories describing each photo and reflect on how this story might describe you as well. Write about that discovery on the same sheet of paper; find other photos from your collection or family album that seem to fit with these, and think about why they go together. You may then want to create a self-portrait that will visually express the qualities in yourself that you described in writing.

Exercise Four: New Additions. Having laid out your taken or found pictures in an arrangement that makes sense, take a quick instant-film picture of yourself and physically place this self-portrait into the arrangement of snapshots where you (the you of today) would best fit in, so that it becomes part of the collage. In what ways does this affect or influence the overall feeling of that collage? What has changed with the addition of your photo as part of the picture?

Exercise Five: Reinterpretations. Gather together some of your favorite snapshots and ask a friend who has not seen them to view them and tell you what they are of and what they are about. Have that friend pretend you aren't there, that he or she has just come upon these pictures in a magazine somewhere as part of a stranger's collection of special snapshots. Have your friend try to create a story from the pictures that makes sense. Ask your friend to try to figure out why each photo was taken, why it was kept, what its significance might be for its photographer, and so forth. You can stop there, or ask your friend to tell you how he or she knows that to be "true," how he or she got that information from that photograph, where in the image this data was visually presented. It will likely be very interesting to hear your friend's version of your photographs and compare it with your own perceptions (whether you discuss this with your friend or not).

Exercise Six: Quick Choice (Two Alternatives). If time for doing exercises is limited, consider doing one of the following quick ones.

A. You have just come in your front door to find your home on fire. You have one minute to select six photos from your entire collection that you can escape with and save. Grab those six and put the others away.

B. You discover that you must move to a much smaller home. In fact it's so small that you can only bring six photos with you when you move there, and you have to pack to leave right now. Choose those six and put the others away. You have one minute to make your selection.

Exercise Seven: The Space Station*. This exercise has to do with making choices based on the meaning your photos have for you. To begin, bring twenty to forty of the photos that are most meaningful to you to the therapist's office. These may include family members, but don't need to. They also don't have to be actual photographs; you can use magazine pictures, greeting cards, postcards, whatever, as long as the pictures are special to you. While you are gathering the collection together, you may wish to reflect on what this choosing process is like and how you are making your decisions. However, although this may be therapeutically informative, it is not the focus of the activity. If there is a photo you wish you could bring but you cannot find it, it doesn't exist, or it belongs to someone else, feel free to sketch a simple representation of it, using only stick figures or symbols, if drawing is difficult for you; try to make this stand-in approximately snapshot size.

It is very important that this exercise be done in total silence, without distractions or interruptions except the therapist's softly spoken instructions. There is to be no other talking until the entire process has been completed. If you are truly confused and cannot continue, request clari-

*As mentioned earlier, this exercise is based on similar versions and variations devised by other colleagues, notably Harbut's (1975) Mars Trip and Stewart's (1980) revision of it.

fication; otherwise there should be no conversation as further instructions limit the experience and interfere with your concentration.

Do each step separately and in sequence. It is important that all of step one be completely finished before reading the instructions for step two, and so on. (If you are doing this on your own without being guided through it, you must try not to look ahead to the next step before finishing the previous one, as advance knowledge will alter your processing of the experience. I realize that this is difficult to do while reading this book, but once you begin using the exercise with clients, follow the steps in sequence because they are essential for good results.) If the narrowing-down forced-choice component is anticipated in advance, it will not be so powerful in actual activation.

Step One: Lay all the photos in front of you so that all of them are visible from where you sit. If it is more comfortable, you may use the floor. No particular order or arrangement is desired; just place them all out there so you can see them all at once.

Step Two: Imagine you have just been told the following: "Congratulations! You have just had your ultimate dream come true! You always wanted to travel in space, and now, out of thousands of applicants, you've been chosen to be the first person to live on the new single-person space station out beyond Mars. It's the new frontier, and you're very happy about this, extremely pleased, very excited, and very much looking forward to the journey. Even though you are to occupy this space station alone and have no further human contact for the rest of your life, not even a satellite phone or computer hook-up, it is still a positively regarded experience for you and you happily agree to go. Now, you have to hurry to pack because you are leaving this evening, and because it's a small spacecraft with a very tight fit, you're only allowed a very small suitcase of personal items. You can only take along a few things such as a change of socks and underwear, a toothbrush, and no more than six photos.

"So quickly make your choices now, in the next ten or fifteen minutes, and put away all the other photos, leaving in front of you only the six you'll take along. Oh, and don't forget: this trip is one-way; you're going to live the rest of your life up there. You're never coming back to Earth or having any contact with its inhabitants ever again. You're never coming back, never ever, but you knew this when you applied, and so that's all right with you. Now select your six photos."

Step Three: Once you have the chosen six photos in front of you, then imagine that you next hear, "Ooops! Did I say six photos? Oh, I'm sorry, the flight manager now tells me it's supposed to be five, not six. So you'll need to end up with a group of five photos instead of six. Your choice now is, if you can only take five photos with you to the Space Station, which five of these six will they be? What you should do is keep that chosen group of five together in front of you, and put that sixth one over to your far left. (Think of it as number six.")

Step Four: Now that you have the five remaining photos out in front of you, imagine that you next hear, "Oh, no! Did I say *five* photos? I'm so sorry, I meant *four.* So you'll need to end up with a group of four photos in front of you instead of five. If you can only take four photos with you, which four of these five will they be? What you should do is keep that group of four together out in front of you, and put that fifth one number five, over to your left, but a bit closer to you than the first one, number six."

Step Five: Next you hear: "By now, I'm sure you are 'getting the picture' of what this exercise is about. What we are doing is reducing this larger group one by one, from 'only four' to 'only three' to 'only two,' until there is only one single photo remaining. In other words, by the end of these steps there would be a line of photos starting with the first one you set aside to your far left—number six; then closer to it, to its right, would be number five, which was just set aside; then numbers four, three, two, and finally, at your far right, number one. This final remaining one would be the one and only photo from that original chosen group of six that would go with you if you could only take one photo to the Space Station. If only two were permitted, these would be number one plus the one immediately to its left, number two. What you will therefore end up with in front of you is a line of six photos that have been emotionally prioritized in order from six to one."

Note to the Therapist: Although these instructions seem simple, this exercise can be an extremely intense experience. It is probably the most powerful exercise in this book. The strong emotions that it inevitably evokes can boil up and erupt with surprising speed and power. If clients wish to talk about what is happening to them, the therapist must decide whether to permit them to interrupt or have them wait to discuss the exercise fully at the end. The therapist should not engage in discussion between the steps unless the client initiates it and the therapist considers the disruption acceptable.

Discussion at the End of This Exercise: First of all, think about how you selected the first twenty to forty snapshots that you brought in (if indeed you kept to this original limit). Then consider how you managed to select the final six that began the narrowing-down part of this exercise. What happened for you in making each choice after that? Contemplate your answers to the following questions and discuss your thoughts, feelings, and discoveries with your therapist (or if working in a group, pair off with a partner and share your comments with him or her).

What were the reasons for your choices? What criteria did you use for selecting or rejecting? How did this feel? Did you do this more from your thoughts or your feelings? Did your mind make the decisions or were these based more on your heart's choices? Were some choices easier to make than others? Which ones, and why? Were your original group more photos of the past, of childhood, relatives, and/or family events, or more in the present or recent past, with friends, lovers, current events and moments? What about those in the final six?

Did you find you "needed" a certain missing photo for a particular placement in your final choices, and you had not brought it, or that doesn't exist? What were the missing ones like and what difference would they have made in your choices? Did you wish that you could "cheat"—that you had one photo with several special people in it so you could squeeze more into each allotted position, or that you could cut and paste two photos together so that they could count as one? Were there any surprises, disappointments, frustrations in your decision process or the actual contents of the snapshots you examined? Did you put in more scenics or pets or objects, or were there mainly photos of people? Did you yourself end up in any of the final six photos chosen?

Regarding the final six photos you ended up with in the first step of the exercise, how might you title that grouping? If a total stranger were to come across these six photos all laid out in a line, what might she or he be able to learn about you from looking at them? What story might that person create to explain the person to whom these were the six most important photos in the world?

Of this final six, which were the most difficult choices to make, and why? If you took along photos of places, why were these so special? If you took along pictures of people, were these who you wanted or were they who you thought you "should" take? Would any of your final choices have to change if the people in the photos you chose or excluded were to find out about what or who you decided to take with you? Were the photos that included people mainly of them, or mainly about your relationship with them?

Which aspect of you and your life does each of the final six snapshots mirror back to you? Were there any memories brought up in response to working with these photos? Were any of these unexpected or connected with particular strong feelings? Have any questions come up for you as a result of doing this exercise?

Try talking directly with each one of your six photos, sharing your thoughts and feelings about how and why it ended up being put where it was. Imagine a dialogue where you can ask or tell those photos anything (or they you). How do you think they would feel, finding out that they ended up in the position that they did (or didn't!). Imagine a dialogue taking place between number one and number two, or any other two; what would this be like?

Think of a significant other in your life, whether this person was included in your top five or not. How do you think this person would have expected you to choose your photos if he or she could look at the group that you brought in for starting the exercise? Do you think this person would have expected you to end up with the final six placed in the order you chose? Imagine this other person doing the same exercise, using their own twenty to forty photos to start. What do you think he or she might have ended up with in that group of six? Do you believe you would have been included somewhere in their top six? Where? Why? How does that feel?

Imagine that instead of doing this as a personal exercise, your entire family had to do this as a unit, starting at the beginning by selecting twenty to forty photos to bring in. What do you think would evolve out of this? Where would the agreements or disagreements be? How would they get solved? What would the top six be like? Whose opinion do you think the photo-choices would most represent? (For more discussion about family applications of this exercise, see Chapter Seven.)

7 Photo Systems

Reviewing Family Albums and Photo-Biographical Collections

My client's purse had been stolen, and she was extremely upset—not about the money and identification she had lost, but about the photographs of her children, husband, parents, and dog that had been inside her wallet. Some of the snapshots could be replaced, but the dog was no longer a puppy, and the children were much older now. She expressed feeling sad and violated. In her words, "When I realized the snapshots were gone, it felt like someone had died."

The photos in that woman's purse constituted a mini-album, as do photos displayed on refrigerator doors, mantelpieces, bedroom dressers, and walls of the house (along with family videos or home movies). What makes each of these an "album," for the purposes of this chapter, is that each grouping means something special to the person who put it together and, in fact, forms a photobiographical narrative of at least part of his or her life.

Family photos in albums are useful as documents that inform family members of their heritage and roots. In looking at album photos together, people often reminisce and tell stories. This is not only usually enjoyable but also educational for others listening; this is an indirect means of learning about the family history and current social network. Hearing such stories over and over again while albums are reviewed gives children and newcomers to the family circle qualitative information about relatives which direct questioning about facts would never produce.

People select which photos of memories they want to make permanent. Photos never taken or never chosen for permanent display dissolve into the unmarked past. If a person is not happy in a relationship or not content with being viewed in certain situations, they are likely not to want permanent visual reminders of those situations. People you are uncomfortable being close to (physically or emotionally) are people whose photos you are not likely to want to keep in your personal life's album. People going through painful or discomfiting times in their lives are not likely to want to permanently record them. For example, if a marriage is in the process of self-destruction, the family may not want to pose happily for a group portrait. Conversely, they may choose to do exactly that to signal a false image of wellbeing to others. One client told me she forced her husband and children to pose for just such a Christmas portrait for her parents because even though divorce was imminent she couldn't face these issues during the holiday season and wanted to present a good image to her friends and relatives.

Spontaneously taken snapshots may offer the best clues to family relationships and interactions. If we look at them in combination with more formally posed pictures, we gain insight into how people wish to be seen by others. And if we then look at how a particular family member has selectively arranged photos to reflect and present the family, we can learn what they think is important for others to know of that group. The underlying assumption here is that each family member's personally constructed album documenting that family will likely be a different version of the family story. Just as an album is more than the sum of all its images and pages, so too is a family much more than just the individual people it happens to contain.

Whereas self-portrait techniques focus on clients' individuality, who they are uniquely, family albums express the connectedness, interdependencies, and complicated causalities from which client individuation and differentiation emerged.

An album is a means of keeping the historical continuity of clients' lives in a way an unorganized collection of photos cannot. Photos of people are kept long after their names have been forgotten; it is a way to keep a family together forever. One client told me, "I stay alive in someone's heart as long as they know who my photo is of." The family album puts the individual into the family context and connects its private and public definition of identity. It is neither totally fact nor totally fiction, but rather a subjective construction by the albumkeeper of the lives of other family members—whose own versions of the family story are likely to be different.

Therapy focuses a lot on personal memories of the past. In telling about their family photos and albums, clients are also telling about themselves. Their explanations reveal their understanding of the paths they have taken. All photo-album explorations are ultimately also self-portrait work; in doing it, clients end up primarily finding out about themselves.

Some people don't have many photos in their lives. Some people don't want to have any, while some clients complain that they didn't get any ("My mother kept them all.") This may have no therapeutic significance unless it is "a difference that makes a difference" in the life or therapy process of the client. If there appears to be some importance to a lack of visual history, I might probe a bit or suggest that the client try to reconstruct what appears to be missing by taking new photographs. (If the client prefers not to, I would pursue a different option.) In any case, it is the client's feeling about the lack of photos that should be explored, before this lack is perceived as any problem.

HOW THIS TECHNIQUE WORKS

In order to use family albums as sources for therapeutic investigations, therapists must have at least a rudimentary understanding of basic systems theory as it applies to family therapy—because each client is a member, no matter how far removed, of a family system whose dynamics have contributed significantly to who that person is and how he or she copes in life.

The basic model for album reviewing with clients is as follows: first the therapist gathers her or his own perceptions and reactions while viewing, then the client's are joined with these. This can be sequential in time or done photo-by-photo as both silently look at, and then discuss, a given image. That is how the technique is done; however, what a therapist looks for will always depend on the client's situation and needs at that time. Therapists need to explore all the various relationships and communication patterns among family members and discover how the alignments and power structures signal and adjust to changes in any of the elements that make up the whole. To help a family we must first identify all its members—including the pets, cars, and so forth—and then chart the relationships among them that mandate behavioral patterns.

Meanings are interwoven among the pages and images of every album.

The individual photographic images can yield information as to who the members of a family are, but the feelings and relationships among the people in those images, and the "accidental" yet likely significant arrangement of the images are of special interest to the therapist.

In most albums photos seem to come in waves: a bunch will be taken of some special event or personal moment, and then there will be relative visual "silence." These ebbs and flows indicate nothing more than life rhythms unless the patterns become noticeably interrupted. Patterns of album keeping are particular to each family; sometimes gaps appear in the chronological presentation that may indicate stressful times, or sometimes people "disappear." Snapshots are put into albums because they stimulate memories rather than show meanings. Vastly different from collections of photographic art, these personally significant images are kept and treasured for the emotional "secrets" they hold. Family members know much better than outsiders what those album photos and their sequencing mean. Family members have privileged knowledge because they have lived with those codes every day of their lives and have shaped their existence by its unwritten rules. The family's fluency with emotional secrets provides them with power to control what gets shown or told to an inquiring "outsider." Sometimes the stories are dressed up or partially censored in the retelling. That editing—conscious or unconscious—frames the public presentation of the family as well as mirrors the thinking process of each person in it. Through the album and the stories that go with it, the client can grasp the family's sense of place—along with ideas of who he or she is, was, and is expected to be. Even if the client wishes to reject or change parts of these, the album can, at least, point to the place where the process can begin.

Album PhotoTherapy techniques not only help reveal clients' background but can also let the therapist learn about the people in their interpersonal network. This natural support group is important in times of clients' physical or emotional need, including, possibly, helping the client while he or she is going through therapy. Finding out the identities of a client's support group can be a necessary component of therapy or of the client's understanding of his or her family system.

Reviewing Albums

Cameras capture the natural rhythmic patterns of those people whose lives are mid-process when that moment was chosen for permanent freezing.

Therefore any ordinary patterns of familial relationships and intergenerational interactions will be visibly captured in these spontaneous photo-documentations of people's daily life. If unconscious dynamics are going on within a family's natural daily living, such as triangulations, cut-offs, alignments and other situations encoding family members' feelings about each other (or their habitual ways of covering their true feelings), then snapshots of them will automatically contain physical representations of these natural occurrences. There could even be said to be a parallel to the collective unconscious in the conceptualizing of a "family unconscious"! But I want to be very clear that, in saying that these are there and available for finding, I do not mean to imply that the therapist can simply go look at the family's personal snapshots and conclusively pronounce discoveries as to their true meanings as if reading from a book.

Rather, after viewing a family's album pages and collected photographs, a therapist can begin to formulate questions based on patterns that seem to be presenting themselves. Bearing in mind that the therapist is as far outside the secrets the snapshots hold as any other nonfamily viewer, the therapist can be trained to observe recurring positionings, relationships, alignments, nonverbal messages, and emotional expressions (or lack thereof) that signal questions that need to be explored with the client or the family.

Kaslow and Friedman (1977, pp. 19–24) have assembled a set of observations of ordinary family photo-taking and album-making patterns, which can be very helpful to therapists planning and implementing Photo-Therapeutic interventions. They found that families most frequently take photos to record important events and "milestones" in the family's life, such as weddings, births, birthday parties, vacations, graduations, anniversaries, ritual gatherings like Christmas or Thanksgiving dinners, and so forth. Conversely, there is usually a sharp drop in the number of pictures taken during periods of stress and family crisis, children's incapacitation, temporary disfigurement, or hospitalization, though sometimes such photos are acceptable if the child is sure to improve soon (for example, from a black eye) or if the condition is a developmental stage (such as loss of baby teeth). (As a personal example, when I was to have corrective surgery on my nose as a teenager, my parents took several photos of me at a mirror so that both face and profile could be seen: it was acceptable for the "before" photos to emphasize my big misshapen nose because there would be "after" shots to illustrate improvement.)

Kaslow and Friedman found that children seem to be photographed most in their early years, when physical appearance changes quickly, and first-born children are usually photographed more than those who follow. If there is something aberrant about the first child—disability or illegitimacy, for example—or if that child is not the sex the parents desired, then the camera's attention may be shifted to the second or "correct" child. As one precocious five-year-old girl once informed me, "There used to be lots of pictures of me in this book until my baby brother was born; now they're all of him. Maybe I was bad."

A child who is in the family temporarily, such as a foster child, may or may not be included in the album. A child who is "going through a stage" that is not approved of, like long-haired boys in the 1960s, may temporarily disappear. Families who take photos, Kaslow and Friedman say, often do it as a family activity and social event, and family attitudes regarding who is important are directly reflected in the size and prominence of photos of people displayed in the home.

Although Kaslow and Friedman's findings reflect only the families they studied, they seem to fit most of my clients' lives, too. Although variations occur owing to cultural, class, or other differences, they tend to be minor. Most cultures value family snapshots and album-keeping.

In sharing contrasting perceptions of images, my interchange with the client can model for them how selectively privileged knowledge about someone can alter our perceptions. I once commented to a client that photos of his father seemed to present a pleasant sort of fellow, and my client exploded in frustration, saying that this was what he was always hearing from people outside the family who could not believe how violent the man was to his wife and children. He then went looking through the album pages to find photos taken spontaneously of his father at home when "his face was not on," and though only a few could be found, he began to show me (using the photos as proof) the differences that only immediate family members were ever privy to. He made the point that those few nonpublic photos were his only validation of his real childhood experience. All the others were constructed from outsider viewpoints, and if he did not have those few snapshots available, he would probably have even begun to doubt it all himself as the years passed and detailed memories faded.

His father was dead and could not now be confronted, but the client could address his anger to those photographs, which gave him permission to say to his father words that had long been festering inside him.

He told his father's photo things he had never dared tell him in person; at least they got said out loud and didn't stay bottled up inside him. Hearing himself say them further validated their truth. Having me listening nonjudgmentally, supporting his right to say those things and have those feelings, reinforced his right to own and reempower his own childhood memories.

To be honest, when I examined the other photos, his father didn't look much different to me from the way he appeared in the "public" ones. I would have been hard put to separate the two versions of him had the client just brought all the snapshots in together in a pile and asked me to sort them. However, he was certain which belonged in which category, being privy to the subtle clues that he could see. Months later, and many improvements along in therapy, we began to look at some parallels that seemed to exist in photos of him with his father and him with his own sons. We began dealing with the parts of his father that he himself seemed to be perpetuating unknowingly.

What brought this to light was the day he was showing his teenage son the older albums and the son kept pointing out how much my client and his father looked alike at the same age. My client, at first very defensive at being physically identified with his father, began to argue with his son about how different the two fathers were; his son, upon hearing for the first time how awful his father's own childhood had been, reflected, "Maybe that's why you suddenly blow up at us, because you wait so long to get angry because you remember what your own dad's anger had been like!" (not an insignificant insight for a fourteen year old!). I took this opportunity to take out my Polaroid camera and ask the two of them to pose, first for a photo where they looked like the older generation father-son relationship, and then for one where they looked decidedly different, showing me and themselves how things in this generation weren't going to repeat the old patterns. I asked them to take the two photos home for further discussion with other family members.

In examining family album pages, I look for patterns and note any that emerge for me—or for my clients, which might well be different. These kinds of questions are helpful: What's important for me to know about this (your) family as I look at these pictures? What must you remember to tell me in explaining these? What might I not understand unless you explain it further?

Are there rules for how one must be to be included? Does the variety of content indicate tolerance of differences on these pages (and in family members)? Is the story of the family presented consistently and regularly, or are there interruptions or omissions? Is emotional intimacy suggested or not? Do there seem to be consistent themes, messages, or feelings expressed, such as who regularly is pictured standing next to, or touching, whom? What are the "peaks" of the family history, the landmarks, the events paid a lot of attention?

One client, on seeing numerous group portraits of his large family together, commented that the people in them were almost never touching. "That's how we are now, too. All separate people going our own way, not very connected to each other." Patterns suggest meaning to those who are sensitized to them.

Applying Systems Theory to Album Explorations

All the major family systems therapy concepts such as triangles, power alignments, boundaries, feedback loops, cut-offs, double-binds, "identified patient," de-personalized roles, and so forth, have been uncovered lurking secretly in the pages of albums. They have been existing like this for decades, embedded as they are inside photos that show slices of each family's "normal life," but rarely before were they ever deconstructed in such a manner (with such a photographically based road map or clue sheet to help open up the secrets). Systems theorists suggest that one way clients tend to "solve" unresolved issues with members of their family of origin is to distance themselves physically (geographically) and/or emotionally. When issues are perceived as irresolvable, and at the same time tension producing, the client may consciously or unconsciously decide that the issue itself should not be dealt with or that the person fused with that specific should be purged from the client's existence. When people are cut off from the client's life, they also often literally disappear from the client's photo collections. Consequently, when disappearances, gaps, and other dissonances turn up in clients' albums, it may help to ask why.

Putting a frame around something (or at least photographic borders) forces an ordering of its contents. Alliances and bonded pairs in a "triangulation" may be uncovered by examining and discussing who always seems to be standing near whom in spontaneous snapshots as well as noting any differences when those same people appear in posed photos. Similarly, the person who is frequently left out of the picture or is often off to the side, unhugged or untouched by others—or who is rarely in the album—could be the "identified patient" or the cut-off person in that family.

Another way to reduce distance in emotional cut-offs is for the client to actually sit with that person and view the family album. An album of photos is a relatively safe focus. It serves to triangulate the attention of both individuals onto the album and permits them to have a closer connection than they are used to having. Communication may thus become less guarded than usual because contrasting memories or opinions about photos can be shared without threat to each other's position.

People who must be or do something to make their appearance in the album acceptable probably find their emotional acceptance in the family equally conditional, and they may become confused over the conflicting expectations they encounter. One client explained his drive for conformity as being based on growing up with alcoholic parents: "Their love was always conditional. We kids were never good enough. With my brothers and sister, I must always be equal and not stand out as being any different or being the lightning rod for extra attention. In our family you couldn't afford to be special or attract attention because it was dangerous to do so. In fact, there are very few photos in our collection of just one of us kids alone; we never dared let each other out of our sight." The tidy story of a family as presented in an album includes numerous nonverbally signaled rules and expectations about acceptability in that album (and that family). A careful probing of its pages with those appearing in them can reveal the family "shoulds" and "oughts" as guidelines embedded in the images that were chosen for inclusion—or rejected.

Pets, and sometimes cars, gardens, hobbies, sports activities, and other subjects of great personal attention, are sometimes considered as being integral parts of the family. Triangulation can occur with two people and a pet just as with three people. Focusing attention on a dog or cat can be a means of diffusing tension between its owners, trying to outdo each other in taking care of the animal, so as to align the pet on "their" side, and so forth. Pets play a large part in the emotional framework of those who live alone (or feel like they do), and they also are often perceived and treated as a child would be. Therefore it is not surprising that photos of pets are often the subject of snapshots in photo albums, desk or wallet displays, and home videos, or even in posed formal portaits.

Albums allow children to see what parents were like during childhood or courtship days, and this can enhance the children's perception of them as more naturally human, with fuller emotional ranges and occasionally humorous whims. In finding out more about the details of their parents' lives, which influenced how they turned out as adults, clients are shown parts of those multi-faceted lives that they may not have previously known about when thinking about the persons only in relationship to themselves. This can bridge to reestablishing contact with those who were previously kept, as one client phrased it, "tightly locked in a labelled box on a shelf in the back corner of my mind." As one client expressed it, "When you asked me to 'be' my father as he appeared in that photograph, to pretend for a moment to take on his identity and expressions as they were shown there, and then to talk in the first person as if I were him about what that period of his life was like, I suddenly grasped the difficulties he had been struggling to live with, and I began to understand him better as a whole person instead of just my being Dad, who was already old when I got to know him."

Album review also allows parents to be perceived as they were at the client's age, so issues prevalent at that life stage can be considered from both points of view. They often turn out to be similar. This can yield new perspectives, as the following example shows:

Two years from finishing high school, and terribly bored with it all, my fifteen-year-old client wanted to drop out. He knew his parents wouldn't approve ("They just think I'm a dumb kid"), but he did seem to have a sensible alternative in mind. He had already secretly applied and been accepted for the local shipbuilding apprenticeship program, and had contacted the local night school about finishing up his degree through their work-study arrangement. Feeling very proud of his (self-described) "untypically thorough" planning, he approached his parents for their required permission, but was devastated to find that his father was furious and uncharacteristically upset with the idea. My client had anticipated his father's approval, as they had discussed his school problems recently, and both parents were clearly hoping for the boy to take some redeeming plan of action.

In our next family session, the son again brought up the idea. He was very upset by his parents' reaction, which he took as personal rejection and lack of trust in his abilities. Luckily, the family had also brought along their photo albums (my earlier request) and I decided to find out what the father had been like at fifteen. I was hoping to explore what was behind this particular crisis.

As the father began to show his son what his own teenage years had been like—the photos of the old farm, the desolate environment, the long walk to school, the one-room schoolhouse, and so forth—he began to share his feelings about those days. While talking about how important his schooling had been to him, he paused in silence for a long time and then told his son, "I guess I was angry with you because to me, school was my *only* chance out of that awful place, and when my own father died and they pulled me out of school at age fifteen, I thought my world and any chance I'd had for escaping it had ended forever. I swore then that any kids I ever fathered would never have to leave school, that they'd never have to suffer what I had because I would understand how important it was for them to stay there. I guess all this got in my way when I heard you say you wanted to drop out. Angry bells started ringing in my head, and it's only now that I finally realize why. It hurt me that school wasn't as important to you as I thought it should be. Tell me again what you're planning and how it makes sense, and this time I'll really listen to you. Maybe we can work something out." With tears in their eyes, they hugged and then began talking.

To produce movement in a client toward more differentiation, therapists would want to have him or her combine self-clarifying and family-separating techniques to help identify which parts of the client are unique and not enmeshed with the family's identity or rules and which of the family origins and contexts are still integrally part of the client (and accept that this is also all right). Albums can reveal a family's tolerance for different behaviors, norms, and degrees of freedom within which members are free to express themselves (for example, in the contrast between formally posed and spontaneous photos).

To discover similarities and differences between clients' individual and family identities (and associated feelings), clients can discuss differences they perceive between photos of themselves alone and of themselves in family groups. They can talk about ways the family portrait presents a single identity as compared with being a photograph of a collection of different individuals. The goal in differentiating is not just how to discover how family members are different, but also to find out (and accept) some of their areas of sameness, without those similarities meaning fusion or lack of individuation.

This type of differentiation/fusion dynamic also affects parents who resist letting their children be whole people rather than extensions of themselves or fulfillers of their expectations. This was clearly demonstrated by a woman who showed me her wallet photos of her daughter and son, who she described as being ages four and eight in the photos. I discussed her children with her (whom she kept referring to as "the girl" and "the boy," and never by name), and only after twenty minutes did I discover that the children were now ten and fourteen. She explained (with no apparent embarrassment) that she preferred the children as their younger selves, because "the boy was beginning to act nasty like his father," and she liked him better when he was younger. She said, "I'm afraid what he's going to grow up to be like!" After hearing that set of fixed expectations, I had the same concerns for his future individuation!

Sometimes people find things in images that have always been there, but were never noticed; then connections and patterns are revealed that had previously been hidden. The following example is a good illustration of this process.

A client I will call Elaine brought me a photo from her personal family album as an example of her childhood and its events (see photo 7.1). "This particular photo has a lot of meaning for me for many reasons," she explained. "I value the closeness of it, the physical placement of the three females (myself at age five, my sister at age eight, and my mother).

Photo 7.1

© 1967 "Elaine's Dad"

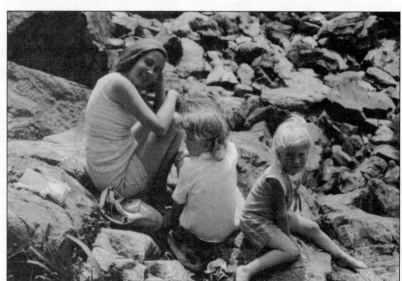

The picture was taken a year before my parents broke up, and it is the only document I have of a 'real' family outing. I also see a lot of affection in my mother's eyes for the photographer—my father—which I have rarely seen in other photos. The three of us—or rather the four of us—appear to be a very close family, which is rather a false view, but still one I really cherished for its idealism."

We explored the image—the people, the setting, the feelings and memories it recalled—attending mostly to these major facets. But Elaine suddenly stopped to stare angrily at what she identified as a folded newspaper on a rock at the far left edge of the image. I had not noticed this detail at all, and even when seeing it, could not determine any relevance.

However, Elaine quickly corrected this: "My rosy view of this scene really changed just now, as I became aware of the newspaper beside my mother. The more I think about the symbolic significance of that newspaper, the more it really bothers me, that my mother may well have not really "been there" with us as I had originally perceived. Generally, she preferred to read than do things with us. This speaks to my desire for a mother who would put her parenting before her intellectual life, as my mother did not. It also speaks to my unarticulated desire for a mother that really loved my father. So my anger was really directed at the newspaper for destroying my perception of the occasion as a happy, intimate family outing." I asked what would happen if the offending newspaper were removed from the photo, and she replied, "It wouldn't be right to take it out as it represented an honest view of the situation." A few months later, Elaine was making a collage of old photos for her mother's birthday gift. She debated for quite some time as to whether to cut the newspaper out, and she ended up doing so, "partly due to the space restrictions of the collage itself, but mostly because I decided to honor *my* vision, realistic or not."

Ideally, I would have liked to have Elaine share her perceptions with her mother, who lived far away, and let them discuss what those times were really like. I thought it might be helpful for Elaine to find out what memories or feelings the photo stimulated for her mother and sister, as their versions of what was going on at that time might give her a different perception. At least, in getting her mother's permission to use this photo for this book, Elaine shared with her the details of the anecdote that would accompany it (not only was this ethically necessary, but I thought it would also spark some good therapeutic conversation).

Her mother responded that there were some errors in Elaine's memory; for example, the paper was the father's, not hers. She explained that she wouldn't read the newspaper there because it was too windy and she would get ink on her hands, which she hates. She added that the place had a special meaning that the girls may not have been aware of: it was the beach where the father and mother had courted. Later, Elaine showed the photo to her father and told him her mother's comments. She reported to me that he responded, "That's not true! We never courted there. This photo was taken at Great Falls on the Potomac, and we courted in North Carolina at the University there."

Even posed photos capture an essence of what is going on in the lives of the subjects. An image on its own may not reveal much, but juxtaposed with others, the nonverbal information can suddenly come into focus. For example, two photos of my parents taken fifty years apart show them pleasantly together in both images (see photos 7.2 and 7.3).

However, when my mother saw the snapshots together, she observed, "Isn't that interesting! First I used to lean on him, and now he leans on me." "Interesting" is such a safe word. Had she been my client in therapy, I would have recommended she explore her feelings further. However, when

Photo 7.2 *(left)*
Photo 7.3 *(right)*

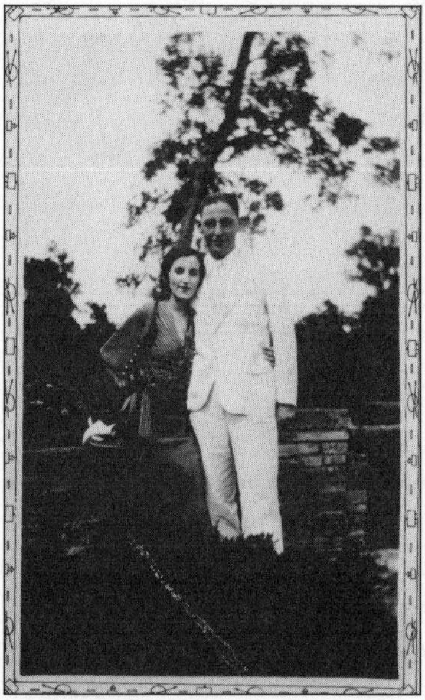

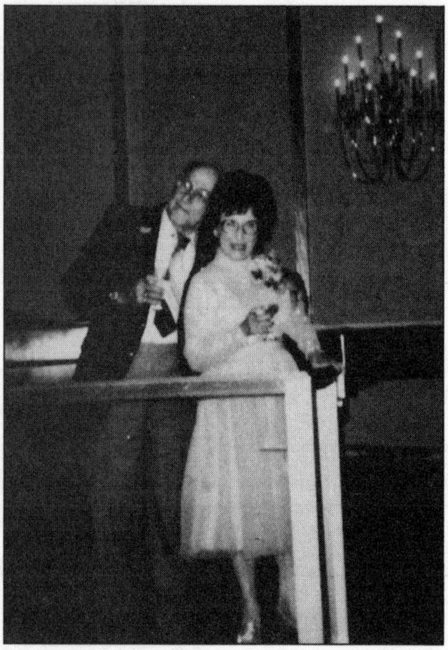

I reflected my mother's words back to her, she said I was reading too much into her comments. Nonetheless, the incident set me to exploring my own family albums. Like other therapists who use PhotoTherapy with clients, I had not really attended to my own family albums as much as I probably should have, and it was time to find out what secrets they held. The results of this exploration are reported as the final illustrative example.

When therapy becomes stressful, or there seems to be too much focusing upon the problems rather than the skills clients have used to survive their crises, album work can serve as a means of looking at the more positive elements of family life, such as those happy times or good qualities that also form part of the family reality. By reconnecting with the many good times shown in photo-memories, people can be reunited with other components of their lives besides the "awful" ones brought forward to therapy, and thus some perspective of the overall balance of life can be gained.

For example, in working with a couple who were having relationship difficulties, I asked them to show me their wedding photos. The pictures helped them think about what had attracted them to each other in the first place. In telling me about each other's desirable points, they became aware of how easy it had been to fall into the trap of always criticizing.

Similarly, I asked parents who were having trouble with their teenager to all look back at childhood photos showing early birthday parties, holiday trips, and the like. The pictures helped them talk about these good times they had shared in the past. I suggested they plan some similar enjoyable times, where arguments wouldn't be allowed to intrude, and I gave them some specific snapshot-taking assignments so that there was a reason to initiate these experiences ("bring the photos of this outing with you to the next appointment"). Out of context, such techniques may seem rather idealized. Readers should recognize that one doesn't just deliver them directly, but works them into the larger conversation during the therapy session. But such suggestions do frequently work surprisingly well as a means of having people pause to redefine when they have been focusing far too disproportionately on negative elements in their lives.

If one of the goals in family therapy is to permit individuals to enlarge their knowledge of the forces and patterns that have shaped them, as well as to improve the quality and depth of relationship with each family member so as to unfuse without such differentiation causing threat or difficulty, then it is also important to consider patterns transmitted through the family from previous generations. Comparing photos from past generations with current ones can reveal unconscious mirroring and repetition that has gone on for years without those involved having any conscious recognition that these trans-generational messages and expectations had been taking place all along.

From a structural perspective, a therapist might be able to find visual "facts" in clients' photos showing multigenerational transmission of family values and behaviors. However, it is much more helpful (and ethical) to have clients take part in this, as their discoveries, and their feelings about those discoveries will provide therapeutic impact. A way to begin is to ask clients to note details they may want to discuss later. What clients notice in terms of patterns, themes, emotional messages, discrepancies, sudden discoveries of previously unnoticed material, or even sometimes people, can be extremely interesting and useful.

One woman, in reviewing her family's photos, said, "I seem to always be in front of my family, and now that I think about it, this makes sense, as I'm very independent of them, and do not really care about the effects upon them of what I do. Now I'm in therapy and I look at the photos of me with my husband, and I see the same pattern: me in front. We're working on lack of intimacy in our relationship and the separation I seem to keep between my feelings and my relationship with him, and now a recent comment of his just suddenly made a lot of sense. He said that when we go somewhere together, I seem to always be walking in front of him, striding off ahead of him, with no knowledge or care as to whether he is back there or not. Ooohh."

I asked her to look more at these photos of her with her husband and her family and note where the hands are, where the gaze is, whose postures duplicate or mirror whose, whether her parents touch or make a lot of eye contact, and if not, when did this stop? One photo she stopped to discuss showed her father standing behind her mother ("of course!"), and resting his hands on her mother's shoulders. When first seeing this she used it as an example of the same "female-in-front" posing, but when she heard her own description of it as being "him holding her back" she described hearing a sudden "whoosh" of realization at the implication of her words. She had uncovered the buried impression that her father had always restricted her mother's emotional growth. "Now I wonder what else is tied in with this style of me always grabbing the front position!"

People who have found their family membership conditional upon their being, doing, or saying things a particular way can use albums as visual maps to trace some of the double messages and double binds they may have been experiencing (often denied by others).

One fellow, who had earlier selected photos of children as his favorite projective images because he was "drawn to the children's innocence and beauty when their life force was vibrant and they weren't yet wise to the street," showed me a photo from his family album taken at his kindergarten graduation party (photo 7.4). "Here I am! The photo has been in the album as long as I can remember, but nobody sees what I see in it. I'm trying to hide from the boy behind me, which doesn't surprise me.

"This picture just validates it all for me. I'm gay, and I believe I always knew I was different, from a very early age, way before I started

Photo 7.4

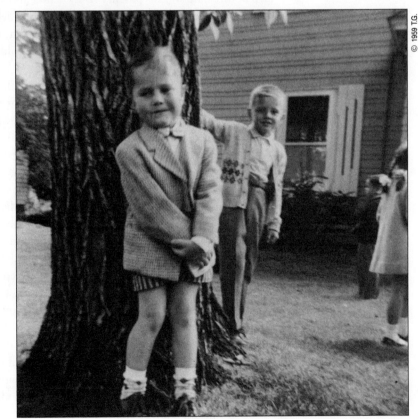

school. I see in this photo the little boy that didn't ever want to play rough, who often was seen and photographed in 'coy and feminine poses,' and my pose in this image was almost as if I was 'cruising' the boy standing behind me. I couldn't stand having dirty hands or clothing. Whenever I got a spot of mud on me I would rush to my mother to have her clean me off. That little boy has always been there, and he is mirrored in me still. I like him a lot, although the family often enjoys reminding me of the little sissy he seems to be in this picture."

Communication systems in families under stress are rife with evasive signals and paradoxical meanings. One man's experience in examining dozens of childhood pictures demonstrated how such double binds and mixed messages can be discovered in photographs. Most of the photos in the family's album were of him alone. Born five years after his sister died at birth, he was his parents' "only" child and was raised as a precious treasure representing everything a child could be to them.

"I became their daughter as well as their son, which complicated the messages and expectations I kept getting," he told me, "You can see this in the way I was always posed year after year as being literally the object of their attention." He said that in addition to all the snapshots, his mother took a formal picture of him every year on his birthday for eighteen years. This regular documentation showed his personal history and, as his many outfits changed from sailor suit to cowboy to more "proper" suits of various styles, the images also constituted not only a personal retrospective but also a sociocultural record of those years in general. One image stood out as particularly significant for him. It was of him with his mother, both smiling, but she was tightly forcing his hands under, which he commented must have been very uncomfortable for him (see photo 7.5).

He says the photo is symbolic of how he was treated and that it illustrates how his mother often subtly tried to block his becoming independent, both physically, as in the picture, as well as emotionally. "My parents had seemed to love me and give me everything, so why was I so angry? Look at this photo! My mother's love was very controlling and ultimately a very crippling love. I see this in the way she is bending my hands as I sat on her lap. I was smiling and she was smiling, but I was being controlled and she was really doing this so we would make a good impression for others. She was invading and manipulating my self and space. I had displaced anger toward her for this action and indirectly to my father for not stopping her manipulation."

Photo 7.5

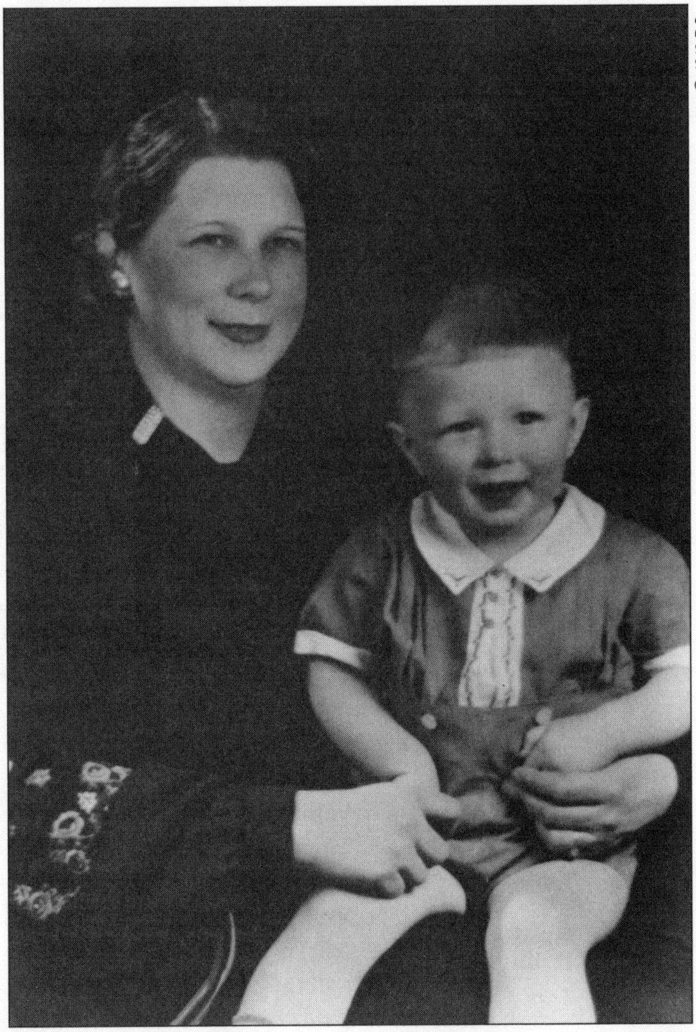

He provided a later example of this (s)mothering: his wedding pictures, in which both his parents placed themselves possessively near the new couple, hovering close to him in particular. He contrasted this with his wife's parents, whose poses signaled a much more relaxed recognition of their daughter's new life and independent relationship.

A therapeutically based review of family photographs can, then, help in many ways to bring to light long-established and well-buried emotional conflicts, especially those having deep roots in family dynamics. As those conflicts become visible and available for conscious examination, they simultaneously become available for therapeutic manipulation to loosen the hold on the client.

The Significance of the Album-Keeper

Whoever controls the family albums controls much of the family history, and thus its "truth," just as the person who defines the rules of any debate will strongly influence its outcome. The album-keeper has the power to make his or her version the "real" one for all viewers, and that person is usually mirroring the family power balance by virtue of their acceptance of him or her as documentor. Whereas the gaze of the photographer creates the photos found in any album, the gaze of the album-keeper constructs the version of these photographic "truths" that is presented for interpretation by the gaze of later viewers. Finding ways for my clients to re-create and reclaim their own versions of their own personal histories has become a major focus of my PhotoTherapy work, particularly with clients in disempowered situations or from traditionally marginalized or excluded populations. I have found that many clients, male and female, heterosexual and homosexual, often need to do a great deal of work around being dehumanized and devalued by either parent. I believe that good psychotherapy must include an attempt to explore the complex nature of the client's relationships with both parents, even though it is the relationship with the mother that is most often the focus in traditional therapeutic models. Family album work can be an effective way of beginning such an inquiry.

Our family album is the place where most of us learned to be the kind of "good children" we were expected to be, and that if we acted or appeared a certain way, we would be included in the photographic records of the family's history. We could see which images of ourselves were acceptable to our parents, or, at least to their public presentation of us, by seeing which ones were permanently fixed in the family history. These idealized images are what we usually return to in nostalgia when we sit down to review our memories for pleasure. Most of us grew up trying to live up to images that others (usually parents) created of us, and trying to meet those nonverbalized expectations that were sometimes subtly presented as conditions to our being accepted or loved.

When reviewing family photos with my own mother for my use in a later section of this chapter, I found it interesting to discover that her memories of a certain photo's details or a certain day's context were often radically different from the reality of it that I myself knew to be true. At a cognitive level I am clear that my own version of these realities are only my own selective constructions of truth, just like anyone else's. However, at a more intuitive/emotional level, both my mother and myself are absolutely certain that the other is remembering incorrectly or distortedly, and that our own version is correct.

It is also worth finding out who is or is not permitted to see a family's albums and other photos. The client's limits of privacy may differ from those of their family's album-keeper (as when mothers embarrass their teenagers by showing naked baby pictures to visitors).

Sometimes the photos' potential therapeutic value lies more in who took the photo or how the subjects felt about that event than in the contents of the image itself. Some members of the family may have strong feelings about being photographed by a particular person, which directly affects their appearance in album photos. The following example demonstrates this.

A teenage boy brought me his album, which included some recent photos of his parents sitting arm-in-arm on a porch swing, smiling. He had told me that they constantly bickered, were never affectionate with each other, and had in fact been separated for two years, so I was surprised. He explained that, when his father had taken him home to his mother's the previous weekend, he had given them each a favorite candy bar as a bribe to let him take just the one photo of the two of them together looking "normal." He had purposely done it outside so that the neighbors would see "that there is still hope." He added, "I told them my psychologist wanted it, and that helped to convince them, but that was just my excuse. I know it's a lie, but I just wanted to have one decent normal picture of my parents for my scrapbook."

There are many ways to take these sorts of deeper-hidden aspects into consideration when activating PhotoTherapy work with family photos. Questions can be designed that touch on these areas in order to precipitate answers which might signal such additional complications. I probe to uncover the process by which a newly taken photo is chosen for addition into the album. What factors influence the decision of whether it is put onto the page or not? Who has the final say if there is disagreement about this? Whose album is it, anyway? What happens to the snapshot if it isn't put into the album?

In other words, what are the unstated rules governing the entry qualifications for album recording (and thus acceptance into the family according to its rules)? Are there any photos in the client's albums which they know to be untrue or distorted? Are there any people whose photos appear who, given the choice, would remove or change them? If the client's album had been put together by someone else instead of the person who made it, or the client could do their own version, what would be different? Does their album show different patterns reflecting the contributions of more than one family photographer, and if so, what do these differences signal? What seem to be the usual patterns for this family? Are these different from the ones listed in an earlier section for the general population, and what are the occasions where this particular album's documenter didn't follow that usual pattern? What may have caused this unexpected divergence from the album's norm; was it external circumstances in the family itself or was this more reflective of changes in the personal life of the album's keeper? How does the client feel about those gaps or deviations from the usual norms occurring in this particular album which keeps their own life? These and other questions found in the Recommended Exercises section can be illuminating in unexpected ways.

Particular Applications: Abuse Survivors and Life Review

PhotoTherapy techniques have been especially useful in two particular areas: helping to uncover and process the less-conscious aspects of emotional, physical, or sexual abuse in a client's past, and in providing a life-review perspective for people facing crises, including impending death, personal problems that seem insurmountable, sudden dependency on others, and so forth.

The common attribution of a quality of truth to photography has proven to be a particularly useful component to PhotoTherapy with abuse survivors. For example, many of these abuse victims, upon reviewing old family photos, find that they were photographed by their offender (often years before the first actual abusive incident) in ways that sexualized their bodies, or that they had been posed with the offender in ways that presented their relationship as a sexually charged one. Such signals are not necessarily obvious to outside observers, but are recognizable to the client who knows the difference between silly poses or joking incidents and those that hide great pain and sadness in their later recognition.

Reviewing albums gives many clients a support that allows them to reencounter parts of their past that they would never risk exploring otherwise. In the album's record of their past, clients will inevitably meet photographs that they know lie or support untruths; photographs whose viewing brings back deep feelings; and photographs taken of them against their will, or in contradiction to the truth as they knew it to be.

Those selective presentations of clients' family lives constructed for public viewing in albums will often not match their inner knowledge of what life at home was really like. Many therapists have guided clients to rephotograph or use collages of found photos to re-create their personal narratives in versions more truthful to their own memories. Old photos can reveal "lost" details of childhood and help them to recognize the true limits of a child's reality and ability. In trying to heal that wounded child within themselves and forgive it for not being able to do more than was humanly possible at a young age, I have found nothing quite so useful as real photographs of the client as a child.

Selective "forgetting" is not always a completely bad thing; "forgetting into the unconscious" may have been the only way a client could survive a time of stress. Until they were strong enough to reconstruct the full story, forgetting gave them a layer of protection against the raw, overwhelming truth. Family albums, which are really only selectively constructed narratives, may not provide the full story to the client. Most clients can benefit by reclaiming their pasts on their own terms, based on their own privileged knowledge about themselves. Clients cannot go back in time and change the historical facts of their lives, but they can go back and clarify those facts or redefine their memories of them and thus alter what they now mean and their emotional potency.

Most therapists involved in treating abuse survivors stress the importance of the adult rejoining the child self in witnessing, giving voice to protest, expressing long-buried and often long-denied feelings, and learning how to comfort and nurture the child's needs within the adult self. PhotoTherapeutically, this frequently is done by focusing on childhood abuse using family photos and/or self-portrait work, often combined projectively with other imagery (see related sections in earlier chapters, particularly the anecdote about the "bleeding" door). Clients often need help to find out that the child self exists, hidden away inside them, before they can give it a voice and feelings. I have helped clients discover what needs to be said (and to whom) by having them rehearse the dialogue whether or not it ever actually takes place in reality. This is because, although there are times when confrontation might be necessary to achieve emotional health, it is potentially so powerful that it could shatter their fragile truce with their past.

Using old family photos, however, to create newer more realistic versions of the past (through collage, rephotographing or photocopying, enhancing with art materials, reconstructing new albums, doing self-portrait work, and so forth) can help to reweave a person's life into a more integrated whole.

Album and photo-biographical explorations have also proven useful when a summary review of the client's life could be therapeutically helpful. The album chronicles the client's evolution from one time or place to another, one family or circle of friends to others, even from being a child to having a child. Reviewing the album, alone or with someone else listening as the client explains the connections, can reconstitute the integrated wholeness that they believe is presented there. Reconstructing connections through individual images evokes the apparent flow and direction of the client's life, retrospectively. This helps make sense of what the client has done and been, much as people perceive motion from the blurred frames of a movie film. No words are needed for this synthesis to occur. People can trace their own visual footprints and find roots, love, friendship, purpose, and continuity that will continue into the future.

WHAT TO DO

Regardless of the theoretical model they espouse, therapists should review as many family photos as possible, not only to "get a better picture" of the people and events that constitute the client's life but also to explore with the client the personal meanings they signal. Beyond that, there are many ways to make use of this information. Some therapists prefer to have clients bring photos and albums in for in-session work. Other therapists prefer to have the viewing and discussing done away from the office, by the client alone or by family members together. I prefer to do both. Each approach can help achieve different goals.

Therapists can make the best use of photo-finding assignments by tailoring them to the therapeutic goals they are working toward. I may ask a client to come back next week with a dozen or so photos they think best illustrate a specific topic; for example, their true childhood, their parents' real relationship, or the rules by which their family operates. I may request they bring in those most significant, those favorite or least favorite, only those which they know to be untrue or tell lies about the family, or the ones they think they would like to redo their own way from their own perspective on the story presented. I may ask for only those photos that they themselves appear in, or only those where they don't, some with siblings or parents or some without.

At first, I scan the album pages lightly and quickly to get a feel for their rhythm and regularities. I want to see who populates the photos, what they are usually doing and where, what kinds of events and moments are documented. Sometimes I do this in silence with the client watching me while I absorb my findings at first glance unfiltered by their interpretations of the images. This initial scanning can be very important in that I will never again encounter any photograph in the client's album as freshly as the first time I view it, so I try to always take the time to note my own first impressions.

Then I begin to talk with the client to get her or his version of the same visual journey in general, or I may tell the client what I am looking for and dialogue about it as I go through the snapshots. I use whichever pattern seems most sensible for my mode of therapy with that particular client having that particular difficulty that day. Either method is fine; neither is wrong.

My perceptions are likely to be different from the client's. That difference, once discussed, may release some significant revelations that the client has been blocked from seeing because of the filters in memory and values or from previous viewings of photos.

Reflective Techniques: What to Look for, and How

First I give the client's album photos an initial brief and silent scan to ground myself in the nature and qualities of their particular imagery. Then, I often start by asking about the client's position in the family, where he or she is in the birth order, how many siblings he or she has, whether grandparents are living, and other questions that give me an idea of the family structure. Uncovering what the client believes or assumes about his or her family of origin is critical to my way of conducting therapy;

it is the client's version of what her or his childhood was like, whether supported by the album or not, that we will eventually encounter as "reality."

I may go backward in time before moving into the present crisis situation, not only to get a larger understanding of the client's life for myself but also because older, more "distant" photos are usually less intense for the client to discuss.

In looking back through albums, clients can be asked to reflect on the following:

What did the family appear to be like before the client was born? How did the client's parents interact with their own parents? What seemed to be different after the client was born?

It can be useful to ask questions like these looking at photos taken before and after the birth of siblings: Does the album seem to show any differences in the way either parent attended to the client? Who held the client most often? Who interacted with, played with, had eye contact with the client (instead of the photographer), and so forth, and what might these differences mean? What were the parents' patterns with brothers and sisters? What might the facial expressions mean in these pictures? Do the parents seem happy, resentful, content or discomfited by the arrival of the new child?

As the client grew older, what events or moments did the family photograph and keep records of? Which were deemed most important? Are there siblings who were photographed more in childhood than the client was? What might be the reasons for this? (Boys more than girls? First-born more than those who followed?) Do there seem to be patterns repeated consistently, and what might these signal? Does one person or child stay pretty much central in the images over time, or is there variety and flexibility regarding who is the "star" of the photo? Are there people who seem to be regularly left out or pushed to the sides? Does this seem connected with any patterns, or particular situations or conditions, or is it there randomly throughout? If the client now has children, are there patterns emerging in the photographs taken of them? If so, how do they compare with those from the client's own childhood?

An example of how such things interconnect can be seen in the experience of one middle-aged client who explored with me a photo from a family gathering when she was eleven (see photo 7.6). She was the final child in a long line of children, and is seen here close to the edge of a group-

Photo 7.6

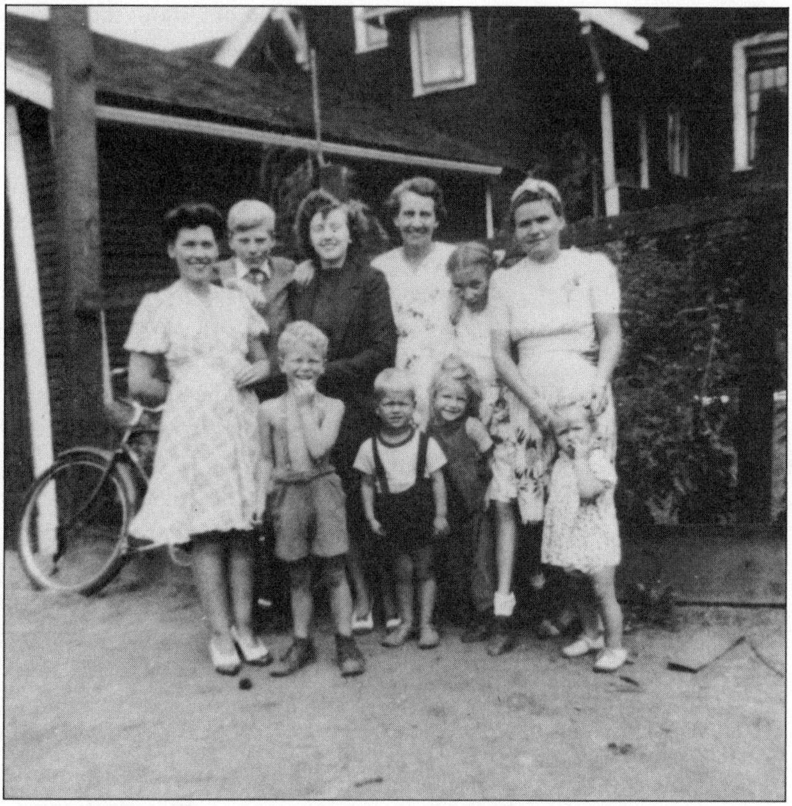

ing that included siblings, nephews, and nieces (some of whom were older than herself).

She observed her face and body in the photo and defined this for me as herself "just barely managing to be seen, struggling massively to not be left out of the picture altogether." She described this feeling as continuing throughout her life and said it suddenly seemed to ring true for her when she realized that the field she had chosen work in made her highly visible in the public eye.

In addition to probing particular images in the linear narrative of the album's pages, I also ask clients general questions about the album, such as, "In looking through these pages, are there any photos that you think should be removed to make the album better or more honest?" "What changes would you want to make now, if you could? Would it matter if anyone was going to find out about these changes? If so, who and why?" "If your album did include those more realistic snapshots you long to see in there, what would happen then?" "Are there any pictures that you see now that you don't remember seeing in there before?" And so forth.

Less general questions can be shaped to aid the search for themes, gender scripts, visual repetitions, transmission of relationship patterns from one generation to the next, and so forth. For example:

What do you notice about who is touching whom, who is facing whom, and/or who appears to be avoiding doing these things? Which people seem always to be together? Which people never seem to be near one another unless forced to pose together?

What or who isn't in the album that ought to be? What photos are there that really should be removed because they are only there for "show" rather than truth?

Do photos of you (the client) and/or other family members vary noticeably, depending on who was taking the picture? Are there some family members who are uncomfortable having their photos taken, and what is the family response to this? Are their feelings respected or are they forced to appear anyway? Are there some members who simply will not let certain others photograph them, and what might this mean?

What rhythms appear in the events that are routinely photographed year after year? Are there certain rituals, ceremonies, parties, holidays, and so forth, that are captured consistently and regularly? Might these be the moments where the family is presented as a single, fused unit and therefore where friction might be anticipated between individuals? If so, are there certain family members who appear in random photos but never in the group ones because of resistance or group exclusion?

Are there time gaps in the regular routine of the family's album-keeping, when no photos were entered or taken? What might that communicate about the family's life at that time? Were there upsets, tragedies, hard times, or other external reasons for the gaps?

Do some people disappear from the album, sometimes reappearing, sometimes not? Is this resulting from reasons forced upon the family by outside sources, such as job transfers, illnesses, divorce, and such, or are these gaps more from internal reasons from the family's emotional signals, such as the person being shunned, their appearance or lifestyle is disapproved of, unresolved differences or consequences of arguments?

It is often interesting to explore who didn't make it into the picture or is in only partially, and what this signifies emotionally or in terms of family politics. If the person reappears later, what might this change signal about them or about the family?

People usually "disappear" from albums because their photographs are no longer included, but they may also be excluded—and rendered nonexistent—in other ways. One man told me that his mother-in-law "doesn't throw out photos—she cuts out the offending person, very carefully removing him or her quite literally from the picture album." I pointed out that, since the holes are left behind on the page, the person's existence is still evident, as a shadow figure in "negative" space. He replied, "She keeps lists, too, like mental scorecards, by which relatives are scheduled 'in' or 'out' of her graces, and it's much the same. By making sure we know about all this, she thinks they are being punished, while in fact she is herself held prisoner by her need to consciously maintain their continued banishment."

Another client told me that when she divorced, her mother carefully cut out all the face and body images of the client's ex-husband from wedding and other family group photos, but saved the photos themselves, "leaving a void that I fear will be very difficult for any new man to fill." And yet another client reported discovering, upon her mother-in-law's death, an old album of wedding pictures of herself and her husband. His mother had scratched out my client's face on every single photo of them together. One adult client, overweight and unhappy with her figure, had gone through her teenage album and cut away her bathing-suited body from all photos of herself, leaving her face, arms and feet behind. Finding things like these in clients' albums cannot help but precipitate useful therapeutic dialogue! Destruction of photos is a type of murder of the psyche. One client told me she became hysterical when she found that her ex-husband had, out of anger, virtually wiped out her personal history: "I had packed my past into two boxes. These held all my photos and letters, and he threw them out for the trash men while I was at the lawyer's dealing with our separation agreement. I will never forgive him."

When a photo has proven to be of particular importance, I may ask questions to find out whether it holds any secrets beyond the information already discussed. For example: "What else should I know about this picture?" "Who else in your family knows this privileged information?" "What would happen if the truth were told?" "Who would you like to have know this information, and can you tell them yourself?" And so forth.

Once I have an understanding of the basic facts of a client's life, I can use them in probing what lies underneath their surface presentation. Probing questions are more associative and less cognitive, and are more likely to produce emotional connections. For example: "In what ways are you similar to the person (or those people) in this picture?" "Which of these people do you like best or least? What are you most drawn to or repelled by in them?" "Does their opinion matter to you?" "Are they welcome to visit unannounced?" "How would you describe the relationships suggested in these photos?" "Why do you think this photo was taken?" "What feelings or memories emerge from seeing it?" "What sorts of changes seem most evident in your family or yourself with the passages of time?" And so forth.

In album review and reconnaissance, I am interested to see what is found there on the pages, how the individual images are combined to produce a narrative of the client's life, whose version of truth this turns out to be, as well as what is not appearing there by choice or accident, along with what this might mean for the client. I use questions as my tools to learn such things, and although a comprehensive list of such questions would be endless to attempt, I hope the above suggestions provide some general types of questions with which to start album-based PhotoTherapy explorations.

Active Techniques: What to Do with What You Find

I often find that what I do with clients' family photos will be a direct outgrowth of what I have encountered earlier in my initial review of the photos with them. In this section I suggest additional creative techniques using particularly selected snapshots. In all cases, if the snapshots themselves are too dear for removal or transporting, then photocopies or even sketches could be substituted.

One activity I have found useful is to have the client use a large sheet of newsprint to draw his or her "family" tree (genogram) and then attach photographs to it. Or I may ask the client to use a long sheet of newsprint or shelf paper to construct a time line, a chronology, of important events in his or her individual life or in the family's life and then match album images to this wherever possible. I have sometimes asked clients, particularly children, to draw their home and then use photos to show me who is there and what they are doing. This can include placing photos in the rooms or windows of the home sketch. I frequently encourage clients to add embellishments with art materials, in order to make use of art therapy components that might also emerge. I also make frequent use of photo-confrontational and photo-interactive dialoguing techniques discussed in previous chapters.

Results from such activities are often prompt and direct. For example, I had a client who kept telling me what an ugly child she had been. She seemed to be fixated on this being the cause of her adult problems, especially as she described her eighteen-year-old daughter as being "beautiful from birth onward." I asked her to make a time line of the years of her life, lay an old album photo of herself at each year's marker, from birth to late teens, and then place beside each one of these pictures a photograph of her daughter at exactly the same age. Several things emerged from this, including her great surprise at how similar she and her daughter looked at each age. She was faced with her labels: her "beautiful" daughter and her "ugly child" self. Saying it was hard to argue with photographic evidence, she began to think about why she had been so invested in maintaining this distorted self-image and to probe a bit more her relationship with her own mother. One assignment she did toward this end was to add photographs from her mother's childhood at each year of the time line.

Combining snapshots with creative artwork or written expression works well with explorations of family dynamics, systems issues, and interconnected feelings. One activity I particularly like is deceptively simple in its early stages. Draw a vertical line down the middle of a large sheet of paper. Then ask clients to place different family members' pictures on either side of the line (one side being positive feelings, the other negative ones, and the midline representing ambivalent or mixed feelings). It is a quick way to have a nonverbal exploration of how clients feel about their family without them having to explain it all in words, though we often then end up discussing the structure they make. The two sides can be labeled to fit any categories, such as people the client trusts or not, feelings of closeness or distance, feelings of similarities or differences, and so forth; the therapeutic focus will determine the labels.

In one case, I had the client use one side for pictures of family members at their best and the other side for them at their worst (in the client's mind). Another time, I had the client use one side for the way the family really is and the other side for how she wished it would ideally be. In this last case, I had the client visualize the dividing line as the barrier blocking such improvement and discuss obstacles to its removal and movement in the positive direction. One client in this exercise grabbed a photograph of her father and pounded it onto the line; no further explanation was needed, although we then spent an hour discussing the "fallout" from her spontaneous act.

In giving families photo-taking, photo-finding (in albums or other places), or photo-collaging assignments, or having them restructure their album, it is useful to note their need for boundaries and enclosures (or lack of them), as these can be covert signals of possible enmeshment or differentiation of the family or its individual members. If a family seems to need to work toward individuation of its members, assignments should be structured so that they end up with photographs of each individual alone, to help disengage and individually distinguish themselves. Conversely, if the goal is to encourage more family engagement and interaction, the assignment could be to return with many photos of the whole family doing album-creating work collectively.

I asked one client to bring in photos of herself at each stage of her life and then use the images to construct her life story. Once it was created, I asked her to use it as a basis for telling me that story. In one snapshot of her parents before their marriage, her mother looked flirtatious and playful. She said, "It is a view of her that I forget was ever part of her life. Suddenly she is human, and even rather sexual. Look at the difference in her holding me when I was first born. Suddenly she looks maternal and responsible."

This client's mother had died soon after her first birthday, and so she had only known her through photos. When her mother became a "fuller" person through our photographic exploration of her childhood and adolescent years, my client began to see her more as a whole person and to think more about what her life had been like. As well, she tried to imagine what her mother's sudden death must have been like for her father. "I had only thought of her before in relationship to me and how I felt about her abandoning me. Suddenly there's much more there. I sure wish I could talk with her."

I suggested she focus on the photos that seemed to attract her and, keeping them in mind, write letters to her mother. Later she returned to tell me she'd started a series of letters much like a journal, and included drawings, poetry, and photos of herself in the pages. "I let her know how I'd turned out and thanked her for letting me be born. I may even show these to my father someday, but for now it's just enough to have done them."

Another way to use family photos to explore and personalize parent-child relationships is to find photos of each parent as he or she was at the age the client is now, and rephotograph that image side-by-side with the client or with a photo of the client, so that comparisons can be made. Talking about what it was like "back then" and "at that age" allows the parent to get back in touch with his or her feelings and beliefs at earlier stages of life. It also lets the child or adult client realize that the parents were once different than they are now, and in fact were once children. Similar work can be done with photos of mother and daughter together or father and son, to look for similarities and differences right now. These explorations can mirror and explore differentiation and individuation issues.

Photos of people clearly show what changes over time and what doesn't. Photos taken each year, over decades, can show how sameness and difference are thoroughly intertwined in people's aging processes. Applications are wideranging and include traditional life-review work as well as therapy in special situations with clients who are, for example, denying health problems such as alcoholism. Such activities can also be helpful in working toward a positive goal, such as health enhancement reinforcement or proof of weight loss.

Using Album Photos in Therapeutic Exercises

This section presents several exercises involving more than just a few images. Its perspective is a bit different in that in these activities the client takes a longer-range perspective on her or his life instead of focusing on specific images and an assigned task.

An example of these more general assignments would be to ask a couple to bring to their next session several pictures from their mutual album that are most important to each of them and also several that they think would be most important to their spouse. These four piles of photos, sometimes with duplicated contents, can precipitate hours of communication between the two clients alone, and even more when the therapist is involved. Spouses are able to compare their choices with those made for them by their spouse; each is able to ask "Why that one?" and other image-based questions, which avoid direct confrontation of challenging each other face-to-face. In explaining their reasons, they base their answers on photographic selections, which cannot be disputed. Each one is presenting her or his opinion. Neither one's choice is necessarily wrong because it is different from the other person's. Such open-ended communication supports each person in a nonthreatened position. Each person is let into the other's value systems and beliefs without either person feeling the need to defend. Although I began this exercise with couples, I have often adapted it for use with any two or three family members who are locked into their separate positions.

Sometimes it is useful for a family to review their family photos all at once, spread out on a large table or the floor. As mentioned earlier, if albums cannot be taken apart in this fashion, it is effective to photocopy the pages and cut out the individual images. In photocopying, pictures can be enlarged for more detailed examination.

When all the photos are seen at once, a general affective quality may present itself. There may be a pervasive feeling suggested, such as a general tone of depression, strength, or some other nonverbal mood. The whole may take on different meaning from the story told by the component parts when sequentially laid onto pages.

Sometimes just spending time gazing at all the photos together, a client will be drawn to a particular image, types of images, or images that carry a theme, and it can help to try to find out why these call to them so much, why these demand their attention whereas others may not. Sometimes unconscious material that has eluded conscious searching presents itself, such as one of my clients suddenly becoming aware of childhood abuse by an uncle when she noticed photographs in which both of them appeared, but in which she never seemed to want to stand close to him. She had seen these images before, but it was only when several of them lay near each other on the table did she notice the discomfort she felt in looking at them.

Important discoveries are often precipitated by activities that force clients to make difficult choices about their photos and the people they represent. The Space Station exercise in Chapter Six is one such activity. The Space Station process can be adapted into a more narrow-focus activity for family photographs. In doing so, it often becomes even more intense, as only family members can be chosen for the final six and then prioritized. Letting go of three or four of these, and thus "rejecting" or abandoning photos of family members, may result in clients experiencing intense grieving for parents and loved ones in a way not previously encountered when doing this exercise with photos of nonfamily. One thing that is driven home when family images are used is that the Space Station exercise is indeed a metaphor for death, dying, leaving others behind, and being left behind. Therefore it can be very useful in situations with clients who have a life-threatening illness such as AIDS or cancer, or with clients who are contemplating suicide without considering the effects on those who would be left behind.

Doing the Space Station exercise in this fashion (using only family photos) one client found that there were no photos of all her family together in one grouping. Another found none of his photos had his father in them because the father had always taken the photos; now that he was dead, all the family had left of him was his occasional shadow. In doing the Space Station exercise using only family photos the discussion is much the same process: trying to find out why each snapshot was included in the original group, how it felt to choose some and leave others behind (and which ones the client may now regret not including), the story of each image (why is it still included now), how the client feels interacting with the picture (and noting its overall tone and feeling). The only difference would be that these are all family members' images being selected or rejected, and thus the feelings around the process may be intensely felt. As one man put it, "My god, it was awful! I had to decide which of my children to discard!"

As mentioned earlier, family album work is useful not only for direct therapy work, but also at an additional level of having clients discover their own personal support networks, which may be useful as resources for them in times of crisis. With a bit of 'network counseling' for all involved, the therapist is often able to withdraw back to an occasional-consultant status instead of being the client's primary dependency object.

The Rings exercise is one way to make such relationships more visible and real to clients, who may be under so much stress that these resources may be temporarily out of their awareness or acceptance. I believe the Rings exercise better informs clients about their own particular core support network of those people most emotionally connected to them, as feelings of guilt or obligation will likely be less involved in choosing snapshots than in the Space Station exercise.

The Rings exercise (details of which are given in the exercises section at the end of this chapter) is simple: the client sits at a large table or on the floor and pretends to be at the center of a series of concentric rings. The ring closest to the client is for the people closest to him or her—those who can be trusted with the client's deepest secrets; those with whom they are comfortable showing vulnerability; the ring furthest out is for absolute strangers.

I usually ask clients to work with four to six ring levels; anything bigger often grows too complex. I permit them to also place people between rings if they feel they need to. Once they understand the framework for the exercise, I then ask them to place snapshots of everyone they know where they belong. (If a photograph includes more than one person, masking tape can be used to block out all but the one person the photo is meant to be 'of.' Conversely, that person can be highlighted by drawing an arrow pointing to the person on a small strip of masking tape.) Their choices and criteria are important. For example, the decision as to how close to put someone can involve feelings about risking commitment and fearing obligation; how easy or difficult it is to make that decision may suggest debate between cognitive and emotional reasoning. This exercise can be done silently and then processed, or accompanied with therapeutic dialogue through all the steps of decision making. Using the Rings exercise, therapists can help clients become more conscious of unfinished business, mutually dependent relationships or expectations, triangulations or other power alliances, and many other underlying hooks to their emotional health.

The Rings exercise can be done at the photo-placing level discussed above or further fleshed out using art materials, found photos, collage, or other techniques discussed in previous chapters. Therapists can also ask the client to arrange subgroups or draw the rings onto a large piece of paper for making clear the interconnections by tying them together by drawing lines or symbols. These kinds of interconnecting substructures clearly emerge visually as primary central resources, and the client could then go on to redo the Rings exercise a different way, by placing any one of these other people at the center instead of themselves, in order to explore that person's perspective and relationship with the same individuals. This would visually demonstrate that these people have their own interrelationships in addition to those primary to the client.

One client told me that it wasn't until she started putting her siblings on particular rings that she became aware of how much more important they were to her than she realized and how her placements pointed out her previously undeclared disapproval of her brother-in-law, by his photo ending up placed out far beyond the final ring, at great distance from his wife (her sister). One man, who had earlier told me that he mainly likes photos showing himself interacting with others who are demonstrating their loving relationships with him, such as friends, lovers, even a favorite dog, also told me that he was rarely drawn to images of himself alone because photos of himself alone made him feel lonely and undesirable, and in fact until recently he did not like being alone at all. Yet when he did the Space Station exercise, most of the photos that made the final count were of his immediate family, and he was not in the majority of the pictures with these individuals.

When he then did the Rings exercise next, he used many of the same images as he had used in Space Station, and ended up with the close inner circle having only a few people in it; in this case none were relatives and several included him in the photo with the chosen person. He explained this by saying that, although he feels his father is his best friend, he didn't make it into his most intimate inner circle because his father is too innocent to hear the truth about his life in all cases, so he must continue to maintain some secrets from him. This man has AIDS and may soon need a support system he can count on for deeply intimate care and trust; it is likely that there may be some conflict between the people he permits to help him and his blood family.

This brings us to my final point about active exercises: doing any one of them in conjunction with any of the others exponentially increases their value to the client. Insight about the self and family relationships increases when the same images provide different information, depending on how they are used. For example, one client doing the Space Station exercise had expressed great anguish over having to choose between his past lover, who had died the previous year, and his new friend—a recent arrival in his life, but one definitely breathing life back into his libido and heart. My client remarked that he had been surprised, when looking for photos to bring me, that there were none of himself with his deceased lover or of the lover alone; there were only some of the lover playing with my client's nephews. Although his lover had been welcomed by most of my client's immediate family, one brother was not very accepting. My client was not surprised to notice he had no photos of this brother in any of his albums.

When my client did the Rings exercise as the next assignment, he found that the two closest rings contained only his family of affiliation and that his family of origin only appeared on rings beyond the first two, some far from him (including one that was pushed off the far side of the table). His new lover did not make it completely into the first ring, but was placed quite near it. He explained, "It's new still. I'll have to spend more time in this relationship before trusting that much again." This example shows how results of two exercises can be woven together to produce new information.

ILLUSTRATIVE EXAMPLE

Unlike the other chapters in this book, this chapter has provided so many detailed examples in previous sections that I think it would be redundant to provide even more client illustrations here. Instead, I am including samplings from an anecdotal personal album review in order to add another layer of understanding for the concepts and techniques this chapter has covered—precisely because it points out, from the photographic examples gathered during one person's lifetime, how family systems theory and photo documentation illustrating its principles are so evidently joined together in real life, in this case my own. My personal album illustrates this section because I know the various people in the photographs and have received the required permissions where necessary. I am not comfortable using my clients' album photos because uninvolved people may find themselves included in this book unexpectedly. Also, I believe a personal firsthand account from someone familiar with the systems perspective can be valuable for readers.

Having studied family systems theory and applied it with individual clients, I decided a few years ago to see what I could find in my own family's albums. I had moved away after university, and so my participation in family photos (and the family itself) became curtailed, except for brief visits or ceremonial holidays, weddings, funerals, and the like. But as I was interested in learning more about my own childhood and teenage years, I hoped that among the many familiar album pages I would find patterns and other visual information that could yield insights.

I found many interesting visual messages that I had not been able to decode previously. I had seen the snapshots before, but had not noticed specific details that took on additional meaning when viewed from my new perspective. In fact, the childhood presented in my albums was not always the one I remembered, or at least not quite that way. While I discovered photographs that validated my personal experience, I also found some whose contents corrected my distorted memories. I shared many of my findings with my parents, particularly my mother, as she is the more introspective one and enjoys such discussions more than my father, who often wondered why we were both spending so much time looking at old pictures.

My parents' comments revealed their touching innocence as to the psychological import of the snapshots, and I realized that had I not been interested in PhotoTherapy myself, I would likely have remained equally naive about the layers of significance these album photos held. I made discoveries about the origins of some of my leftover feelings and learned quite a bit about my parents as vulnerable, emotional, human beings, apart from their roles as my mother and father. I also encountered some unfinished business, unresolved issues, emotional "hooks," and uncommunicated needs that should have been dealt with long ago.

I explained to my parents that I wanted to "go public" with some of the family stories because I thought they would be useful illustrations of the effectiveness of PhotoTherapy techniques. They gave their assent as long as I would make it clear that, to quote my mother, "What you are saying isn't necessarily true, because you were a child and didn't see things as they *really* were" [emphasis mine]. Perhaps I didn't, but perhaps the eyes of a child see differently, though not necessarily always incorrectly. Therefore, readers need to keep in mind that these personal examples are from *my* childhood perspective, and are not necessarily the "truth" in any objective sense. Nor am I implying that any problems that I perceived at that time were consciously intended by the individual being discussed in relation to them.

However, what I perceived and remembered is and was *my* truth, and for the purposes of therapy, it cannot be discounted or invalidated by others whose perspectives were different or who see my reality as distorted. For example, what may have been deemed appropriate physical discipline or reasonable personal criticism at one time may now be considered humiliation or even child abuse. So without disputing my parents' versions of what happened and why, I present my stories as my own version of what the family photographs have revealed to me, and more importantly, validated for me, about the way my childhood "really" was. I present these not to signal that my parents are somehow "to blame" for what happened in my life, or are responsible for all my current attitudes, beliefs, or values, but only to note that our mutually interactive patterns (as captured in all those spontaneously taken snapshots of us) are all partially responsible for creating this. *Together* we are all "to blame" for who I have become, so to speak, because we are the family who produced each other by developing together and inseparably.

My childhood was relatively uneventful and not particularly unhappy, in general, although I took the angst of my teenage years terribly seriously. Apart from some rather insensitive physical and emotional discipline by my father (which he viewed to be proper at the time), it was far more positive than most childhoods I've heard about from my clients. However, it wasn't the ideal one constructed nicely in our family album, either.

Looking for Patterns

Spontaneously taken snapshots can only capture what already exists. Therefore, a study of all the photos in my family album would show what my relationships with my family, relatives, and friends were usually like. To find these, I looked many times through all the photographs until distinct patterns seemed to emerge in their contents.

Readers will have to simply accept my word that my examples and the photographs shown here are truly representative of what consistently appears in my family album. Issues of reliability and validity like this must be addressed in serious PhotoTherapy research. If patterns are claimed to exist, there should be supporting evidence that any samples used are truly typical. If only one photograph is used to illustrate something specific, it can well support its own proof individually, but generalizations or extrapolations from it should be made very cautiously, especially if no additional photographs can be provided to support claims made about it.

In my family's photos, I found many striking patterns. For example, on the many dozen pages documenting my first few years, about half of the photographs were of me alone, and approximately another 40 percent were of me with my mother. In these she was almost always holding me, touching me, and seeking direct eye contact with me rather than with the camera being held by my father. The word that comes to mind is "nurturing" (see photo 7.7).

Of those of me with my father, in nearly all of them, he is holding me awkwardly to his side while searching for my mother's gaze inside the camera. It is clear to me that he is not comfortable (see photo 7.8). Their "photographic gazes" were radically different, and this contrast continues even now. For my father, this might represent his discomfort at being photographed rather than at holding his child, but this cannot be ascertained forty years after the fact. Having lived as his child, however, I am fairly experienced with his lack of ease in parenting and would guess the second option to be the correct one.

Indeed, my individual relationships with each of them were very different. Consequently, no album reviewer would ever see spontaneously-taken

Photo 7.7 ***(left)***
Photo 7.8 ***(right)***

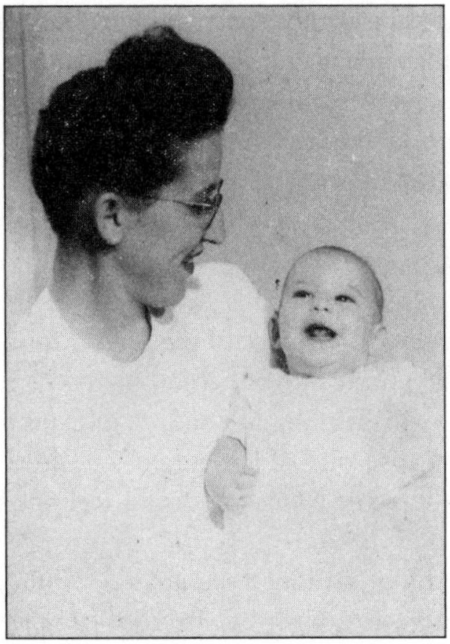

photos of me relating to my father as I did to my mother, as these situations never happened in the first place for any camera to be able to come along and capture naturally. While most photos of my mother and me show us emotionally engaged with each other and usually touching, I could find no photographs of my father and me spontaneously interacting or of my voluntarily touching him. Though not unfriendly, we seemed to be only posing for the picture.

In itself, this means nothing apart from documenting our ordinary daily behaviors. It just documents that my father and I didn't have much "quality time" together, not necessarily out of choice, but partly because he worked long hours and so wasn't around much, and partly because he wasn't really prepared for parenting. Moreover, fathers were not expected to be involved with child rearing. In my first decade playing at home, doing homework, going to the doctor, attending Brownies and school meetings, and the like, he was pretty much out of the picture. This was

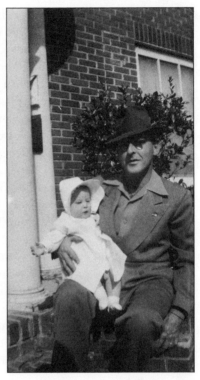

literally reflected by his not appearing very often in photos on album pages, unless my mother had him pose for a snapshot of the two of us.

Photographs of us taken by others would show us in different arrangements if the photographer gave directions for an "ideal family pose." However, when we were being photographed formally but allowed to position ourselves as we wished, another interesting pattern seemed to emerge. I use the word "seemed" here, because few photographs of the three of us together were ever taken. This pattern can be seen in photos 7.9 and 7.10 and is repeated in three more of the seven I found in the entire collection.

Repeatedly, I am shown behind my two seated parents, a reversal of the traditional positioning of children in front of their parents. This may have been because one of my parents decided on the arrangement. In any case, the images bring up strong feelings for me and carry several messages.

For one thing, although we are all smiling, I sense myself being on guard, wanting them both out in front of me where I can keep my eyes on them (and perhaps to have some control over how they could affect me). Also, the pose seems to communicate reverse dependency; I seem to be taking care of them, even at an early age. My only reaction to this thought is that they had great expectations for my future accomplishments and geared their lives toward my happiness and success. Therefore, much

Photo 7.9 ***(left)***
Photo 7.10 ***(right)***

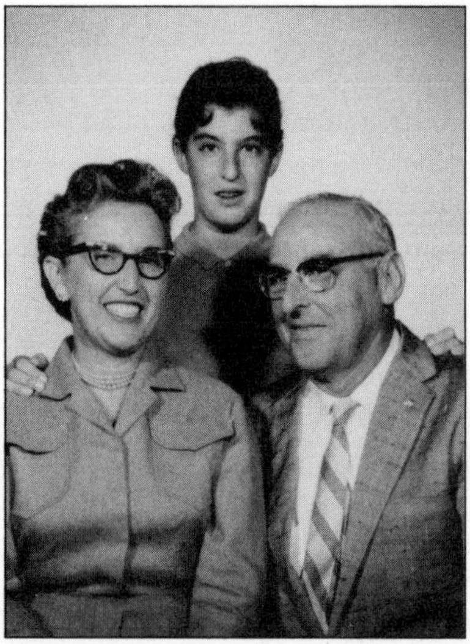

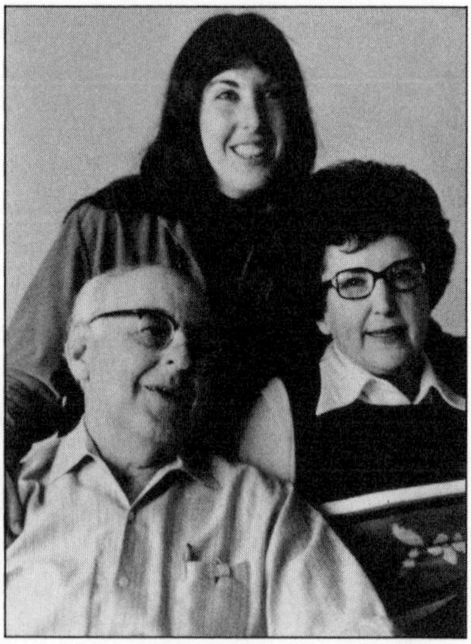

of their approval and acceptance had conditions attached, and thus I may also have been "lived through" a bit. After all, I was their only child.

My mother's response to my telling her these perceptions was that I was overreacting and that they were seated this way simply because they were older and deserved to be seated comfortably. But my version is still the reality of my life in those days *for me,* though I recognize that it is only one of many possible perceptions of our family dynamics, and that my parents strongly disagree with my interpretation.

Many other patterns emerged for me out of the snapshots taken during my childhood, but one was particularly striking. From about age two until I entered school, I seem to have been regularly photographed in close association with the family car (see photos 7.11 and 7.12). I am not certain whether one should read this as the car being my almost-sibling, whether I was being displayed for posterity as a treasure among other significant possessions and status symbols, or whether there was some plan to document my growth relative to the car. My parents' reactions

Photo 7.11 *(left)*
Photo 7.12 *(right)*

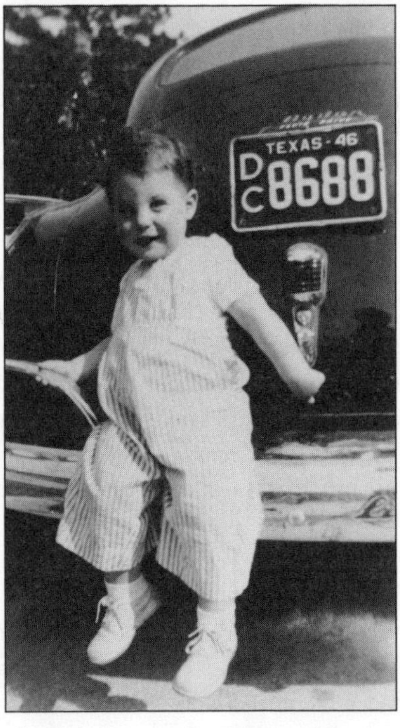

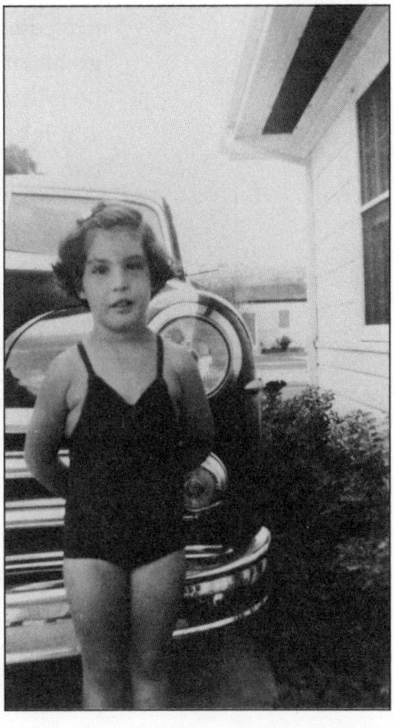

to this pattern was, "It was a new car and we liked taking pictures of you, so we put you together." My memory of most weekends was of my father outside washing and waxing his car while I played in the backyard and my mother attended to house chores. He had no hobbies, such as sports or reading, and she had little time for any, so perhaps these pictures also symbolically represented my relationship with him.

Generational Transmission

My four grandparents had no photographs of their ancestors. They were immigrants to the United States who had left all their traditional roots and community behind. There were only a handful of photographs of my parents that documented them or their immediate family in group portraits. This is the meager totality of my photographic heritage, and most of those who could have provided further details died decades ago. Yet, generational parallels nevertheless persist in the hidden, unconscious transmission of patterns.

One of the best examples of this kind of "secret" generational connectedness that I found was my discovery in a storage closet of a photograph of my mother's mother taken when she was in her late thirties. I literally came face to face with our striking resemblance. I put her photograph beside my own face and asked my husband to take a picture of the two of us "together" (see photo 7.13).

When I viewed the resulting photograph, I was surprised at feeling a sudden surge of strength and power arising from my sense of connection with her. This strong, resilient woman, who had walked her children out of Russia by herself (having never before been out of her family's village), suddenly emerged as an integral part of me, and I discovered that she and I were likely similar in our determination to overcome great odds. I later found out (four years after I started working with people who have AIDS) that she had spent years caring for the dying. This connection may be accidental, but it is validating and reaffirming for me.

Triangulation Dynamics

In systems theory I learned to examine how the arrival of the first baby affects the relationship of its parents, and how its assuming of primary position between its mother and father creates a triangulation of emotional

Photo 7.13

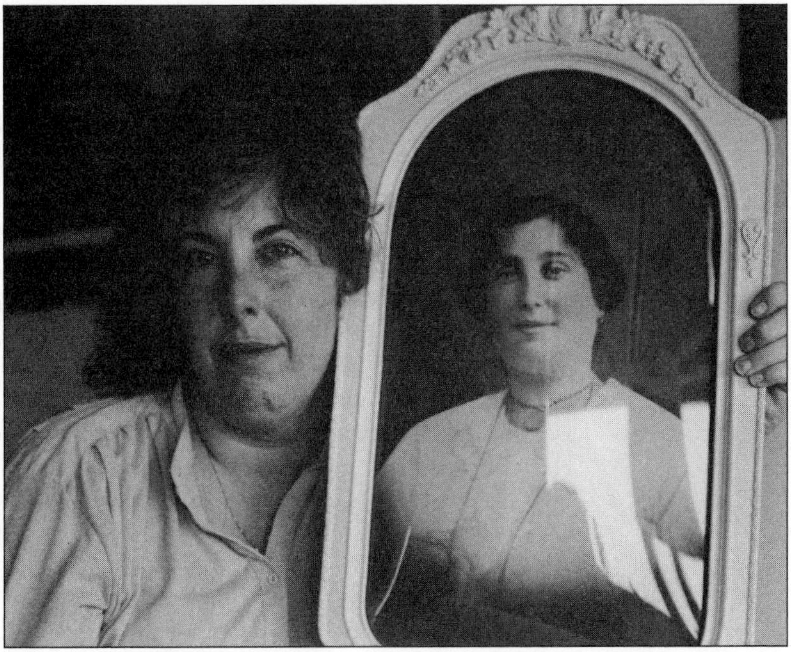

interactions which can influence the rest of all three lives. Rarely is this particular triangle equal in relationship in all three directions. Frequently the realignment forces redefining of power dynamics, role shifts, attentional focus, and the repositioning of one of the three persons as a new 'outsider.'

I am the only child in my family. But several years before my birth, my mother had a child who would have been my brother. He died shortly after his birth. I believe I was never told of this child until I was in my teens, although my mother says she just figured that I had known. My father never talked about his need or desire for a son; however, he "playfully" called me "Junior" until I reached puberty, and I innocently answered to the nickname, not realizing any potentially deeper significance.

Before I was born, my father had had my mother to himself for more than a dozen years and was not overjoyed with this colicky, demanding baby. Though definitely happy to have a child, my father was rather overwhelmed by me—a frenetic squally infant—and his discomfort evolved into a distant and brusque style of fathering, not uncommon in those days.

After my arrival, his wife was no longer solely his own. She began to divert a great deal of attention to my needs (and hers as well). It was not until adulthood that I heard the defensive explanations that his harsh temper and lack of understanding feelings were probably rooted in his own unhappy and occasionally abusive childhood, as well as in his belief that children were too often spoiled by emotional tenderness.

All I knew as a child was that I was fearful of his moodiness and quick temper, and had a "survivor's" desire not to get too close or risk showing any weaknesses. There were many times in my childhood where I felt (probably correctly) that my father saw me as a rival for my mother's attention. He competed with me for her affection in several ways, including treating me differently when she was around to witness and protect. In the triangle thus formed we were frequently adversaries (especially as I seem to have inherited his stubbornness!), and as the adult, he had most of the power to sabotage, humiliate, and otherwise disempower me, without my having any awareness about what really was going on.

My mother, however, was a rock of physical and emotional security and comfort. We spent a lot of time together, formed very close bonds, and she shared all my secrets. Although she could also be strict, her discipline was always tempered with love rather than sarcasm or revenge. She was a very good friend to me throughout my childhood (and still is), and we shared a lot of time together in pleasant moments and quiet comfortable silences, developing a lifetime of open communication through words, unspoken communications, and lots of reassuring touching. I was not afraid of her, nor of getting too close for comfort. Instead, when wounded, I would seek her help—quite the opposite of my interactions with my father.

Examples of this triangulation can be found in many places in my own photo albums. A particularly outstanding illustration can be seen in a snapshot taken of myself and my mother in my kitchen, with my father looking on from behind us, trying to also be noticed yet invisible to both of us, and with very little luck of being able to break through our tightly circled arms (see photo 7.14).

In this small slice of time, a majority of my childhood's emotional structure is presented "for all to see" as still evident. Even now, this is the family pattern: my father still finds himself frequently left out of what my mother and I are deeply involved in sharing (in the case of this photo, a giggle at her joke). My husband's camera captured a moment of us being "as we always are," and there is our triangle, still alive and operating.

Photo 7.14

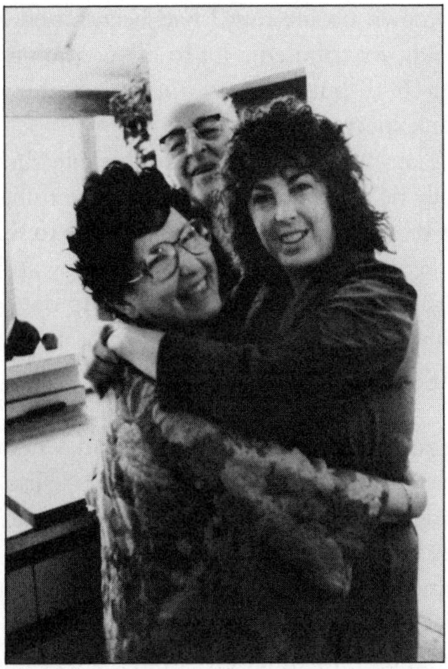

If I had been asked by a therapist to look back through all the photos in our family collection and find the one photograph that best expresses what our life together was like, I have little difficulty in deciding that this snapshot would be my choice. It says much more than the proverbial thousand words about my relationship with my parents, from early childhood through the present time.

Gender Roles and Expectations

From my earliest years, I was a tomboy and encouraged by both parents to aim for a university education and a job—in addition, of course, to being married and probably also a mother. My childhood was somewhat nontraditional in that, after I began school, my mother either worked outside the home as my father's office manager or brought in extra work to do at home to help with finances. Since she worked full time, the expectations regarding my future accomplishments didn't seem particularly unusual, although I was aware that my girlfriends' mothers didn't seem to be setting their own daughters' aims quite so high. Later when I began to study the construction of sexuality and sex-role conditioning, the light began to dawn on me that I had been raised as both a boy and a girl, which likely contributed a lot to my becoming an independent and self-confident child, but this was still both a blessing and a curse upon my own later expectations.

Some of my memories are double-edged, such as asking my father to carefully tie the waist-bow on my yellow ruffled-organdy dress and later the same day asking him to show me how to walk a beam at a construction site he was wiring. I remember my joy at finally being permitted to wear fingernail polish, and also my jump out of a tree onto the back of the neighborhood bully, who I tried to beat up, breaking my newly grown nails. My father took me to stock car races at the local track, and we especially enjoyed brutal demolition derbies, much to my mother's disgust. He and I regularly watched the Friday night wrestling matches with great pleasure; she despised my murderous shrieks. I always thought I had developed rather "naturally" into self-confident, assertive, self-liking personhood, but now in searching my albums for clues I also believe I find my parents' unconscious needs and attitudes expressed as subtle influences on what I was permitted or encouraged to do. I was given much more freedom than many other girls, but I didn't know this was uncommon. I aimed high because no one told me I might not succeed.

I discovered numerous snapshots that demonstrate this bipolar gender role identity. Two of the most obvious, to me, are photos 7.15 and 7.16, taken during the same year, roughly forty years ago.

To this day, I can remember the minutes surrounding the first. I had clearly been told, "Let me get a picture of you as a nice young lady" and had been shown how to curtsy. Awkwardly dropping to one knee (onto a rough pebble, which hurt, and is probably the reason I remember the moment), I held my frozen grin for what seemed ages until the shutter snapped. Another time, I was told I could have my photo taken any way I wanted. I remember being ecstatic that I was wearing my cowboy suit (definitely not cow*girl,* mind you), and took the stance that was my preferred identity of the moment. Even today, I treasure this image of myself standing tough and strong, as a cowboy would (which is what I was planning at that age to grow up to be).

The moment was important enough to embed itself in my subconscious. How it affected my later growth in assertiveness I cannot state in words, but I'm sure it's there in the tapestry. These two images have become almost iconic for me, as I am now both of these little girls, grown

Photo 7.15

Photo 7.16

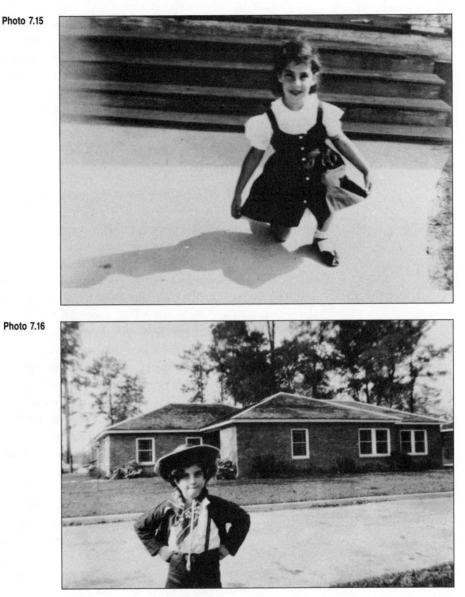

up and synthesized as one now, but clearly knowing both my male and female aspects. This to me is a component of mental health, and also, I think, a clue as to why I am comfortable with people of any sexual orientation. I think my parents' unconscious influences on my childhood identity laid the pattern for who I have become and what I like about myself, although none of this was conscious to me before my PhotoTherapy album-searching began a few years ago.

Emotional Intimacy or Distancing

Reviewing family albums from a systems perspective would suggest a lot of attention be paid to who is close to, facing, touching, or at least appearing to be in emotional contact with, whom. This is not to suggest that these things have direct one-to-one correlation of meaning from such positionings, but rather that they can be used to probe the feelings associated with the visually-captured relationships. My family album holds numerous snapshots that substantiate the close and almost exclusive bond between myself and my mother. (See photo 7.17.) However, the few that exist of me with my father show little direct interaction or emotional engagement. These relationships were consistent throughout my childhood.

By the time I was a teenager, my relationship with my father had become severely strained and emotionally destructive. In particular, we had very different understandings regarding his physical disciplining of me, and although now I no longer doubt that he loved me during those years, I didn't believe it at the time. His ways of expressing anger, jealousy, and disapproval during my younger years were offensive, as well as dangerous to my physical and emotional health. As a result, as a teenager I tried to avoid him as much as possible.

I thought I had hidden these feelings quite well, but one snapshot to me blatantly expresses my resistance to trust or intimacy with him. Photo 7.18 was originally supposed to be of me alone, but he rushed over to intrude into "my" picture.

I look at this picture and again experience a feeling of personal violation, feelings of being overpowered once again. My spontaneous attempt to avoid contact seems obvious to me. The top half of my body is recoiling from his head moving in toward my chest, and to me, my finger looks like a gun.

My parents passed right over this one when viewing the photos from that visit, as it didn't signal anything out of the ordinary to them. But

Photo 7.17

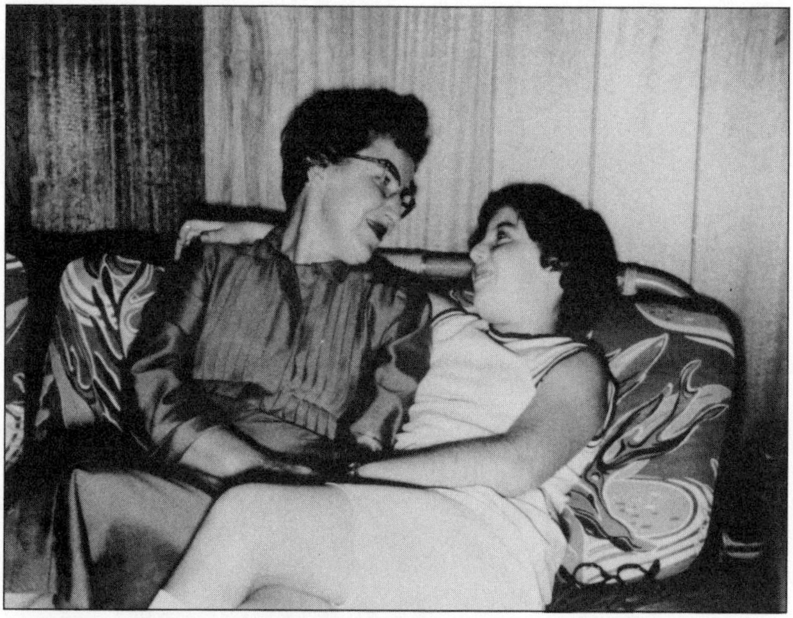

I have rarely seen such a clear, spontaneous statement of personal boundaries and their violation as this photo makes (for me). This photograph gives me a sick and fearful feeling, yet the gun metaphor reassures me that I am able to protect myself because now I am the stronger one. All this resulted from an accidental intrusion into a moment of photographic spontaneity. Had my father not rushed to force himself into my photographic relationship with my husband (the photographer), whose male/son attention he has long coveted, and had I not been holding something in my hand that gave my fingers that "gun" position, I might not yet have come to terms with some of the feelings this snapshot evoked.

Personalizing Roles

Knowing my parents only as my parents, until my study of family systems theory led me back to exploring who they were as individuals, I really had not thought much about their lives apart from my own. Finding out what their own childhoods and adolescences had been like was enjoyable, and I discovered details I had never known about in their explanations of each old photograph. For example, I never knew they had both played

Photo 7.18

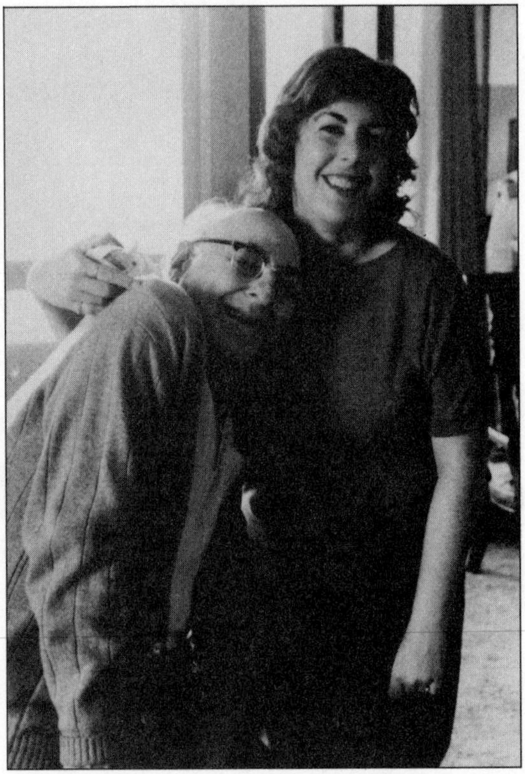

accordion or that my mother had had a pet goat when she was young. Seeing them as flirtatious lovers was a real shock: my mother on her bicycle could have been a pinup, and seeing my father as a shirtless young man, I suddenly realized she might actually have been physically attracted to him rather than just finding him acceptable to her parents. With the photos to stimulate talk about the past, my parents have entertained me with many stories I had never heard before.

SAMPLE EXERCISES

Overall general findings and feelings resulting from looking at all the client's album and photo-biographical snapshots has been well discussed in previous pages, and selections of questions have been given for journeying through clients' albums with them. I have already stressed that attention be paid to overall themes, trends, and consistencies that emerge in images taken over many years, in many locations, and usually across several generations. I have suggested looking at patterns in family interactions, roles, and relationships, as well as chronological or contextual information presented within these snapshots.

Therefore, I am assuming that, by this point in this book, readers are fully aware of the kinds of questions to use in beginning album explorations and thus I provide here only two sample exercises: one is reflective and can be used when contemplating family members' photos, and the other more active one is the Rings exercise discussed earlier.

Reflective Exercise: Family Photo Interaction

This two-part exercise is designed to have the client encounter an individual family member as a unique individual in addition to his or her role. This means learning about numerous less-known aspects of the person's life and about his or her range of feelings and experiences, and generally exploring beyond what is commonly known of the person in his or her usual roles. There are several ways to do this; for example, the client could select a particular individual and review all photos of that person's life up to the present moment, observing how she or he has externally changed, and trying to comprehend any inner accompanying changes which may have precipitated or followed the actual physical changes. Clients can be asked to explore these observations and try to "tune in" to the visual signals to such inner realities. If possible, clients should then discuss their findings with the person in a low-key non-threatening conversational situation.

Although such reflective exercises can theoretically be done as homework assignments, I much prefer that my clients do them in my presence so that I can observe any nonverbal behavior on their parts and also be available for spontaneous discussion, which may be lost if we wait for a delayed retelling. (As these exercises can be done without removing photographs from album pages, they make good starter assignments.)

Clients are asked to look at snapshots of their family's past, starting as far back as they would like, and then to think about or discuss with the therapist answers to questions such as those listed below. Clients can respond silently, or by writing down answers or by voicing their thoughts. (Repeat the following sequence for each family member.)

Look at a photo of a particular family member. Study the image slowly, quietly; examine the many details and the whole of it. Get a feeling for this image and write down (or say aloud) your answers to the following questions:

1. What are the first three things that come to mind as you look at this photo?
2. What other people or places come to mind?
3. Describe three feelings, thoughts, or memories that come up in response to the photo. Try completing these sentences: "When I look at this photo, I think ____." "I feel ____." "I remember ____." "I find myself wanting to say ____."
4. What are some things you would like to tell the person in the photo? Think about why this conversation has not happened yet, and try to express what you have always wanted to tell that person but for some reason never could or would.
5. What are some things you have always wanted to ask or find out from this person, but never could or would?
6. What is something you would like to have this person tell (or ask) you? Why it is that this conversation has not happened yet? What would it take (what would have to change) for this to happen?
7. Who do you think may have taken this photo and for what reasons? Did they get what they wanted in the result? Would you have taken it this way? Do you want to rephotograph it now? How might it be different if you did it?
8. What would you like to see this photo get up and do or say? To you?
9. Who in the family is or was this person's favorite, and why?
10. What would you title this photo?
11. What gift might you give this photo?
12. Would you want to be in a photograph with this person, and why or why not?
13. What, if anything, seems to be missing in this photo? What would need to be added to make it more complete?
14. Is this photo a true depiction of that person, or does it lie in some way?
15. Would this person be permitted to have a photograph (that you like) of yourself, and why or why not? If not, what would have to change before they could?

To delve further, consider any or all of these questions:

Is there any family member whose photo you did not bring along and what might this be about? If there is a particular photo that makes you feel a certain way, address it directly through open-ended questions such as these: "When I see this picture (person), it makes me angry, because ____." Then say what the subject would have to do for the anger to go away. Then try the exercise again, but instead of saying "*You make me angry when you do or say ____*," say "*I feel hurt*." What does the difference feel like?

If art materials are available, try to draw (within a similar frame proportion as the person's photo) a "snapshot" portrait that would better express your knowledge of, and feelings about, this person. Try to create a more honest picture than the photograph.

Holding the photograph in your mind, try mentally enlarging the borders of the image. Pretend you can pull the edges apart to see what else was in the scene from which this photograph was taken. Perhaps set the image down on paper and draw in the rest of it.

If clay or plasticine is available, hold some and manipulate it while you study the snapshot and contemplate the feelings that emerge.* Do this for several minutes, and then set down the material. Do not stop to analyze what you have created. Pick up more clay or plasticine and move immediately to the next photo. Once all photos have been done, focus on the clay objects: what emerged nonverbally? How does this add to your understanding of the family?

Active Exercise: The Rings

In contrast with the exercise above, where clients simply look at and respond to certain family photographs, other exercises require the client to be more actively involved with creating or rearranging new versions of their family snapshots. Some of this may be fairly simple to suggest, such as telling the client to go make new photographs of images in their album that aren't satisfactory in their original form, redoing them as if they were the original photographer, or to photograph what is missing from their album, and so forth.

*This exercise is adapted from one demonstrated by Jean-Luc LaCroix (Professor of Social Work at the Université du Montréal) at the Family Therapy Mental Health Conference at the University of British Columbia, May 1987.

As the text of this chapter has already suggested, in addition to taking new snapshots clients could work with existing photos (or photocopies of them) on large sheets of paper or newsprint, expanding them with further elaboration by means of additional artwork or writing, as if the photos illustrated the pages of a newspaper or book. Clients could be asked to pick a few images that are especially significant for them and use a photocopier to enlarge, shrink, or crop them as desired. These could even be rearranged or collaged into a "truer" individual, family, or group portrait.

Or, clients might be asked to arrange one photo of each family member onto a sheet of newsprint so that the overall proportions and alignments visually convey the actual interpersonal relationships of those family members. If the client has access to a darkroom or an enlarging type of photocopier, they could even try "blowing up" the family into sizes proportional to their power or influence, amount they are loved or disliked, their good or bad qualities, or other aspects that exist in the client's opinion, and visually represent these concepts in collage or sculptural form.

Other active exercises involve more complex assignments, such as those suggested in the Rings exercise below, where the client is given the following instructions:

Lay out in front of you all the photos of each person in your immediate family, your friends, acquaintances, and pets, if you wish, so that you can see all of them at once. Pick the one that best represents each individual and put the others away. Now you should be sitting facing one photo of each person. Imagine yourself at the center of a circle, with concentric rings around you.

Imagine these rings as being resting places for your snapshots. Each ring level is generally defined below. Put each snapshot where it seems to fit best in relationship to these definitions, and feel free to place people between the rings, as they may be in-between the descriptions given below. If some seem to "go with" others that are in the same ring category, feel free to cluster them in spatial relationships near each other, expressing the connections among them. The following definitions of the ring levels are for your use; feel free to redefine them if other meanings seem to fit better for you conceptually.

The ring closest to you is very close. Only a few people in your life can get that close to you. They have to be very special to be this close, as these are the only people who are allowed to know absolutely everything about you, the people from whom you keep no secrets and with whom you have no fear of being vulnerable or taking risks.

The second ring is for people who are very close to you, but from whom you still wish to maintain some secrets or keep some boundaries that they are not welcome to cross. Though close to you, these are people with whom you still need to have a few barriers to protect your vulnerability, as you just don't want to have them know you that well yet.

The third ring is for people you know and like, and definitely feel connected with, but whom you wouldn't really call "close." They are close enough through family or friendship ties that you like to be around them, but they don't quite fit into the closer bonds of those at ring levels one and two. If there was an emotional crisis in your life, you might not share that burden with these people.

The fourth ring is for casual acquaintances or family members you don't feel very close to. These are often the people you feel should be included, but you don't want them too close.

The fifth, and further rings, are for those not in the inner circles. Perhaps you'll space them on ring levels defined by your own parameters, but be sure to put all your photos somewhere within this ring framework.

This exercise may be done on a table or on the floor; however, it can also be done on large sheets of newsprint if materials are available. The photos can be spread out on top of the paper and their places marked (or their outlines traced or contents sketched), and the client can further elaborate their relationships with each other, and with the client, through additional drawing, writing, and collaging. The client may also find it useful to draw lines connecting each person's snapshot with those others they have connections with.

In debriefing this, the therapist may have clients talk their way through each decision or feeling or, instead, do the entire process in silence and then discuss the finished creation. Both methods have benefits and limitations, and therapists need to be fluent with both options in order to choose the best one for the client.

In thinking back about the sorts of things that went through your mind (and feelings) as you placed each person, consider these exploratory questions:

- Did you find people's places shifting in relationship to you or each other as you added others to the overall scene? What precipitated these moves?
- Did you have a hard time with some placements? Which ones, and why?

- Pretend there is a conversation going on between each of these photos and you. What is being communicated and what feelings, thoughts, or memories arise in association with this discussion?
- Were you surprised to find out which people turned out to be emotionally the closest? Were these mainly blood relatives, friends, or a mixture of both?
- If you had to return the snapshots, and could only use a symbolic image to mark each person's place on the rings, what symbol or image would you choose for each one?

Imagine that each of your immediate family members or close friends did this exercise with the very same photos you used. Pick a family member you like most (and/or least) and do the exercise from his or her perspective.

- What did you learn about this person from this experience?
- Compare where this person probably placed you on the rings and where you placed him or her on yours. What thoughts and feelings emerge for you when you do this?

If you also did the Space Station exercise in Chapter Six, how did your top six photos in that one compare with the photos in the rings nearest you in this one? If you used the same snapshots for both exercises, what differences emerged and what contrasting feelings were evoked?

8 Using PhotoTherapy to Promote Healing and Personal Growth

A machine that can freeze time, a way to make that fleeting moment permanent, exactly as it happened, eternally unchanged. It all seems so simple: point the mechanical object (the camera) at a scene, and it will capture the image in front of the lens, duplicate the scene in front of it, objectively, and with none of the distortion that we find in paintings and drawings. From the age of scientific reason and objectivity of the previous century arrived this fantastic possibility that a machine could finally document the world as it really is, its beauty and truth untainted by human interference and its image untouched and unfiltered by the frailties and pitfalls of human perception or intervention.

This book has, I hope, demonstrated how faulty such presumptions proved to be. I have aimed to show how personal and private our photographic realities are. With photographs, time literally stops and external spatial reality in some ways ceases to exist. Each snapshot is simultaneously a moment taken from all moments and yet part of them all. Observer and observed are to me part of the same thread of life, which is itself unobservable, yet we attempt to stop it all with the click of a shutter. This is what PhotoTherapy is all about: when a person interacts with the snapshot, even just by looking at it or pressing the shutter to create it spontaneously, he or she "changes the picture" altogether.

An ordinary snapshot gives form and structure to our deepest emotional states and unconscious messages. It serves as a bridge between the cognitive and the sensory, between the inner self lying below conscious awareness and the self able to be known to us, and between the self we are aware of inside and that self we are seen as by others. It can also connect the past with the present, forming a multilevel interlocking matrix and preparing us to continue this onward to time beyond the present moment. It joins the physical world with the psychic one, the reality we are aware of with that which only presents itself after the fact in connections or patterns visible only in retrospect.

In reviewing our personal photographs we learn things about ourselves that we were not at all conscious of when we took the pictures—things that later seem obviously visible were latent or embedded at the moment we captured them. This is why I refer to them as "footprints" of our minds and "mirrors" of our lives; they are visual markers that let us know not only where we have been but also, perhaps, where we might be going, even when this is not yet conscious to us.

Given all of this, it is easy to see how even ordinary snapshots can be good tools for illuminating areas of unconscious thought and feelings that were previously not accessible through words or conscious investigation. PhotoTherapy techniques as presented in this book can be used to bring information that we have forgotten, buried, and defended ourselves against into the realm of the knowable and recognizable, especially the information we hold without words and cannot tell with words. They reconnect us with the details of our lives that were originally recorded as sensory impressions and, as well, with remembered information whose relevance we do not recognize until visual stimuli help us make associations to it. A personal snapshot is both an intellectual and an emotional property, possessed not because of its appearance alone, but also because of what its appearance has been unconsciously constructed to mean.

Personal photography gives new meaning to the well-worn saying, "out of sight, out of mind" and reinforces the claim that most people use a predominantly visually-based language to express themselves. It becomes clear that any language we use to try to communicate our inner thoughts, feelings, or memories can at best be only representational and metaphoric. What we see and know inside our mind can never be directly observed. Our language reflects our cognitive mapping strategies and the values inherent within them; it is itself a map, even its visual language components.

In this book I have tried to explain and demonstrate how ordinary snapshots have the power to communicate far beyond any words, how they are perceived by most of us to represent (and re-present) reality, the emotional truth, and the unarguable proof of a split-second slice of time.

Each moment captured on film, when viewed later, appears to us as if in the present, as if it were "right now," and we reexperience all its feelings, memories, and messages embedded in it—as well as later associated ones—as if they were happening right now.

In providing the theoretical rationale for, and then demonstrating the techniques of, PhotoTherapy as a tool for therapists, I have tried to explain and show how ordinary snapshots can be used to get in touch with feelings, information, and memories from "then" in order to understand their influence "now." Carefully designed questions are the chief tool with which we can help our clients bring part of their unconscious to conscious awareness.

Photographs can gently remind you, safely confront or inform you from the past, and speak, both for you and to you. They can help you find out more about what you want from life and where you may be heading. Through PhotoTherapy work, we learn about the facts of our lives and also about those usually out-of-conscious-awareness elements, such as our inner values from which we operate and form opinions, judgments, interpretations, and expectations. We gain insight into our feelings and why they are the way they are; our own unique personal symbols, which have private and even secret meanings for us; and how we construct our own lives. We begin to comprehend the various effects of our family, gender, society, culture, and other such factors on what we think are our own perceptions. Using photo-based questioning techniques we all can learn more about those hidden, mysterious, and otherwise "quiet" places that are at the core of self-knowledge and our communications with others.

PhotoTherapy has been presented not as a closed, fixed model, with rules about how to do it "right," but rather as a set of flexible tools with which to construct a process tailored to each client's individual needs and goals. I have shown not only how much can be done therapeutically using a snapshot in someone's hand (or mind), but also how much more can be done using this artifact as a beginning to facilitate additional process. It is not just the snapshot, but also the planning, posing, snapping, viewing, keeping, giving, associating, treasuring, and imagining that go along with it that provide such freedom to express, explore, and experience.

People learning to use PhotoTherapy techniques must be aware of the significance of what is precipitated during the client's process of interaction with a given image (encountering, remembering, imagining, and changing it). Views of the self from inside out and outside in are enhanced when personal snapshots are used to help focus. Photos of us and by us provide insight and outlook; photos from the inside out (by us) and from the outside in (of us) present us to ourselves. Self-portraits present both, simultaneously, and album snapshots do both, with a time delay between the two, but in the final analysis they are all the same in that they are useful tools for seeing ourselves better.

Projectives teach that how a person views photos reflects how he or she defines the world and other people, and that thoughts, feelings, memories, and many other things are stored in codes that sometimes only visual cues can unlock. Self-portraits are perhaps the most powerful photos for individual learning and for differentiation of a mature and aware self, and exploring and confronting one's self-image can be some of the most important and valuable PhotoTherapy work a client can do. Photos of the client give numerous external correlations with which to match inner self-concepts, and photos taken or collected by clients are self-constructs in phenomenological ways in that all the photos clients take are in some ways indicators of what matters to them. Family album photos and other biographical snapshots illustrate the selective reality of a family, constructed to withstand time; inside its contents people are frozen forever together, along with a lot of information about the dynamics of their relationships and their feelings about it all. It quickly becomes obvious that PhotoTherapy is not just about what snapshots show, but also about what can be done with them to further explore their secrets.

I have attempted to show how the process of doing PhotoTherapy lies most of all in knowing how to design questions that use the snapshot as a catalyst to access, release, and often actually transform unconscious, buried, overdefended, or "forgotten" information and emotions inside of clients. Such material, consciously or unconsciously "held captive," must be freed up and worked with as part of the healing and learning process of the therapy itself. The key lies in learning how to ask questions based on the photograph-as-stimulus that will lead to the inner explorations desired, the knowledge of what to ask when, and how, in order to join clients in discovering more about themselves.

Being competent with PhotoTherapy techniques requires an open inquiring mind and a willingness to expand your possibilities as a facilitator. It requires enlarging your repertoire of probing techniques to include nonverbal and visual components and to accept that you and your client are exploring that person's life together on a road that neither of you can yet see. Skill in PhotoTherapy is manifested in your ability to ask questions that stimulate the client into unconscious and previously protected depths below their conscious awareness or ability to recall or reexperience. You must be comfortable with concepts such as selective perception, situationally based reality, synchronicity, egocentrism and ethnocentrism, and be fluent enough with your own theoretical underpinnings to recognize where these things may be affecting your communications with your client. You must be able to accept that there can be more than one correct possibility in any given situation and that often these are found to be coexisting in mutual contradiction, paradox, or denial, right in front of you, or inside you. And you have to be at ease enough with receiving and accepting all this that it does not significantly interfere with your helping your client's progress.

For most people who stop to consider how photographs really do freeze slices of time, there is a sense of wonder and awe at the magic that permits taking a moment from the ever-moving flow and process of time and stopping it into a brief instant that can last forever. That power is part of the emotional connectedness and unconscious understanding that people's relationships with their snapshots give them; it certainly can also be a powerful tool in helping them focus inward on themselves and their lives. Literacy is primarily visual, and visual literacy is so primary that photos become the logical solution to the search for a language of communication. People from all cultures and socioeconomic backgrounds take, keep, and treasure pictures. Most have photos of themselves, significant others in their lives, and places that have special meanings. Someone once told me they understood photographs as being poems without words and called them visually frozen music.

Whatever the metaphor, people's ordinary snapshots have strikingly important lives (and secrets). They permit people to explore this predominantly nonverbal terrain in a predominantly nonverbal manner. Thus they are effective keys that unlock doors to previously hidden information, feelings, and memories. They permit us to connect the verbal with the visual, and both of these with the emotional, and in explaining the connection, be able to bear witness to our own life's story and its importance. Using PhotoTherapy techniques people can "get a picture" of their life that is worth far more than the proverbial thousand words. It has been said that the best test of something's value is to imagine life without it, so I tried to imagine a world where there never has been any photography and no one had ever thought to invent it. What fantasies I could dream up for such a tool, what amazing promises it could offer—but none better than what already exists.

In closing, I would like to encourage both therapists and clients to go have fun with your snapshots and albums, go explore the secret lives they have beyond what you've usually seen, and their messages to you and about you. I hope that after reading this book you can never again look at your own photos in quite the same way as before. Use them now as a way to begin looking deeper into yourselves and as catalysts to conversations long overdue, to improve understanding of, and communication about, your feelings. Find in them clues to your own uniqueness as well as your own roots. But be warned: once started, there is no end to the journey; it is the getting there that is the "all." To arrive at the place from where we started and to know it again, for the first time (to paraphrase T. S. Eliot), is certainly part of it, but even more important therapeutically is the journey itself. And, please feel free to write me to let me know what happens along the way!

References

Akeret, R. U. (1973). *Photoanalysis: How to interpret the hidden psychological meaning of* personal *photos.* New York: Simon & Schuster.

Amerikaner, M., Schauble, P. & Ziller, R. (1980). Images: The use of photographs in personal counseling. *Personnel and Guidance Journal, 59,* 68–73.

Anderson, C. M. & Malloy, E. (1976). Family photographs: In treatment and training. *Family Process, 15* (2), 259–264.

Atkins, R. (1989). Photographing AIDS. In J. Z. Grover (Ed.), *AIDS: The artists' response* (pp. 26–31). Ohio State University: Hoyt L. Sherman Gallery.

Bandler, R. & Grinder, J. (1975). *Structure of magic* (vols. 1 & 2). Palo Alto, CA: Science & Behavior Books.

Bandler, R. & Grinder, J. (1979). *Frogs into princes: Neuro-linguistic programming.* Moab, Utah: Real People Press.

Bayer, J. (1977). *Reading photographs: Understanding the aesthetics of photography.* New York: Pantheon.

Brenneman, J. (1990). *PhotoTherapy with adolescent violent offenders: A photo-journal approach.* Unpublished manuscript, State of Colorado Division of Youth Services.

Brody, J. (1984, July 17). Photos speak volumes about relationships. *New York Times,* pp. 21–25.

Note: In case of difficulty locating any of the sources listed, the author can be contacted for assistance at PhotoTherapy Centre, 1107 Homer St., Suite #304, Vancouver B.C., Canada V6B 2YI.

Burckhardt, J. (1990). *Photodrama: A therapeutic intervention to assist subpersonality integration* (Vols. 1 & 2). Doctoral dissertation, Menlo Park: Institute of Transpersonal Psychology.

Burgin, V. (Ed.). (1982). *Thinking photography.* London: Macmillan Education.

Carpenter, P. K. (1986). *Using expressive communication through photography to facilitate self-awareness: A handbook for educators.* Master's thesis, California State Polytechnic University (Pomona).

Coblenz, A. L. (1964). Use of photographs in a family mental health clinic. *American Journal of Psychiatry, 121,* 601–602.

Cohen, J. (1983, January 10). Abstract photocatharsis. *Maclean's,* p. 44.

Combs, J. M. & Ziller, R. C. (1977). Photographic self-concept of counselees. *Journal of Counseling Psychology, 24*(5), 452–455.

Comfort, C. E. (1985). Published pictures as psychotherapeutic tools. *Arts in Psychotherapy, 12*(4), 245–256.

Cooper, J. (1984). *Photo therapy in the field of child care.* Unpublished manuscript, University of Victoria, British Columbia.

Cosden, C. & Reynolds, D. (1982). Photography as therapy. *Arts in Psychotherapy, 9* (1), 19–23.

Craig, L. (1991). *Photography as therapy with emotionally disturbed adolescents.* Unpublished manuscript.

Crimp, D. (with A. Rolston). (1990). *AIDS Demo/Graphics.* Seattle: Bay Press.

Doughty, R. (1988). *Inner landscapes: Reading photographs which describe our lives.* Unpublished manuscript, Capilano College, Vancouver.

Duval, S. & Wicklund, R. A. (1972). *A theory of objective self-awareness.* New York: Academic Press.

Elias, M. (1982, December 22). Photo albums hide secrets. *USA Today,* pp. D1–D2.

Entin, A. D. (1979). Reflection of families. *Phototherapy, 2*(2), 19–21.

Entin, A. D. (1980). Family albums and multigenerational portraits. *Camera Lucida, 1*(2), 39–51.

Entin, A. D. (1981). The use of photographs and family albums in family therapy. In A. Gurman (Ed.), *Questions and answers in the practice of family therapy* (pp. 421–425). New York: Brunner/Mazel.

Entin, A. D. (1983). The family as icon: Family photographs in psychotherapy. In D. Krauss & J. L. Fryrear (Eds.), *Phototherapy in mental health* (pp. 117–134). Springfield, IL: Charles Thomas.

Erickson, M. H., Rossi, E. & Rossi, S. (1976). *Hypnotic realities.* New York: Wiley.

Evans, C. (1989). *Innovative projects program: Photography–Thoughtfulness, fantasy, and future.* Unpublished manuscript, University of British Columbia.

Fenjues, P. (1981, November 20). Understanding the family may be a snap. *Chicago Sun Times,* pp. 16–17.

Fenster, G. (1989, November 18). *Art therapy with HIV positive patients: Mourning, restitution, and meaning.* Paper presented at the 20th Annual Conference of the American Art Therapy Association, San Francisco.

Festinger, L. (1957). *A theory of cognitive dissonance.* Stanford: Stanford University Press.

Fryrear, J. L. (1980). A selective nonevaluative review of research on photo therapy. *Phototherapy, 2*(3), 7–9.

Fryrear, J. L. (1982). Visual self-confrontation as therapy. *Phototherapy, 3*(1), 11–12.

Fryrear, J. L. (1983). Photographic self-confrontation as therapy. In D. A. Krauss & J. L. Fryrear (Eds.), *Phototherapy in mental health* (pp. 71–94). Springfield, IL: Charles Thomas.

Gallagher, P. A. (1981). *Photography for handicapped children: Techniques and adaptations.* Unpublished manuscript, University of Kansas.

Glass, O. (1991). *Everyday life photography: A picture of existence.* Unpublished master's thesis, Lesley College Graduate School.

Goffman, E. (1963). *Stigma: Notes on the management of spoiled identity.* Englewood Cliffs, N.J.: Prentice-Hall.

Gooblar, M. (1989). *PhotoTherapy literature review.* Unpublished manuscript, University of British Columbia.

Gosciewski, W. F. (1975). Photo counseling. *Personnel & Guidance Journal, 53*(8), 600–604.

Graham, J. R. (1967). The use of photographs in psychiatry. *Canadian Psychiatric Association Journal, 12,* 425.

Grover, J. Z. (1989a). Visible lesions: Images of the person with AIDS. *Afterimage, Summer,* 10–16.

Grover, J. Z. (Ed.) (1989b). *AIDS: The artists' response.* Ohio State University: Hoyt L. Sherman Gallery.

Hagarty, J. (1985, March 7). Pictures bring life into focus, counselor says. *Winnipeg Free Press,* p. 30.

Hall, E. T. (1973). *The silent language.* Garden City, NY: Doubleday.

Harbut, C. (1975). *Mars trip still photo assignment.* Unpublished paper, Northern Illinois University.

Hathaway, N. (1984). The camera's always candid. *American Way* (American Airlines, *April,* 160–163.

Hogan, P. T. [*see also Turner*]. (1981). Phototherapy in the educational setting. *Arts in Psychotherapy, 8*(3), 193–199.

Hopper, D. (1990). Young man with autism takes photographs that intrigue. *Autism Society of Canada, 9*(3), 13–15.

Howard, B. (1989). *Epitaphs for the living: Words and images in the time of AIDS.* Dallas: Southern Methodist University Press.

Howie, P. (1989, November 18). *Art therapy with HIV seropositive patients: Issues for the therapist.* Paper presented at the 20th Annual Conference of the American Art Therapy Association, San Francisco.

Jung, C. (1971). *The spirit in man, art, and literature.* Princeton: Princeton University Press.

Kaslow, F. W. & Friedman, J. (1977). Utilization of family photos and movies in family therapy. *Journal of Marriage and Family Counseling, 3*(1), 19–25.

Krauss, D. A. (1979). *The uses of still photography in counseling and therapy: Development of a training model.* Doctoral dissertation, Kent State University.

Krauss, D. A. (1983). Reality, photography and psychotherapy. In D. A. Krauss & J. L. Fryrear (Eds.), *Phototherapy in mental health* (pp. 40–56). Springfield, IL: Charles Thomas.

Krauss, D., Capizzi, V. M., Englehart, T., Gatti, A. & Reed, P. (1983). Adjunctive use of still photographs in the partial hospitalization program of Cuyahoga Valley Community Mental Health Center, 1979–1983. *Phototherapy, 3*(4), 15–17.

Krauss, D. A. & Fryrear, J. L. (Eds.). (1983). *Phototherapy in mental health.* Springfield, IL: Charles Thomas.

Lambert, M. (1988). *Improving self-esteem through photo/videotherapy: A graduate project.* Unpublished manuscript, University of Houston at Clear Lake.

Landgarten, H. (1981). *Clinical art therapy: A comprehensive guide.* New York: Brunner/Mazel.

Landgarten, H. (1987). *Family art psychotherapy: A clinical guide and casebook.* New York: Brunner/Mazel.

Lankton, S. (1980). *Practical magic: A translation of basic neuro-linguistic programming into clinical psychotherapy.* Cupertino, CA: Meta Publications.

Lesy, M. (1976). Snapshots: Psychological documents, frozen dreams. *Afterimage, 4*(4), 12–13.

Lesy, M. (1980). *Time frames: The meaning of family pictures.* New York: Pantheon.

Levey, P. (1987). *Death of the Puella: Self-portrait photography.* New York: SoHo Gallery Exhibition Brochure.

Levey, P. (1988). *Self-portrait photography as a form of therapy with women.* Master's thesis, Antioch University.

Levey, P. (1989). Death of the Puella: Photography by Patti Levey. *Versus, 1*(2), 11–13.

Levey, P. (1991). The camera doesn't lie. In L. M. Wisechild (Ed.), *She who was lost is remembered: Healing from incest through creativity* (pp. 49–71). Seattle: Seal Press.

Levinson, R. (1979). Psychodynamically oriented phototherapy. *Phototherapy, 2*(2), 14–16.

Lipovenko, D. (1984, September 4). Photos shed light on emotions. *Globe and Mail: Science & Medicine,* p. 16.

Loellbach, M. (1978). *The uses of photographic materials in psychotherapy: A literature review.* Master's thesis, George Williams College.

Lusebrink, V. (1989). Art therapy and imagery in verbal therapy: A comparison of therapeutic characteristics. *American Journal of Art Therapy, 28*(1), 2–3.

McDougall-Treacy, G. (1979). The person-as-camera experience. *Phototherapy, 2*(2), 16–18.

Mann, L. (1983). *An album of albums: Phototherapy with schizophrenic adults.* Master's thesis, Lesley College Graduate School.

Marino, A. & Lambert, M. (1990). *Expressive Therapies Center: We make a difference for you and your family.* Houston: Expressive Therapies Center.

Martin, R. (1987). Phototherapy: The school photo (Happy days are here again). In P. Holland, J. Spence & S. Watney (Eds.), *Photography/Politics: Two* (pp. 40–42). London: Commedia/Photography Workshop.

Martin, R. (1990). The "pretended family" album. *Feminist Art News, 3*(5), 22–24.

Martin, R. (1991). Unwind the ties that bind. In J. Spence & P. Holland (Eds.), *Family snaps: Meanings of domestic photography* (pp. 209–221). London: Virago Press.

Martin, R. & Spence, J. (1985). New portraits for old: The use of the camera in therapy. *Feminist Review, 19,* 66–92.

Martin, R. & Spence, J. (1986). Photo therapy: New portraits for old, 1984 onwards. In J. Spence, *Putting myself in the picture: A political, personal, and photographic autobiography* (pp. 172–193). London: Camden Press.

Martin, R. & Spence, J. (1987). New portraits for old: The use of the camera in therapy. (Updated from 1985 article.) In R. Betterton (Ed.), *Looking on: Images of femininity in the visual arts and media* (pp. 267–279). London: Pandora.

Martin, R. & Spence, J. (1988). Phototherapy: Psychic realism as a healing art? *Ten:8, 30,* 2–10.

Medina, S. (1981, August 17). "See and tell" color photography. *Time,* pp. 34–35.

Morgan, W. (1974). Snapshot anniversary. *Popular Photography, 10*(28), 127.

Morganstern, C. (1980). In the mind of the beholder: "See and tell photography." *Lens On Campus,* 2(1), 8–10.

Muhl, A. M. (1927). Notes on the use of photography in checking up unconscious conflicts. *Psychoanalytic Review, 14,* 329–331.

Nath, J. (1981). *Phototherapy in the education of the mentally handicapped child.* Unpublished master's thesis, University of British Columbia, Department of Special Education.

Newberry, B. (1990). *Exhibition brochure.* Grants Pass, OR: Wiseman Gallery Publication.

Nierman, J. (1989). Creative healing for sexual abuse survivors (The art of recovery: Patti Levey). *Recovery, 12,* 9.

Nucho, A. O. (1988). *The psychocybernetic model of art therapy.* Springfield, IL: Charles Thomas.

Palmer, V. E. (1990, October 7). Arts program a form of treatment. Mesa, AZ: *Tribune,* p. 6.

Peck, L. (1990). *Photoexplorations and the family album.* Master's dissertation, Birmingham Polytechnic, School of Art.

Poli, K. (1979). Photoprobes. *Popular Photography, 85*(3), 91–94.

Probus, L. (1988). *The psychosocial consequences of AIDS.* Master's dissertation, University of Louisville: Department of Expressive Therapies.

Probus, L. (1989, November 18). Using art therapy in counseling the psychosocial issues of the AIDS patient. *Paper presented at the 20th Annual Conference of the American Art Therapy Association,* San Francisco.

Proudfoot, D. (1984, February 26). Phototherapy: Images can open a door to the unconscious. *Toronto Sun,* p. B-3.

Ray, G. (1990). Living with AIDS: Collaborative portraits. *Gallerie: Women Artists' Monographs, 1*(4).

Reid, M. (1985). My use of photographs in therapy. *Phototherapy, 4*(3), 10–12.

Rhyne, J. (1984). *The Gestalt art experience: Creative process and expressive therapy.* Chicago: Magnolia Street.

Rhyne, J. (1990). Gestalt psychology / Gestalt therapy: Forms / Contexts. *American Journal of Art Therapy, 29*(1), 2–8.

Riley, S. (1985). Draw me a paradox: Family art psychotherapy utilizing a systemic approach to change. *Art Therapy, 2*(3), 116–125.

Riley, S. (1988). Adolescence and family art therapy: Treating the "adolescent family" with family art therapy. *Art Therapy, 5*(2), 43–51.

Riley, S. (1990). A strategic family systems approach to art therapy with individuals. *American Journal of Art Therapy, 28*(3), 71–78.

Robotham, R. (1982, October). Camera at work: Pictures that unlock the psyche. *Life,* pp. 15–22.

Roskill, M. (1989). *The interpretation of pictures.* Amherst: University of Massachusetts Press.

Roskill, M. & Carrier, D. (1983). *Truth and falsehood in visual images.* Amherst: University of Massachusetts Press.

Rosner-David, I. & Sageman, S. (1987). Psychological aspects of AIDS as seen in art therapy. *American Journal of Art Therapy, 26*(1), 3–10.

Sevitt, C. (1983, May 4). Baycrest's photographers still in the picture. *Toronto Star,* p. B-3.

Sheehan, A. (1988). Here's looking at you, kid: What family photos reveal. *Child, 3*(6), 106–115.

Sherkin, S. (1989). Photo therapy: Ink blots of the '80s. *Photo Life, January/February,* 31–36.

Smith, M. (1989). *The use of photographic images as a therapeutic modality.* Unpublished manuscript, University of Louisville.

Smith, M. (1990). The use of photographic images as a therapeutic modality. *Student Art Therapy* (University of Louisville). *1 (Spring),* 4–5.

Sobol, B. (1982). Art therapy and strategic family therapy. *American Journal of Art Therapy, 21*(3), 43–52.

Sobol, B. (1985). Art therapy, behavior modification, and conduct disorder. *American Journal of Art Therapy, 24*(2), 35–43.

Spence, J. (1978). Facing up to myself. *Spare Rib, 68,* 6–9.

Spence, J. (1980). What did you do in the war, mummy? Class and gender in the images of women. In T. Dennett, D. Evans, S. Gohl & J. Spence (Eds.), *Photography/Politics: One* (pp. 2–10). London: Photography Workshop.

Spence, J. (1983). *War photos: The home front.* Unpublished thesis.

Spence, J. (1986). *Putting myself in the picture: A political, personal, and photographic autobiography.* London: Camden Press.

Spence, J. (1989). Disrupting the silence: The daughter's story. *Women Artists Slide Library Journal, 29* (June), 14–17.

Spence, J. (1991). Soap, family album work, and hope. In J. Spence & P. Holland (Eds.), *Family snaps: The meanings of domestic photography,* (pp. 20–27). London: Virago Press.

Stewart, D. (1978). *Photo projects manual.* Sycamore, IL: Photo Therapy Press.

Stewart, D. (1979a). Photo therapy comes of age. *Kansas Quarterly, 2*(4), 19–46.

Stewart, D. (1979b). Phototherapy: theory and practice. *Art Psychotherapy,* 6(1), 41–46.

Stewart, D. (1980). The use of client photographs as self statements in Photo Therapy (Doctoral dissertation, Northern Illinois University). *Dissertation Abstracts International, 8020*–780.

Tomaszewski, I. (1981, October 13). Getting a picture of the mind. *Vancouver Sun,* p. B-1.

Trusso, J. (1979). Some uses of instant photography in holistic therapy. *Phototherapy,* 2(1), 14–15.

Turner-Hogan, P. [*see also Hogan*]. (1980). *The use of photography as a social work technique.* Unpublished manuscript, San Jose State University.

Tyding, K. (1973). Instamatic therapy. *Human Behavior, February,* 30.

Walker, J. (1980). See and tell. *Phototherapy,* 2(3), 14–15.

Walker, J. (1982). The photograph as a catalyst in psychotherapy. *Canadian Journal of Psychiatry, 27,* 450–454.

Walker, J. (1983). The photograph as a catalyst in psychotherapy. In D. A. Krauss & J. L. Fryrear (Eds.), *Phototherapy in mental health* (pp. 135–150). Springfield, IL: Charles Thomas.

Walker, J. (1986). The use of ambiguous artistic images for enhancing self-awareness in psychotherapy. *Arts in Psychotherapy, 13*(3), 241–248.

Walker, J. & Cohen, P. (1984, May). *The creative elderly.* Paper presented at the International PhotoTherapy Symposium, Toronto.

Wallace, A. (1979). *The theory and practice of Photo Therapy.* Unpublished master's thesis, Lesley College Graduate School.

Watney, S. (1987). *Policing desire: Pornography, AIDS, and the media.* Minneapolis: University of Minnesota Press.

Weal, E. (1979). Photo psychology. *Innovations, 6*(3), 13–15.

Weiser, J. (1975). PhotoTherapy: Photography as a verb. *The B.C. Photographer, 2,* 33–36.

Weiser, J. (1983a). Using photographs in therapy with people who are "different." In D. A. Krauss & J. L. Fryrear (Eds.), *Phototherapy in mental health* (pp. 174–199). Springfield, IL: Charles Thomas.

Weiser, J. (1983b). Using PhotoTherapy to help: A study of Debbie. *Montage: Kodak's Educator's Newsletter, 83*(1), 4–5.

Weiser, J. (1984a). PhotoTherapy: Becoming visually literate about oneself. In A. D. Walker, R. A. Braden & L. H. Dunker (Eds.), *Visual literacy: Enhancing human potential* (pp. 392–406). Blacksburg: Virginia Polytechnic State University Press.

Weiser, J. (1984b). PhotoTherapy: Becoming visually literate about oneself, or, "Phototherapy? What's phototherapy??" *Phototherapy, 4*(2), 2–7.

Weiser, J. (1984c). Brief field reports: Using PhotoTherapy to help—A study of Debbie. *Phototherapy, 4*(2), 8–9.

Weiser, J. (1985). Training and teaching photo and video therapy: Central themes, core knowledge, and important considerations. *Phototherapy, 4*(4), 9–16.

Weiser, J. (1986a). Ethical considerations in PhotoTherapy training and practice. *Phototherapy, 5*(1), 12–17.

Weiser, J. (1986b). Ethical considerations in PhotoTherapy training and practice. *Video-Informationen, 9*(2), 5–10.

Weiser, J. (1988a). "See what I mean?" Photography as nonverbal communication in cross-cultural psychology. In F. Poyatos (Ed.), *Cross-cultural perspectives in nonverbal communication* (pp. 245–290). Toronto: Hogrefe.

Weiser, J. (1988b). PhotoTherapy: Using snapshots and photo-interactions in therapy with youth. In C. Schaefer (Ed.), *Innovative interventions in child and adolescent therapy* (pp. 339–376). New York: Wiley.

Weiser, J. (1989). *Getting a better picture—family systems therapy using family snapshots and albums.* Unpublished paper presented at the 20th Annual Conference of the Art Therapy Association, San Francisco, Nov. 18.

Weiser, J. (1990). "More than meets the eye": Using ordinary snapshots as tools for therapy. In T. Laidlaw, C. Malmo & Associates (Eds.), *Healing voices: Feminist approaches to therapy with women* (pp. 83–117). San Francisco: Jossey-Bass.

Wilcox, M. E. (1990). The secret lives of snapshots: Photo albums can unlock a wealth of information about you and your family. *Canadian Living, November,* 115–121.

Williams, D. (1987). *PhotoTherapy: Humanistic helping.* Unpublished master's thesis, West Georgia College.

Wolf, R. I. (1976). The Polaroid technique: Spontaneous dialogues from the unconscious. *International Journal of Art Psychotherapy, 3*(3), 197–201.

Wolf, R. I. (1977). The use of instant photography in the establishment of a therapeutic alliance. *Convention Program,* American Art Therapy Association, 20–22.

Wolf, R. I. (1978). The use of instant photography in creative expressive therapy: An integrative case study. *Art Psychotherapy, 5:1,* 81–91.

Wolf, R. I. (1982). Instant Phototherapy: Some theoretical and clinical considerations for its use in psychotherapy and in special education. *Phototherapy, 3*(1), 3–6.

Wolf, R. I. (1983). Instant Phototherapy with children and adolescents. In D. A. Krauss & J. L. Fryrear (Eds.), *Phototherapy in mental health* (pp. 151–174). Springfield, IL: Charles Thomas.

Wolf, R. I. (1990). Visceral learning: The integration of aesthetic and creative process in education and psychotherapy. *Art Therapy, 7*(2), 60–69.

Yankovich, S. (1990). PhotoTherapy groups with persons with AIDS. *Personal communication.* Calgary.

Zabar, S. (1987). Photo-expressive activities in the health care environment. *Phototherapy, 6*(1), 2–6.

Zakem, B. (1977a). Phototherapy: A developing psychotherapeutic approach. Unpublished manuscript. Chicago: Ravenswood Community Mental Health Center.

Zakem, B. (1977b). Newsline: Photographs help patients focus on their problems. *Psychology Today, 11*(4), 22.

Zakem, B. (1983). Phototherapy intervention: Developing a comprehensive system. In D. A. Krauss & J. L. Fryrear (Eds.), *Phototherapy in mental health* (pp. 201–210). Springfield, IL: Charles Thomas.

Zakem, B. (1984). Bringing images to mind. *World book science year* (offprint), 100–113.

Zakem, B. (1990). *An exploratory study using a still photographic project as a humanistic broad focus psychosocial clinical assessment tool.* Doctoral dissertation, The Fielding Institute.

Ziller, R. C. (1989). Orientations: The cognitive link in person-situation interaction. *Journal of Social Behavior and Personality, 3*(1), 1–9.

Ziller, R. C. (1990) *Photographing the self: Methods for observing personal orientations.* Newbury Park, CA: Sage.

Ziller, R. C. & Lewis, D. (1981). Self, social, and environmental percepts through auto-photography. *Personality and Social Psychology Bulletin, 7,* 338–343.

Ziller, R. C., Rorer, B., Combs, J. & Lewis, D. (1983). The psychological niche: The auto-photographic study of self-environment interaction. In D. A. Krauss & J. L. Fryrear (Eds.), *Phototherapy in mental health* (pp. 95–115). Springfield, IL: Charles Thomas.

Ziller, R. C., Vera, H. & Camacho de Santoya, C. (1981). Frederico: Understanding a child through auto-photography. *Childhood Education, 57*(5), 271–275.

Recommended Readings

Adamson, E. (1984). *Art as healing.* London: Coventure Press.

Ammerman, M. S. & Fryrear, J. L. (1975). Photographic enhancement of children's self-esteem. *Psychology in the Schools, 12*(3), 319–325.

Appel, A., Jr. (1983). *Signs of life.* New York: Knopf.

Arnheim, R. (1966). *Toward a psychology of art.* Berkeley: University of California Press.

Arnheim, R. (1969). *Visual thinking.* Berkeley: University of California Press.

Arnheim, R. (1974). On the nature of photography. *Critical Inquiry, 1*(September), 149–161.

Arnheim, R. (1986a). *New essays on the psychology of art.* Berkeley: University of California Press.

Arnheim, R. (1986b). The two faces of Gestalt psychology. American Psychologist, 41(7), 820–824.

Arnheim, R. (1988). *The power of the center: A study of the composition in the visual arts.* Berkeley: University of California Press.

Aronson, D. W. & Graziano, A. (1976). Improving elderly clients' attitudes through photography. *The Gerontologist, 16,* 259–264.

Bacher, F. (1977). *Tension: A book about family relationships.* Rochester: Visual Studies Workshop Press.

Barkan, J. L. (1978). Candid camera renews zest for life. *Innovations, Spring,* 37–38.

Barthes, R. (1957). *Mythologies.* New York: Hill & Wang.

Barthes, R. (1981). *Camera lucida: Reflections on photography.* (Richard Howard, Trans.). New York: Hill and Wang.

Becker, H. S. (1974). Photography and sociology. *Studies in the Anthropology of Visual Communication, 1*(1), 3–26.

Becker, H. S. (1981). *Exploring society photographically.* Chicago: University of Chicago Press.

Belloff, H. (1985). *Camera culture.* New York: Basil Blackwell.

Berger, J. (1972). *Ways of seeing.* New York: Penguin.

Berger, J. (1980). *About looking.* New York: Pantheon.

Berger, J. & Mohr, J. (1982). *Another way of telling.* New York: Pantheon.

Berner, J. (1975). *The photographic experience: Awakening vision through conscious camerawork.* New York: Anchor Press.

Bernhardt, A. J., & Gilman, S. L. (1987). The depiction of the insane and some clinical implications. *Phototherapy,* 6(2), 4–14.

Betensky, M. (1977). The phenomenological approach to art expression and art therapy. *The Arts in Psychotherapy,* 4(2), 173–179.

Betterton, R. (Ed.) (1987). *Looking on: Images of femininity in the visual arts and media.* London: Pandora.

Birenbaum, R. (1980, October 7). Pictures of stillborn help ease postpartum grief. *Medical Post,* p. 25.

Blinn, L. M. (1986, June). Japanese family photos: Propositions about family identity. *Conference Program,* Fourth International Conference on Visual Sociology/Anthropology.

Blinn, L. M. (1987). Phototherapeutic intervention to improve self-concept and prevent repeat pregnancies among adolescents. *Family Relations, 36,* 252–257.

Bodner, B. A. (1975). The eye of the beholder: Photography for deaf preschoolers. *Teaching Exceptional Children, Fall,* 18–23.

Bolen, J. S. (1979). *The Tao of psychology: Synchronicity and the self.* San Francisco: Harper & Row.

Bowen, M. (1972). Toward the differentiation of a self in one's own family. In J. Framo (Ed.), *Family interaction: A dialogue between family researchers and family therapists.* New York: Springer.

Bowen, M. (1978). *Family therapy in clinical practice.* New York: Jason Aronson.

Braden, S. (1983). *Committing photography.* London: Pluto Press.

Brookman, P. (Ed). (1990). Shooting back: Photographs by and about the homeless. *Curatorial Booklet,* Washington Project for the Arts Exhibition.

Brunswick, E. (1945). Social perception of traits from photographs. *Psychological Bulletin, 42,* 535–536.

Bunnell, P. (1972). Taken from life. In D. P. Vanderlip (Ed.), *Photographic Portraits.* Philadelphia: Moore College of Art.

Burt, B., Ball, K. & Malchiodi, C. (1989, November) *Reminiscence and life review using art therapy with the elderly.* Paper presented at the 20th Annual Conference of the American Art Therapy Association, San Francisco.

Butler, R. (1963). The life review: An interpretation of reminiscence in the aged. *Psychiatry, 26,* 65–76.

Byers, P. (1964). Cameras don't take pictures. *Columbia University Forum,* 9(1), 27–32.

Cameron, J. R. & Plattor, E. E. (1971). *The leaf not the tree—Creative workshop two: Working with words, photographs, and tape recordings.* Toronto: Gage Educational.

Campbell, D. T. & Burwen, L. S. (1956). Trait judgments from photographs as a projective device. *Journal of Clinical Psychology, 12,* 215–221.

Campbell, J. (1972). *The masks of god: Primitive mythology.* New York: Viking.

Canfield, J. & Wells, H. C. (1976). *100 ways to enhance self-esteem in the classroom: A handbook for teachers and parents.* Englewood Cliffs, NJ: Prentice-Hall.

Chalfen, R. (1974a). Review of Akeret's "Photoanalysis." *Studies in Visual Communication, 5,* 57–59.

Chalfen, R. (1974b). *Seven billion a year: The social construction of the snapshot.* Unpublished manuscript.

Chalfen, R. (1975). Cinema naivete: A study of home moviemaking as visual communication. *Studies in Visual Communication,* 2(1), 47–54.

Chalfen, R. (1987). *Snapshot versions of life.* Bowling Green: Popular Press.

Cimons, M. (1978, November 6). Photos introduce the world: Helping a blind man see. *Los Angeles Times,* pp. 1, 4.

Close-Holden, S. & Crooks, R. (1988, February 19). *Communication through photography: A bridge to literacy.* Paper presented to the Ottawa Board of Education Media Center.

Coe, B. & Gates, P. (1977). *The snapshot photography: The rise of popular photography 1888–1939.* London: Ash and Grant.

Collier, J., Jr. & Collier, M. (1986). *Visual anthropology: Photography as a research method.* Albuquerque: University of New Mexico Press.

Corbit, I. E. & Fryrear, J. L. (1985). Visual transitions: Metaphor for change. *Phototherapy, 4*(3), 5–9.

Cornelison, F. S. & Arsenian, J. (1960). A study of the response of psychotic patients to photographic self-image experience. *Psychiatric Quarterly, 34,* 1–8.

Craven, G. M. (1975). *Object and image.* Englewood Cliffs, NJ: Prentice-Hall.

Crean, S. (1989). The female gaze—Women's bodies, women's selves: Reclaiming an artistic identity. *Canadian Art, Summer,* 21–22.

Danet, R. B. (1968). Self-confrontation in psychotherapy reviewed. *American Journal of Psychotherapy, 22,* 245–258.

Darrow, N. R. & Lynch, M. T. (1983). The use of photography activities with adolescent groups. *Social Work with Groups, 11*(A), 43.

Davis, P. (1986, June). The man who undressed men (Bruce Weber). *Esquire,* pp. 338–347.

deBono, E. (1970) *Lateral thinking: A textbook of creativity.* New York: Penguin.

deBono, E. (1973). *Po: Beyond yes and no.* New York: Penguin Books.

Dennett, T., Evans, D., Gohl, S. & Spence, J. (Eds.). (1979). *Photography/Politics: One.* London: Photography Workshop.

Devenyi, D. (1980, September). Photographer's eye: The perception machine. *Photo Life,* pp. 28–29.

Diamond, H. (1976). On the application of photography to the physiognomic and mental phenomena of insanity. In S. Gilman, (Ed.), *The face of madness: Hugh W. Diamond and the origin of psychiatric photography.* Secaucus, NJ: Citadel Press. (Original work read before the Royal Society, May 22, 1856).

Dinklage, R. I. & Ziller, R. C. (1989). Explicating cognitive conflict through photo-communication: Images of war and peace among German and American children. *Journal of Conflict Resolution, 33*(2), 309–317.

Dondis, D. A. (1973). *A primer of visual literacy.* Cambridge, MA: MIT Press.

English, R. W. & Palla, D. A. (1971). Attitudes toward a photograph of a mildly and a severely mentally retarded child. *Training School Bulletin (VINEL), 68*(1), 55–63.

Entin, A. D. (1982). Family albums: Icons of the family. *Phototherapy, 3*(1), 7–10.

Evans, C. (1992). *Photoworks.* Toronto: Lugus Productions.

Evans, G. S., Fryrear, J. L. & Corbit, I. E. (1989). Visual transitions as therapy. *Art Therapy,* 6(2), 57–66.

Ewald, W. (1983, May). A testimony to love: Touching words and pictures from the children of Appalachia, where hardship is a way of life. *Psychology Today,* pp. 52–54.

Ewald, W. (1985). *Portraits and dreams: Photographs and stories by children of the Appalachians.* London: Writers and Readers Publishing.

Fischer, J. (1961). Art styles as cultural cognitive maps. *American Anthropologist, 63,* 79–93.

Foley, V. D. (1974). *An introduction to family therapy.* New York: Grune & Stratton.

Forbes, R. (1979). *Click: A first camera book.* New York: Macmillan.

Fordham, F. (1953). *An introduction to Jung's psychology.* New York: Penguin.

Fox, H. M. (1957). Body image of a photographer. *Journal of the American Psychoanalytical Association, 5,* 93–107.

Freund, G. (1980). *Photography and society.* Boston: Godine.

Frieze, I. H. & Ramsey, S. J. (1976). Nonverbal maintenance of traditional sex roles. *Journal of Social Issues, 32*(3), 133–141.

Fryrear, J. L., Kodera, T. L. & Kennedy, M. J. (1981). Self-recognition ability in mentally retarded adolescents. *The Journal of Psychology, 108,* 123–131.

Fryrear, J. L., Nuell, L. R. & Ridley, S. D. (1974). Photographic self-concept enhancement of male juvenile delinquents. *Journal of Consulting and Clinical Psychology, 42*(6), 915.

Fryrear, J. L., Nuell, L. R. & White, P. (1977). Enhancement of male juvenile delinquents' self concepts through photographed social interactions. *Journal of Clinical Psychology, 33*(3), 833–838.

Fryrear, J. L. & Stephens, B. C. (1988). Group psychotherapy using masks and video to facilitate intrapersonal communication. *The Arts in Psychotherapy, 15*(3), 227–234.

Galassi, P. (Ed.). (1981). *Before photography: Painting and the invention of photography.* New York: New York Graphic Society.

Gallagher, P. A. (1983). Social skills and photography: A unit of study for adolescents with behavior problems. *The Pointer (for all Educators and Parents of Exceptional Children), 27*(3), 42–45.

Gardiner, H. (1982). *Art, mind, and brain: A cognitive approach to creativity.* New York: Basic Books.

Garner, G. (1977). A psychologist observes photography: An interview of Dr. Stanley Milgram. *Camera 35, 21*(8), 26–28, 62, 64.

Gassan, A. (1972). *A chronology of photography.* Athens, OH: Handbook Co.

Gassan, A. (1979). The documentary dilemma. *Kansas Quarterly, 11*(4), 125–130.

Gassan, A. (1986). *Summary report on father-daughter incest research using photographs and the Semantic Differential.* Athens, OH: A. Gassan.

Gasswint, C. D. (1968). Changes in self-concept as a function of immediate self-image confrontation. (Doctoral dissertation, University of Oklahoma). *Dissertation Abstracts International: 29.* (University Microfilms No. 1839-B)

Gerace, L. (1979) The use of family photographs as a communications process: A summary. *Phototherapy, 2*(1), 7–8.

Gersheim, H. (1965). *A concise history of photography.* New York: Grosset & Dunlap.

Gill, N. T. & Messina, R. (1973). Visual self-confrontation and the self-concept of the exceptional child. *Florida Journal of Educational Research, 15,* 18–36.

Gilligan, C. (1982). *In a different voice: Psychological theory and women's development.* Cambridge, MA: Harvard University Press.

Gilman, S. (1976). *The face of madness.* Secaucus, NJ: Citadel Press.

Gilman, S. (Ed.) (1982). *Seeing the insane.* New York: Brunner/Mazel.

Goffman, E. (1976). Gender advertisements. *Studies in the Anthropology of Visual Communication, 3*(2), 37–41.

Goldman, J. (1976, June 28). The camera confronts death. *Village Voice,* p. 120.

Gombrich, E. H., Hochberg, J. & Black, M. (1972). *Art, perception, and reality.* Baltimore: Johns Hopkins University Press.

Gordon, L. (1987, May 15). Art used as therapy by cancer patients. *Los Angeles Times,* pp. 18–19.

Green, J. (Ed.). (1974). *The snapshot.* New York: Aperture.

Gregory, R. L. (1966). *Eye and brain: The psychology of seeing.* New York: World University Library.

Griffith, J., Miner, L. & Strandberg, T. (1975). *Classroom projects using photography. Part one: For the elementary school level.* Rochester, NY: Eastman Kodak.

Grover, J. Z. (1988). Beyond the family album: The autobiography of Jo Spence. *Afterimage,* Feb. 8–10.

Grover, J. Z. (1990). Photo therapy: Shame and the minefields of memory. *Afterimage, 18*(1), 14–18.

Grundberg, A. & McCarthy-Gauss, K. (1987). *Photography and art: Interactions since 1946.* New York: Abbeville Press.

Güenther-Thoma, K. (1984, May 18). *Photo groups in a German prison for women.* Paper presented at the International PhotoTherapy Symposium, Toronto.

Güenther-Thoma, K. (1987). Emotional and sensory experiences with photography. *Phototherapy, 6*(2), 25–26.

Güenther-Thoma, K. & Katz, H. (1986). *Fotografie hinter gittern* [Photography behind bars]. Frankfurt: Dezernat Schule und Bildung.

Guerin, P. (Ed.). (1976). *Family therapy: Theory and practice.* New York: Gardner.

Gutman, J. M. (1982). *Through Indian eyes: 19th and early 20th century photography from India.* New York: Oxford University Press and International Center for Photography.

Haber, R. N. & Hershenson, M. (1973). *The psychology of visual perception.* Troy, Mo.: Holt, Rinehart & Winston.

Haley, J. (Ed.) (1967). *Advanced techniques of hypnosis and therapy: The selected papers of Milton H. Erickson, M.D.* New York: Grune & Stratton.

Haley, J. (1973). *Uncommon therapy: The psychiatric techniques of Milton H. Erickson, M.D.* New York: Norton.

Hall, E. T. (1969). *The hidden dimension.* Garden City, NY: Doubleday Anchor.

Hall, E. T. (1976, July). How cultures collide. *Psychology Today,* pp. 66–74, 97.

Hall, E. T. (1977). *Beyond culture.* Garden City, NY: Doubleday Anchor.

Hall, E. T. (1984). *The dance of life.* Garden City, NY: Doubleday Anchor.

Hall, J. A. (1983). *Jungian dream interpretation.* Toronto: Inner City Books.

Hare-Mustin, R. T. & Marecek, J. (1988). The meaning of difference: Gender theory, postmodernism, and psychology. *American Psychologist, 43*(6), 455–464.

Hattersley, R. (1971). *Discover yourself through photography.* New York: Association Press.

Hattersley, R. (1980, February). Thirty ways photography is good for you. *Popular Photography,* pp. 87–127.

Hazen, B. S. (1971). *Happy, sad, silly, mad: A beginning book about emotions.* New York: Grosset & Dunlap.

Hedges, R. E. (1975). Photography and self-concept. *Audiovisual Instruction, 17*(5), 27–28.

Hedges, R. E., Nicoletti, D. J. & Tydings, K. (1972). *Self-directed children's photography.* New York: Photo-Lix.

Henley, N. M. (1977). *Body politics: Power, sex, and nonverbal communication.* Englewood Cliffs, NJ: Prentice-Hall.

Hevey, D. (1989). Liberty, equality, disability. *Ten:8, 35,* 2–15.

Hiley, M. (1983). *Seeing through photographs.* London: Gordon Fraser.

Hillman, J. (1981). *Archetypal psychology: A brief account.* Dallas: Spring Publications.

Hirsch, J. (1981). *Family photographs: Content, meaning, and effect.* New York: Oxford University Press.

Hoffman, M. (Ed.). (1978). *Minor White: Rites and passages.* Millerton, NY: Aperture.

Hogan, P. T. (1981). The uses of group PhotoTherapy in the classroom. *Phototherapy,* 2(4), 13.

Holland, P., Spence, J. & Watney, S. (1987). *Photography/Politics: Two.* London: Commedia Publishing Group and Photography Workshop.

Holzman, P. S. (1969). On hearing and seeing oneself. *Journal of Nervous and Mental Disease, 148*(3), 198–209.

Hunsberger, P. (1973). *Collaboration: A new approach to photography.* Unpublished manuscript.

Hunsberger, P. (1979). A self-led activity group within a day treatment program for chronic mental patients. Unpublished manuscript, Boston University.

Hunsberger, P. (1984). Uses of instant-print photography in psychotherapy. *Professional Psychology: Research and Practice, 15*(6), 884–890.

Husband, R. W. (1934). The photograph on the application blank. *Personnel Journal, 13,* 69–72.

Isherwood, S. (1988). *The family album: A workbook to accompany the Channel 4 program "Opening up the Family Album."* London: Broadcasting Support Services.

Jacobi, J. (1973). *The psychology of C. G. Jung.* New Haven: Yale University Press.

Johnson, B. & Entin, A. D. (1985). The family as subject: Photographs by Emmet Gowin and David Levinson. *Exhibition Catalogue,* Richmond, VA: Chrysler Museum.

Johnson, D. R. (1987). The role of the creative arts therapies in the diagnosis and treatment of psychological trauma. *The Arts and Psychotherapy, 14*(1), 7–13.

Jung, C. (1952). *Symbols of transformation.* New York: Bollingen Foundation.

Jung, C. (1964). *Man and his symbols.* New York: Dell.

Jung, C. (1969). *The archetypes and the collective unconscious.* Princeton: Princeton University Press.

Jury, M. & Jury, D. (1976). *Gramp: The extraordinary record of one family's encounter with the reality of dying.* New York: Penguin.

Kaslow, F. W. (1979). What personal photos reveal about marital sex conflicts. *Journal of Marital and Sex Therapy, 5*(2), 34–141.

Kempler, B. (1987). The shadow side of self-disclosure. *Journal of Humanistic Psychology, 27*(1), 109–117.

Kent, S. & Morreau, J. (1985). *Women's images of men.* London: Writers and Readers Publishing.

Kepes, G. (Ed.). (1966). *Sign, image, symbol.* New York: George Braziller.

Kiell, N. (1965). *Psychiatry and psychology in the visual arts and aesthetics: A bibliography.* Madison: University of Wisconsin Press.

Kimelman, M., Tomkiewicz, S. & Maffioli, B. (1983). Le photodrame en institution psychiatrique: Reflexions sur l'image corporelle [The photodrama in the psychiatric institution: Reflections on the corporal image). *L'Evolution Psychiatrique, 48*(1), 73–109.

King, G. (1984). *Say "Cheese": Looking at snapshots in a new way.* New York: Dodd Mead.

Kotkin, A. (1978). The family photo album as a form of folklore. *Exposure, 16*(1), 4–8.

Kozloff, M. (1974). The territory of photographs. *Artforum, 13*(3), 64–67.

Krauss, D. A. (1980). A summary of characteristics of photographs which make them useful in counseling and therapy. *Camera Lucida, 1*(2), 7–12.

Krauss, D. A. (1981). Photography, imaging, and visually referent language in therapy: Illuminating the metaphor. *Camera Lucida, 1*(5), 58–63.

Lafferty, T. (1981). *The use of the photograph in art therapy. Unpublished master's thesis,* New York University.

Laidlaw, T., Malmo, C. & Associates (Eds.). (1990). *Healing voices: Feminist approaches to therapy with women.* San Francisco: Jossey-Bass.

Langsan, N., Levinson, R. & Teller, A. (1975). *Photography in the classroom: A workbook.* Chicago: Illinois Arts Council.

Larson, S. (1982). Photography for adolescent E.D. students. Unpublished manuscript, University of Kansas.

Laughlin, S. (1981). *Family histories: approaches to the past—A handbook of workshops and projects for youth.* Spencer, IN: Stone Hills Area Library Services Authority Publication.

Lesser, R. & Margello, A. (1970). Instant color photography for teaching deaf children. *Medical Biology Illustrated, 20*(2), 95–99.

Levine, S. K. (1988). Image abuse and the dialectic of interpretation. *The Canadian Art Therapy Association Journal, 3*(2), 18–26.

Lewis, M. I. & Butler, R. N. (1974). Life review therapy: putting memories to work in individual and group psychotherapy. *Geriatrics, 29,* 165–173.

Lindley, D. A., Jr. (1979). Photography and the way of the self. *Kansas Quarterly, 2*(4), 11–17.

Lofgren, D. E. (1981). Art therapy and cultural difference. *American Journal of Art Therapy, 21,* 25–30.

Lucie-Smith, E. (1984). *Movements in art since 1945.* London: Thames & Hudson.

Lyons, N. (Ed.). (1966). *Photographers on photography.* Englewood Cliffs, NJ: Prentice-Hall.

Malcolm, J. (1980). *Diana and Nikon: Essays on the aesthetic of photography.* Boston: Godine.

Maluta, B. & Hutton, J. (1983). *The Calgary "Alternatives Centre" program.* Unpublished manuscript, Cambyr Counseling Agencies, Calgary, Alberta.

Mann, S. (1988). *At twelve: Portraits of young women.* New York: Aperture.

Martin, R. (1990a). Dirty linen: Photo therapy, memory, and identity. *Ten:8, 37,* 1–10.

Martin, R. (1990b). How does the lesbian gaze. *Outlook, Autumn/ Winter,* 12–16.

Martin, R. (1991). Don't say 'Cheese', say 'Lesbian'. In J. Fraser & T. Boffin (Eds.), *Stolen Glances: Lesbians Take Photographs* (pp. 95–105). London: Pandora.

Martin, R. & Spence, J. (1987). *Double exposure: The minefield of memory (The school photo revisited)*. London: Photographers Gallery (Photographs in Context Monograph No. 5).

McConeghey, H. (1986). Archetypal art therapy is cross-cultural art therapy. *Art Therapy, 3*(3), 111–114.

McGoldrick, M., Anderson, C. M. & Walsh, F. (Eds.). (1989). *Women in families: A framework for family therapy.* New York: Norton.

McIsaac, M. S. (981). Student produced photographs: Bridging the gap between language and aesthetics. *Camera Lucida, 4,* 3–9.

McKim, R. H. (1972). *Experiences in visual thinking.* Pacific Grove, CA: Brooks/Cole.

McKinney, J. P. (1979). Photo counseling. *Children Today, 8*(1), 29.

McKinney, J. P., Seagull, A. & Turner, K. (1979). Fostering emotional growth through photography. *Academic Psychology Bulletin, 1* (1), 69–71.

McNiff, S. (1987). The interpretation of imagery. *Canadian Art Therapy Association Journal, 3*(1), 8–16.

McNiff, S. (1988). The shaman within. *The Arts and Psychotherapy, 15*(4), 285–291.

McNiff, S. (1989). *Depth psychology of art.* Springfield, IL: Charles Thomas.

Meer, B. & Amon, A. (1963). Photo preference test (PPT) as a measure of mental status for hospitalized psychiatric patients. *Journal of Consulting Psychology, 27*(4), 283–293.

Mehrabian, A. (1981). *Silent messages: Implicit communication of emotions and attitudes.* Belmont, CA: Wadsworth.

Meiselas, S. (1974). *Learn to see: A sourcebook of photography projects by teachers and students.* Cambridge, MA: Polaroid Corporation.

Metz, C. (1980). The perceived and the named. *Studies in Visual Communication, 6*(3), 56–68.

Metz, C. (1981). Perception and photography. *Camera Lucida, 1*(3), 5–19.

Milford, S., Fryrear, J. L. & Swank, P. (1983). Phototherapy with disadvantaged boys. *Arts in Psychotherapy, 10*(4), 221–229.

Milford, S., Swank, P. & Fryrear, J. L. (1981). *Enhancement of self-esteem, social skills, and grooming in institutionalized adolescent boys through photography.* Unpublished manuscript, University of Houston at Clear Lake.

Milgram, S. (1977, January). The image-freezing machine. *Psychology Today,* pp. 50–54, 108.

Milgram, S. & Banish, R. (1977, January). City families (Frozen on film). *Psychology Today,* pp. 59–65.

Miller, J. R. & Erb, L. (1978). Atlanta's Georgia-Hill photography club. *Phototherapy, 1*(4), 2–4.

Miller, M. F. (1962). Responses of psychiatric patients to their photographed images. *Diseases of the Nervous System, 23*(1), 296–298.

Mills, J. L. (1982, November 19). *Men and women speak different body language.* Paper presented to the International Visual Literacy Association, Vancouver.

Minton, C. (1983). Uses of photographs in perinatal social work. *Health and Social Work, 8*(2), 123–125.

Musello, C. (1979). Family photography. In J. Wagner (Ed.), *Images of information: Still photography in the social sciences* (pp. 101–118). Beverly Hills, CA: Sage.

Musello, C. (1980). Studying the home mode: An exploration of family photography and visual communication. *Studies in Visual Communication,* 6(1), 24–41.

Naiman, D. L. (1977). Picture perfect: Photography aids deaf children in developing communication skills. *Teaching Exceptional Children,* 9(2), 36–38.

Naitove, C. (1980). Arts therapy with sexually abused children. In S. M. Sgroi (Ed.), *Handbook of clinical intervention in child sexual abuse* (pp. 269–308). Boston: Lexington.

Nath, J. (1979). Ronnie and the magic of photography. *B.C. Teachèr, 1,* 112–114.

Nath, J. (1983). Phototherapy and self-esteem. *B.C. Teachers' Federation Newsletter,* 4–5.

Nath, J. (1984). The use of still photography as learning assistance for the language handicapped in the classroom. *Phototherapy,* 4(1), 15–17.

Nathan, D. J. (1978). The use of self-confrontation through photography or videotape as a therapeutic method for changing self image and aiding weight maintenance in formerly obese adults (Doctoral dissertation, University of Miami). *Dissertation Abstracts International, 39:11,* 6659A.

Nelson-Gee. E. (1975). Learning to be: A look into the use of therapy with Polaroid photography as a means of recreating the development of perception and the ego. *Art Psychotherapy, 2,* 159–164.

Newhall, B. (1978). *The history of photography.* New York: New York Graphics Society.

Nicoletti, D. J. (1971). An investigation into the effects of a self-directed photography experience upon the self-concept of fourth grade students. (Doctoral dissertation, Syracuse University.) *Dissertation Abstracts International, 32:11-A.* (University Microfilms No. 6213)

Norfleet, B. (1988). Studio photographers and two generations of baby raising. *Photo Communique, 10*(1), 14–23.

Okura, Y., Ziller, R. C. & Osawa, H. (1986). The psychological niche of older Japanese and Americans through auto-photography: Aging and the search for peace. *The International Journal of Aging and Human Development,* 22(4), 247–259.

Oudejans, M. (1986). Drawing with light: The effects of photographic techniques on society. *Journal of Visual Verbal Languaging, Spring,* 55–62.

Parker, R. & Pollock, G. (Eds.). (1987). *Framing feminism: Art and the women's movement, 1970–1985.* London: Pandora.

Patterson, F. (1979). *Photography and the art of seeing.* Toronto: Van Nostrand Reinhold.

Perls, F. S. (1969). *Gestalt therapy verbatim.* Moab, Utah: Real People Press.

Perls, F. S. (1973). *The Gestalt approach: Eye witness to therapy.* Palo Alto, CA: Science and Behavior Books.

Phillips, D. (1986). Photography's use as a metaphor of self with stabilized schizophrenic patients. *Arts in Psychotherapy, 13*(1), 9–16.

Platt, L. A. (1984). Experience exchange: Photography project gives old and young new perspective. *Aging, 34*(6), 30.

Pollock, G. (1990). *Vision and difference: Femininity, feminism, and histories of art.* London: Routledge.

Polster, E. & Polster, M. (1973). *Gestal therapy integrated.* New York: Brunner/Mazel.

Poyatos, F. (1983). *New perspectives in nonverbal communication: Studies in cultural anthropology, social psychology, linguistics, literature, and semiotics.* New York: Pergamon.

Poyatos, F. (Ed.). (1988). *Cross-cultural perspectives in nonverbal communication.* Toronto: Hogrefe.

Pribram, K. (1971). *Languages of the Brain.* Englewood Cliffs, NJ: Prentice-Hall.

Propp, D. (1974). *Awareness through photography.* Vancouver, BC: S/S/P Publications.

Ragan, J. (1982). Gender displays in portrait photographs. *Sex Roles, 8*(1), 33–43.

Ritchin, F. (1990). *In our own image: The coming revolution in photography—How computer technology is changing our view of the world.* New York: Aperture.

Robins, L. L. (1942). Photography. *Bulletin of the Menninger Clinic,* 6(3), 89–91.

Rosenblum, B. (1978). *Photographers at work: A sociology of photographic styles.* New York: Holmes & Meier.

Routh, R. (1977, May). *Photography as therapy.* Paper presented to International Visual Literacy Association Annual Convention, Los Angeles.

Ruben, A. G. (1978). The family picture. *Journal of Marriage and Family Counseling, 4*(3), 25–27.

Ruby, J. (1976). In a pic's eye: Interpretive strategies for deriving significance and meaning from photographs. *Afterimage, 3*(9), 5–7.

Ruby, J. (1981). Seeing through pictures: The anthropology of photography. *Camera Lucida, 1*(3), 19–32.

Ruby, J. (1982a). Images of the family: The symbolic implications of animal photography. *Phototherapy, 3*(2), 2–7.

Ruby, J. (1982b). An anthropologist looks at photography in Juniata County, Pa. *Photographica, 14*(3), 5–7.

Ruby, J. (1984a). Postmortem portraiture in America. *History of Photography, 8*(3), 201–222.

Ruby, J. (1984b). Photographic view companies: The camera leaves the studio. *Pennsylvania Heritage, 10*(4), 26–31.

Ruby, J. (1987, June). *Photographs, memory, and grief.* Paper presented at the Foundation of Thanatology Conference, Columbia-Presbyterian Medical Center, New York.

Samples, B. (1980). *The metaphoric mind: A celebration of creative consciousness.* Reading, MA: Addison-Wesley.

Samuels, M. & Samuels, N. (1975). *Seeing with the mind's eye.* New York: Random House.

Sandel, S. L. & Johnson, D. R. (1987). *Waiting at the gate: Creativity and hope in the nursing home.* New York & London: Haworth Press.

Satir, V. (1972). *Peoplemaking.* Palo Alto, CA: Science & Behavior Books.

Scalingi, V. (1988). Feature: Focus on photography. *A Positive Approach, September/October,* 18–19.

Scharf, A. (1975). *Art and Photography.* Baltimore: Penguin.

Scheflin, A. E. (1972). *Body language and social order: Communication as behavioral control.* Englewood Cliffs, NJ: Prentice-Hall.

Schudson, K. R. (1975). The simple camera in school counseling. *Personnel and Guidance Journal, 54*(4), 225–226.

Schwarz, H. (1985). *Art and Photography: Forerunners and Influences.* Rochester: Visual Studies Workshop.

Searle, L. (1979). Language theory and photographic praxis. *Afterimage, Summer,* 26–34.

Sedgwick, R. (1980). The use of photoanalysis and family memorabilia in the study of family interaction. *Corrective and Social Psychiatry Journal, 25*(4), 137–141.

Segal, R. (1984). Symbolic and metaphoric communication and phototherapy. *Phototherapy, 4*(1), 7–14.

Segall, M. H., Campbell, D. T. & Herskovits, M. J. (1966). *The influence of culture on visual perception.* Indianapolis: Bobbs-Merrill.

Sekula, A. (1975). On the invention of meaning in photographs. *Artforum, 13*(5), 36–45.

Seskin, M. (1978). Photobiography: A phenomenologically based approach to human story and personal insight. (Doctoral dissertation, California School of Professional Psychology). *Dissertation Abstracts International, 38:9-B.* (Microfilms No. 4481-B)

Shavelson, L. (1986). *I'm not crazy, I just lost my glasses: Portraits and oral histories of people who have been in and out of mental institutions.* Berkeley: De Novo Press.

Shore, A. (1989). Themes of loss in the pictorial language of a nursing home. *The Canadian Art Therapy Association Journal, 4*(1), 16–32.

Sinclair, L. (Ed.). (1989, May 8). Photography: The cultural impact. (Transcript of the radio program "Ideas.") Montréal: Canadian Broadcasting Corporation.

Smith, J. R. (1978). Taking portrait photographs of children in therapy. *Phototherapy, 1*(4), 1–2.

Sontag, S. (1966). *Against interpretation.* New York: Farrar, Straus & Giroux.

Sontag, S. (1977). *On photography.* New York: Farrar, Straus & Giroux.

Spence, J. (1984). Public images/private functions: Reflections on High Street practice. *Ten:8/(Face Values), 13,* 7–17.

Spence, J. (1986). Photo therapy. *Venue, 14*(101), 48–49.

Spence, J. & Holland, P. (Eds.) (1991). *Family snaps: Meanings of domestic photography.* London: Virago Press.

Spence, J. & Roberts, D. (1986). *Things my father never taught me: A dialogue between lovers.* Unpublished manuscript.

Spire, R. H. (1973). Photographic self-image confrontation. *American Journal of Nursing, 73*(7), 1207–1210.

Spitzing, G. (1985). *Foto psychologie—Die subjective seite des objektivs* [Photo psychology—the subjective site of the objective]. Weinheim, Germany: Beltz.

Spoerner, T. M. (1981). Look, snap, see: Visual literacy through the camera. *Art Education, 34*(3), 21–24.

Sponseller, D. B., et al. (1979, April). *Photographic feedback effects on preschool exceptional children's self-concept and social competence.* Paper presented at the Annual International Convention of the Council for Exceptional Children. Dallas.

Steinbauer, M. (Ed.). (1988, November). 150 Years of photography: Pictures that made a difference. *Life* (anniversary issue), p.10.

Stewart, D. (1979). Photo therapy and contemporary therapy theories: Gestalt therapy. *Phototherapy, 2*(1), 16–18.

Sulzberger, C. F. (1955). Unconscious motivations of the amateur photographer. *Psychoanalysis, 3,* 18–24.

Sussman, G. (1987). Two classroom projects: Self-concept enhancement and video-poetry project. *Phototherapy, 6*(2), 23–24.

Sutman, F. X. (1977). Self-esteem and vocabulary through photography. *Science and Children, 14*(4), 17–18.

Szarkowski, J. (1966). *The photographer's eye.* Boston: New York Graphic Society.

Szarkowski, J. (1973). *Looking at photographs: 100 pictures from the collection of the museum of modern art.* Boston: New York Graphic Society/Rappaport.

Tamashiro, R. T. (1971). Using photography to amplify self-esteem in the primary grades. *Educational Perspectives, 10,* 7–12.

Tartakoff, K. (1989). My stupid illness. [Exhibition brochure (and Newsletter for the Children's Legacy).] Denver: Gallery 44.

Teller, A. (1979). Some questions for photo therapy. *Phototherapy, 2*(2), 12–13.

Thomas, L. (Ed.). (1979). *Photography and language.* San Francisco: NFS Press.

Titus, S. L. (1976). Family photographs and the transition to parenthood. *Journal of Marriage and the Family, 38*(3), 525–530.

Toman, W. (1969). *Family constellation: Its effects on personality and social behavior.* New York: Springer.

Turner, P. (1977). Photographs: Demands and expectations. In J. Bayer (Ed.), *Reading photographs: Understanding the aesthetics of photography* (pp. 77–80). New York: Pantheon.

Vacheret, C. (1985). Photolangage et thérapie (Expression et Signe) (Photolanguage and therapy: Expression and signaling). *Psychologie Médicale, 17*(9), 1353–1355.

VanVliet, K. (1977). Creativity and self-image: An odyssey into poetry through photography. *Art Psychotherapy, 4*(1), 89–93.

Vardell, M., McClellan, L. & Fryrear, J. L. (1982). A structured group phototherapy program and its use with adjudicated adolescent girls. *Phototherapy, 3*(2), 8–11.

Vogel, R. (Ed.). (1969). *The other city: In photographs and words, four teenage boys explore the city close to them.* New York: David White.

Voss, S. H. (1968). The use of photography to study children's perceptions of themselves and others (Doctoral Dissertation, University of Florida). *Dissertation Abstracts International, 29:3-A.* (University Microfilms: 822)

Wagner, J. (Ed.). (1979). *Images of information: Still photography in the social sciences.* Beverly Hills, CA: Sage.

Walker, J. (1981, Aug.), *"See and tell"– Comparative survey: Mexico and New York.* Paper presented at the American Psychological Association Annual Convention, Los Angeles.

Walker, J. (1984). *The Walker Visuals (Kit): An aid in psychotherapy.* Toronto: Therapeutic Images.

Watzlawick, P. (1978). *The language of change: Elements of therapeutic communication.* New York: Basic Books.

Weaver, P. L. (1983). Photography: A picture of learning. *Phototherapy, 3*(4), 6–12.

Weaver, P. L. (1985). Was Ansel Adams a phototherapist? *Phototherapy, 4*(3), 13–16.

Webster, F. (1980). *The new photography: Responsibility in visual communication.* London: John Calder.

Weiser, J. (1981). *Using photo albums in therapy with "Special Needs" families.* Unpublished manuscript, with contributions by Dr. Alan Entin.

Weiser, J. (1982, August). *Projective uses of photographs taken or selected by clients.* Paper presented at the Annual Convention of the American Psychological Association, Washington, DC.

Weiser, J. (1990). Round things don't have any straight lines, or, Looking for the feminist requires "systems" thinking. *The Arts in Psychotherapy, 17*(3), 265–267.

Weiss, R. & Enter, S. (1975). *Creating environments and personal awareness through the use of Polaroid cameras.* Unpublished manuscript, Bronx-Lebanon Hospital.

Weissman, N. & Heimerdinger, D. (1979). *Self-exposures: A workbook in photographic self-portraiture.* New York: Harper & Row.

Wejaparn, P. (1978). A comparative study of the pictorial perception of American and Thai elementary school pupils (Doctoral dissertation, University of Washington). *Dissertation Abstracts International, 39 (3-A),* 1308.

Wessells, D. T. (1985). Using family photographs in the treatment of eating disorders. *Psychotherapy in Private Practice, 3*(4), 95–105.

White, M. (1957). What is meant by "reading" photographs. *Aperture, 5*(2), 48–50.

White, M. (1962). Varieties of responses to photographs. *Aperture, 10*(3), 116–128.

White, M. (1966). Equivalence, the perennial trend. In N. Lyons (Ed.), *Photographers on photography* (pp. 168–175). Englewood Cliffs, NJ: Prentice-Hall.

White, M. (1969). Extended perception through photography and suggestion. In H. Otto & J. Mann (Eds.), *Ways of Growth* (pp. 34–48). New York: Viking Press.

Wikler, M. E. (1977). Using photographs in the termination phase. *Social Work, 22*(4), 318–319.

Williams, R. D. & Williams, R.C.M. (1981). Photography as a bridge between institution and community: A preventive intervention. *Phototherapy, 2*(4), 8–12.

Williams, V. (1986). *Women photographers: The other observers, 1900 to the present.* London: Virago Press.

Wolz, C. (1980). Equivalent: Window or mirror. *Camera Lucida, 1*(1), 13–18.

Woychik, J. P. & Brickell, C. (1983). The instant camera as a therapy tool. *Journal of the National Association of Social Workers,* 316–317.

Young, V. & Wright, E. N. (1973). *The tree looked lovely, so I took its picture: Visual awareness in children's photographs* (Research Rep. No. 117). Toronto: Board of Education.

Yovel-Recanati, J. (1989). *PhotoTherapy for patients with spinal cord and head injuries at a rehabilitation center.* Unpublished master's thesis, Lesley College Graduate School.

Zakem, B., Kunka, J. & Cardone, L. (1977). Exploratory analysis of the uses of the TAT and personal photography pilot project. Unpublished manuscript. Chicago, IL: Ravenswood Hospital.

Zakia, R. (1975). *Perception and photography.* Englewood Cliffs, NJ: Prentice-Hall.

Zeigler, B. (1976). Life review in art therapy with the aged. *Art Therapy, 15*(2), 46–54.

Zeiller, B. (1985). Le photodrame: un appoint thérapeutique aux perturbations de l'image du corps chez l'adolescent (Photodrama: A therapeutic approach with disturbance of body image in adolescents). *Psychologie Médicale, 17*(9), 1351–1352.

Ziller, R. C. (1975). Psychology and photography. *The B.C. Photographer, Fall,* 7.

Ziller, R. C., Cowart, J. & Smith, D. (1975). The photograph: An image of the photographer's information processing. *Human Behavior, 33,* 17–19.

Ziller, R. C. & Rorer, B. (1985). Shyness-environment interaction: A view from the shy side through auto-photography. *Journal of Personality, 53*(41), 626–639.

Ziller, R. C. & Smith, D. E. (1977). A phenomenological utilization of photographs. *Journal of Phenomenological Psychology, 7*(2), 172–185.

Zwick, D. S. (1978). Photography as a tool toward increased awareness of the aging self. *Art Psychotherapy, 5*(2), 135–141.

Zwick, D. S. (1981). Photo Therapy as an adjunct to group process: A project review of "Fostering adolescent social interest: A photographic approach." *Phototherapy, 2*(4), 3.

Index